Will You Be The HIV-Negative?

Sex	Age	Date	Lab	Test	Result
M	50	3/93	Vanderbilt University	HIV and AFB	Positive
		4/93	The Medical Laboratory	P24	Negative
M	29	1/93	St. Vincent Hospital	HIV Antibody screen	Positive. Repeatedly reactive.
		4/93	The Medical Laboratory	P24	Negative
M	41	11/92	Mayo Medical Laboratories	HIV antibody, Western Blot Assay	Positive. Reactive at p17, p24, p31, gp41, p51, p55, p66, gp160.
		3/93	The Medical Laboratory	P24	Negative
M	40	8/92	Bartholomew County Hospital	HIV Antibody	Positive
		9/92	The Medical Laboratory	P24	Negative
M	29	1/93	Anonymous AIDS Antibody Clinic	HIV Antibody	Positive
		2/93	The Medical Laboratory	P24	Negative
M	28	9/89	Not shown	HIV Antibody	ELISA Assay positive. Western Blot Analysis positive.
		4/93	The Medical Laboratory	P24	Negative
M	37	2/90	SmithKline BioScience Lab	HIV Antibody Screen	This specimen was found to be repeatedly reactive by the HIV ELISA screen. A western blot analysis is being performed for further evaluation of this result.
		2/90	SmithKline BioScience Lab	Western Blot	P24 reactive P31 non-reactive GP41 reactive GP120/160 reactive
		7/93	Nichols Institute	P24	Positive (On program only two weeks)
		11/93	Mayo Medical Laboratory	P24	Negative
You **You**		**Now** **In**	**Six Weeks**		**Positive** **Negative!**

53 CURED Cases–All Who Used This Method

Cure, not treatment, is the subject of this book. In 1991 I discovered the source of HIV. Once the source became clear the cure became obvious. But would it work? After curing 53 cases in a row, I could wait no longer to present these findings. Some of these cured cases have already become reinfected, as would be expected without ongoing vigilance. There are things we must do as a society to remove these sources of infection before we are all ill.

You May Not Have Time

to read this entire book first if you are sick with AIDS. You may wish to skip the part about how HIV infection is caused and go directly to the *HIV Curing Recipe*. Order your supplies (see *Sources*). Follow the recipe exactly; it was carefully worked out for you. It takes 5 days to be cured of HIV regardless of how ill you are. After you have eliminated the virus, you can turn your attention to getting well from AIDS (*Part 2*). Read the case histories to see how easy it is to stop even terminal AIDS (*Part 3*). Learn from them to avoid mistakes.

Does this mean you can cancel your appointment with your clinical doctor? No, it does not. Although you will not need AZT and other HIV-specific drugs after you test negative, you may need antibiotics and life support systems. It could take you two years to get completely well.

Remember that doctors are kind, sensitive, compassionate people. They want the best for you. They have no way of knowing about the true cause and cure of HIV/AIDS since it has not been published for them. I chose to publish it for you first so that it would come to your attention faster.

The Cure For HIV And AIDS

Published in the United States by ProMotion Publishing, 10387 Friars Road Suite 231, San Diego, CA 92120, (800) 231-1776.

ISBN 0-9636328-3-3

Library of Congress Card Catalog Number 87-70299

10 9 8 7 6 5 4 3 2

This book is one of a set of two books. The other book is titled *The Cure For All Cancers*, by the same author.

Disclaimer To the Reader:

Please understand that we cannot be responsible for any adverse effects believed due to the use of information in this book. The author has provided safe dosage information wherever appropriate, but everyone is different. Use common sense when trying any treatment.

Acknowledgments

I would like to express my sincere gratitude to **Dr. Frank Jerome, D.D.S**. for the loan of his parasite slide collection. If he had not made a slide of *Fasciolopsis buskii* in his student years and if he had not stored his slides carefully for three decades, finally to loan them to me in a generous offer, none of these discoveries would have been made. Furthermore, most of these HIV/AIDS patients could not have regained their health without his development of a new metal-free dentistry. Thanks are also due to his wife, **Linda**, for her patience and willingness to listen to new ideas. And a very special thank you is due to **Mary L. Austin, Ph. D.** for her daily support and who, at the age of 97, has an amazing open-mindedness. Another special thank you goes to my son, **Geoffrey**, whose computer expertise and help with instrumentation and editing were indispensable and very much appreciated.

Preface

From Time Immemorial Healthy People Have Held Sick People Hostage.

The Witch Doctor, Medicine Man and Woman, Herbalist and Clinician are all alike in this respect. They wish to keep information surrounding illness and wellness to themselves and away from the common person so that a profession of medicine can grow and become lucrative. The Herbalist did not tell which herbs could relieve colds or bring on a woman's menstrual period (birth control) for fear that the people in need would get them for themselves and not need (nor pay) the Herbalist. The modern medical profession overlooks information on prevention; it tries to make self-help and simple treatments illegal. All for the same purpose: to build and aggrandize their profession. This seems inappropriate, especially where communicable or wide-spread illness is involved. This example is taken from a text on herbology:

> This [bath] is a safe and sane procedure and will prove most beneficial to those who are obese and desire to reduce safely. In combination with the internal treatment with decoction of *Fucus*, this course is worth considerable to very stout people, and should not be sold too cheaply. It is a grave mistake to put this scientific treatment in the same class as the many advertised nostrums on the market. It is also a mistake to let your patient know what you

are using. If any do make this mistake, he will lose his client who will straight away go to a drugstore for supplies.[1]

I believe hostage-holding of the sick is immoral, fundamentally unethical, and needs to be stopped.

Besides the moral issue, there is a practical issue. It would benefit society much more if the sick person were quickly rescued and helped back to productivity. A healthy society benefits each of us immensely. Likewise, an ill society injures us immensely, even when it is half a planet away. With this book, I hope to give away as many secrets as I can about the cause and the cure of low immunity, AIDS and the HIV virus, letting the truth come first and "professional concerns" come last.

The human species can no longer afford to make a business out of illness. Global travel reduces our planet to the size of our backyards. In order to keep our own backyards clean, the neighbors must keep theirs clean. So it is with keeping our bodies free of viruses, bacteria and parasites. We *all* must be free of them. The concept of health as a narrow professional concern is obsolete.

This book is intended as a gift to humanity. I make a plea to the public and private sector of the medical community not to suppress this information but to disperse it regardless of embarrassment or liability from the simplicity and newness of the cure, provided only that it meets your standard of truth.

---

[1] *Advanced Treatise in Herbology*, Dr. Edward E. Shook, Trinity Center Press, 1978, p. 172.

Contents

Detailed Contents

Figures

HIV is a *virus*.

AIDS is a *condition*.

Sometimes they occur together.

Sometimes they occur separately.

HIV stands for Human Immunodeficiency Virus

AIDS stands for Acquired Immune Deficiency Syndrome.

Part One: The HIV Virus

<u>This</u> is the source of the HIV virus

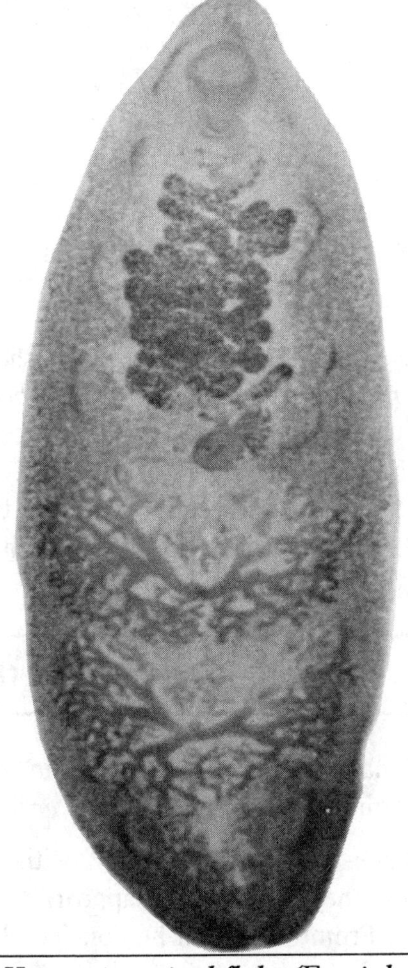

Fig. 1 Human intestinal fluke (Fasciolopsis buskii)

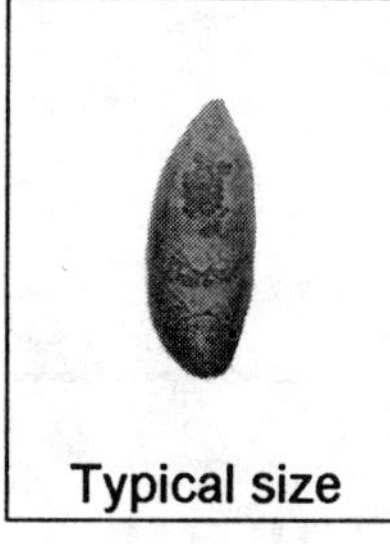
Typical size

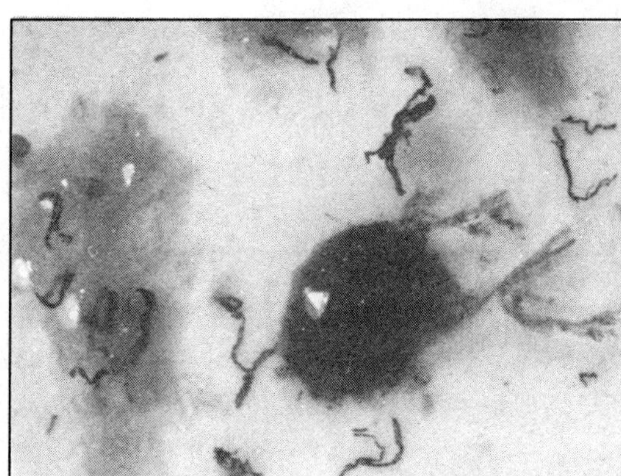
Five flukes, in various stages of decay, expelled from bowel. They float. "Black hairy legs" are strings of eggs.

This parasite typically lives in the intestine where it might do little harm, causing only colitis, Crohn's disease or irritable bowel syndrome, or perhaps nothing at all. But if it invades a different organ, like the liver, uterus, kidneys or thymus, it does a great deal of harm. If it establishes itself in the thymus, it causes HIV/AIDS! It only establishes itself in the thymus in some people. These people have *benzene* in their bodies. All HIV patients (100%) have both benzene and a stage of the intestinal fluke in their thymuses. The solvent benzene is responsible for letting the fluke establish itself in the thymus. In order to get HIV, you must have both the parasite and benzene in your body.

The HIV virus belongs to this fluke.

Many of us have this fluke parasite in our intestines. Humans are the natural host for this parasite.

When this fluke is killed, together with its eggs and microscopic stages, the HIV virus disappears from the human body in 24 hours. From this it can be concluded that the virus belongs to the parasite. The virus must have the fluke to survive.

IT IS NOT DIFFICULT

to kill this parasite and all its stages.

In fact, the intestinal fluke and all its millions of eggs and microscopic stages can be killed in 5 days. Read the case histories to follow the fate of the HIV virus.

AIDS IS A CONDITION

AIDS reflects the condition of the *thymus*. When the thymus gland cannot "make" enough T cells,[2] your immunity is lowered.

The Thymus and AIDS

The "T" in T cells comes from the word *THYMUS*.

The thymus is located under the top of your breast bone. It is just below the thyroid gland.

To find these glands:

1. Look in the mirror and turn your head from side to side.

---

[2] T-cells are actually made in the bone marrow, but go to the thymus to be given instructions as immunity-defenders.

2. Notice a V-shape is formed at the front of your neck as you do this. Put your finger in the hollow at the bottom of this V. Your thyroid gland is on both sides of this V.
3. Move downward from this hollow about 1½ inches to a raised flat area shaped like a baseball plate. This is the top of your breastbone (sternum). Your thymus is under this, stretching down and up, depending on its size.

What could be happening to the thymus that prevents it from making enough T cells? **It is being invaded by the intestinal fluke.** The thymus is a small gland and the intestinal fluke is a large parasite! The thymus has a lot of work to do and the flukes are eating its food and leaving their wastes in it. It is like having a moose invade your kitchen!

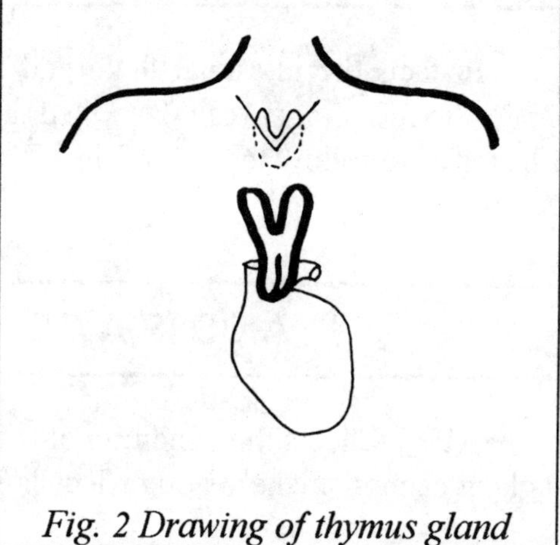

Fig. 2 Drawing of thymus gland

Why is this fluke, which belongs in the intestine (hence its name), suddenly invading the thymus? Does the fluke travel from the intestine to the thymus? Is there something about the thymus that attracts it? As you read the case histories a fascinating story is revealed.

The real culprit is benzene.

Benzene

Benzene is a *solvent*. It is an extremely toxic solvent. We would not expect to find benzene anywhere in our environment. It is even monitored in gasoline. It is prohibited in dry-cleaning fluids and rubber cement. How could it be present in your body?

BENZENE IS THE CAUSE OF AIDS

What is a solvent? A solvent is a substance that can dissolve grease. There are many solvents used in industries but none dissolves grease as fast as benzene.

The living body is made of greases! Fats and oils make the brain and spinal cord and nerves and the protective covering of every living cell!

Benzene accumulates in the thymus!

Different toxins accumulate in different organs. If you accidentally drink some wood alcohol, which is another solvent, it goes to your pancreas first. This organ makes your insulin and regulates your blood sugar. People with "low blood sugar" or chronic fatigue actually do have wood alcohol in their pancreas. How did they get it? Wood alcohol is a pollutant in carbonated beverages, artificial sweetener and many other foods. At first your body can detoxify it; this is when your body is young and strong like a child's. But as you keep drinking the wood alcohol, the pancreas wears out, the wood alcohol begins to pile up there and do a lot of harm. It weakens the pancreas so much that any parasite can live there. The immunity of the pancreas is being lowered. Bacteria, viruses, metal dissolved from tooth fillings, chemicals from the air you breathe and food you eat can now find a home in your pancreas. Is it any wonder that this leads to diabetes? Wood alcohol also accumulates in the eyes. Sometimes they burn and itch. Now the eyes let parasites in to multiply, like *Toxoplasma* from cats. The eyes also let in toxins from food and environment and we call it **allergies**. The real culprit is wood alcohol!

The most common parasite in the pancreas is *Eurytrema*, the pancreatic fluke of cattle. All persons with diabetes have wood alcohol accumulated in the pancreas and a big population of pancreatic flukes growing there. There is also mercury and gold present, from tooth fillings and gold crowns! Cattle carry this parasite and fresh raw milk always carries infective stages in it. Eating rarely cooked hamburger would certainly give it to you!

Just as wood alcohol accumulates in the pancreas and eyes, benzene accumulates in the thymus and bone marrow.

If you eat the tiniest bit of benzene, it goes directly to your thymus. If you rub the tiniest bit of benzene into your skin, it is found in the thymus a half minute later! Of course, your white blood cells immediately begin to eat it up and get it out of the thymus, but damage has already been done! No tissue can have benzene in it without being damaged.

Benzene damages the thymus so much that everything else is allowed to land there, too. The mercury from metal tooth fillings, the tin from stannous fluoride, the bismuth from Pepto Bismol,™ the gasoline you pumped into your car, can all be found in your thymus after benzene damage has been done. It is as if the front and backdoors to your house have been opened, letting in all comers.

Is it any wonder that the thymus can't turn out T cells when it is full of bits of your toothpaste, your hand lotion, your hair spray, your soap, junk food and beverages? Before the benzene damage, these loitering chemicals would have been escorted to the liver, to the kidney and out of your body. Now they are caught by the thymus and remain stuck there, accumulating to higher and higher levels. The T cell production falls lower and lower.

Meanwhile, the bacteria and viruses, which are hidden in our bodies, have been quietly waiting. Waiting for their chance to come out of hiding. Waiting for their chance to grow and multiply as all living things must do to survive. When the T cell level falls low enough, they seize their opportunity. Look at the long list of pathogens (bacteria and viruses) in many of the case histories that have come out of hiding. Your body is a huge warehouse of pathogens and parasites. You have accumulated them in a lifetime. Chicken pox, mumps, measles, strep, eye infections, flu, colds! Each one of these is <u>still</u> in your body somewhere! Nothing ever disappears. It just waits. But they are carefully bottled up. Some are put into capsules. They won't come out of their capsules until they know they will be safe from your immune system T cells. Some are in a latent form or dormant state in which they patiently wait for your T cell count to go down. Then they emerge. Some come from hiding under rotten teeth, like *Clostridium tetani* and *Staphylococcus aureus*. Some come from hiding in the nerve centers, like *Herpes 1* and *2*. Some come from the digestive tract like *Salmonella* and *Shigella*. Some come from the lung like *Pneumocystis carnii*.

We are accustomed to thinking that we "pick up" our infections. Indeed, we do keep picking up new strains. But we already have in us all the bacteria and viruses that could make us very ill if our immunity drops. They are not making us sick <u>now</u> because our immune system does not let them multiply. They are not dead but simply "bottled up" in various places. Most of them did not even make us sick when we originally picked them up because our immune system was strong at that time, too.

Now that the T cell count is gradually going down, this Pandora's box of pathogens is opening, letting out one after another, until the body is seething with infectious organisms.

Yet, the human body is large and strong. It will put up a good fight. It may take ten years before it begins to lose the battle. Now it is called *AIDS*, Acquired Immune Deficiency Syndrome. Acquired from polluting the thymus with hundreds of bits of garbage dumped on the body and into the body, but mostly from benzene. This garbage was thought to be "progress." We are led to believe that "new, improved" lotions and detergents are "better". When we see this label on a package we automatically reach for it. It may indeed, be doing a "new, improved" job on the dishes because cobalt is added to make spots invisible but the cobalt is doing a "new, more toxic" job on your body. "New, improved" taste in your coffees and herb tea blends may be due to adding flavor extracts to them, which also adds the solvents used in extracting! "New, improved" taste in cereals may be due to added flavors, which are extracts, again bringing solvents to these foods.

SIMPLER IS BETTER

The less that is done to a food, the less chance there is to pollute it. But, of course, such matters should not be left to chance. Processed foods should be monitored in the grocery store for all the toxins that might be there.

Parasites Plus Benzene

Let us review for a minute:

1. The HIV virus is an infection of the parasite, Human intestinal fluke. It is not a human virus. It only infects us incidentally when we host this parasite in us.
2. Benzene in our bodies weakens the thymus gland where our T cells are made, causing AIDS

When the thymus has benzene accumulated in it, fluke parasites are attracted to it, just as the toxins and pollutants are.

There are many fluke parasites. In addition to *Fasciolopsis buskii*, the human intestinal fluke, there are three other very common flukes: sheep liver fluke, pancreatic fluke of cattle, and human liver fluke.

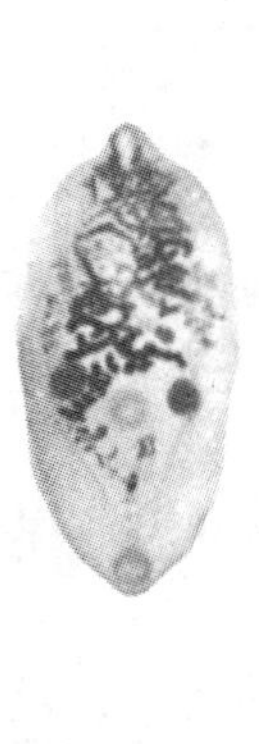

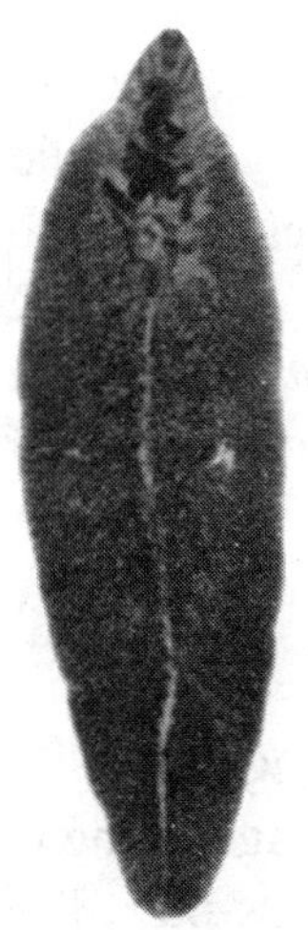

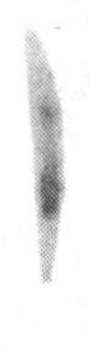

L to R: pancreatic fluke (causes diabetes); sheep liver fluke (causes "universal allergy syndrome"); and human liver fluke.
Fig. 3 Three other common flukes.

There are many more flukes that parasitize us. There is *Prosthogonimus*, a fluke of chickens and *Paragonimus Westermanii*, the lung fluke, and *Cryptocotyle*, a fluke of sea gulls, and *Platynosomum*, cat liver fluke.

If we have a few of these, they don't make us very sick. But when they have a population explosion, swarming in one of our organs, we get sick. Solvents cause such population explosions. Solvents dissolve away the egg shells forcing them all to hatch. Hatch in your body! Normally, this would not happen. The eggs produced by the adult, thousands every day, are passed into the intestine to exit with the bowel movement. But if they are forced to hatch before they exit, they swim away, into your body!

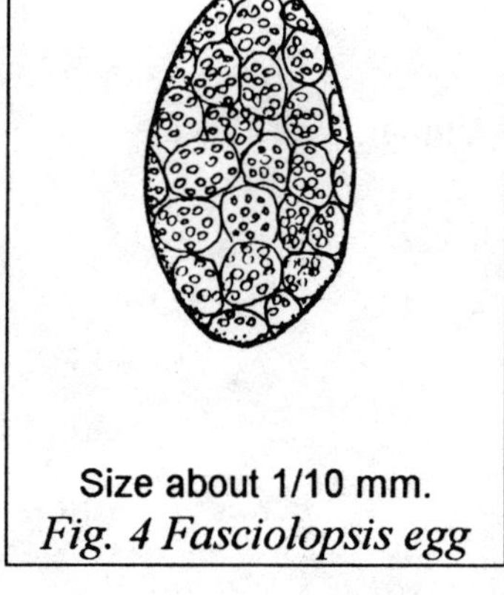

Size about 1/10 mm.
Fig. 4 Fasciolopsis egg

Flukes

To understand HIV you should understand the basic facts about the human intestinal fluke. Its scientific name is *Fasciolopsis buskii*. Fluke means "flat", and flukes are one of the families of flatworms. It is as flat as a leaf. The parasite is not unknown, it has been studied since at least 1925.[3]

This parasite has stages that it must go through to keep reproducing. The first stage is the *egg*. The adult produces millions of eggs. They pass out of us with the bowel movement.

[3] C. H. Barlow, *The Life Cycle of the Human Intestinal Fluke, Fasciolopsis buskii* (Lancaster) Am. J. Hyg. Monog. No. 4, 1925.

The adult, though, stays tightly stuck to our intestine (or liver, causing cancer, or uterus, causing endometriosis, or thymus, causing AIDS, or kidney, causing Hodgkin's disease).

Most of us get little lesions in our intestines from time to time. These tiny sores allow the eggs, which are microscopic in size, to be pulled into the blood stream (other parasite eggs get into the blood this way too).

Some of these eggs actually hatch in the intestine or in the blood. The microscopic hatchlings are called *miracidia* and are the second stage. They swim about with their little swimmer-hairs. And of course, the liver whose job it is to dispose of toxins will receive them and kill them as the blood arrives from the intestine. They have no chance to survive in normal people.

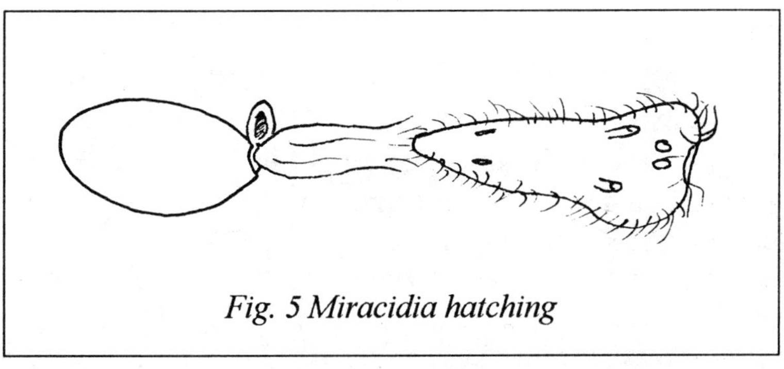

Fig. 5 Miracidia hatching

Flukes and Solvents

BUT SOMETHING SPECIAL HAPPENS TO PEOPLE WHO HAVE SOLVENTS IN THEIR BODIES. The liver is unable to trap and kill these tiny fluke stages. These baby-stages are actually allowed to make their home in the liver and other tissues. It is as if the immune system has no power to kill them. The flukes begin to multiply in people with solvents in their bodies! The miracidia (hatchlings) start to make little balls inside themselves, called *redia*[4]. But each redia (ball) is alive! It pops itself out of the miracidia and begins to reproduce itself. 40 redia can <u>each</u> make 40 more redia! And all of this out of <u>one</u> egg!

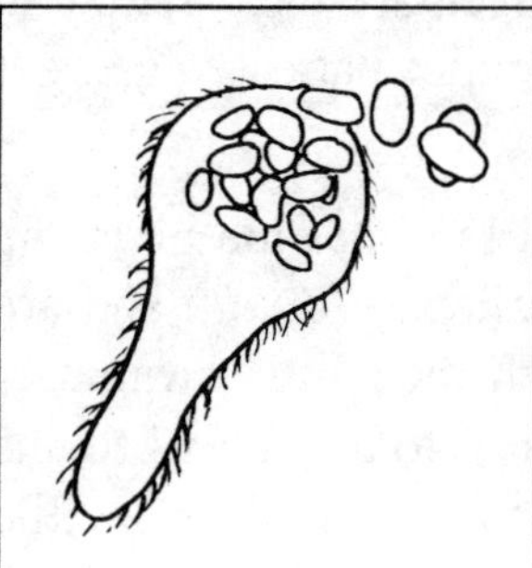

Fig. 6 Miracidia expelling "mother" redia

This parasite is laying eggs and producing millions of redia right in your body! These redia are swept along in your blood, landing in whatever tissue lets them in. Smokers' lungs, breasts with benign lumps, prostate glands full of heavy metals, a thymus loaded with benzene are

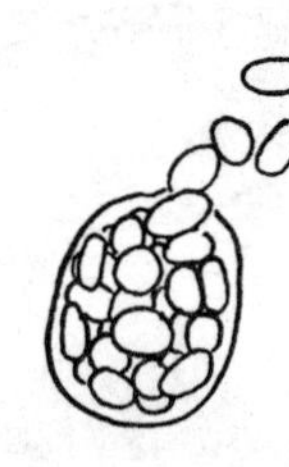

Fig. 7 "Mother" redia bearing "daughter" redia

[4] The Latin names are *rediae* (plural) and *redia* (singular). I have used simplified spelling, "redia", for both the singular and the plural, more like English usage.

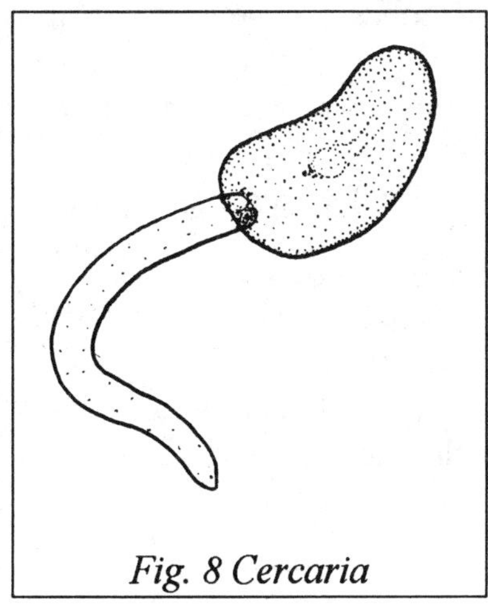

Fig. 8 Cercaria

examples of tissues that give the redia their landing permits[5].

Multiplying continues at a hectic pace, generation after generation. Redia are nesting in numerous organs. Suddenly they change their shape. They sprout a tail and can swim again. Now they are called *cercaria*[6].

The cercaria only need to find a place to attach. After they glue themselves to your tissue, their tails disappear and they begin to grow a "cocoon".

Now they are called *meta*cercaria. Normally, this would

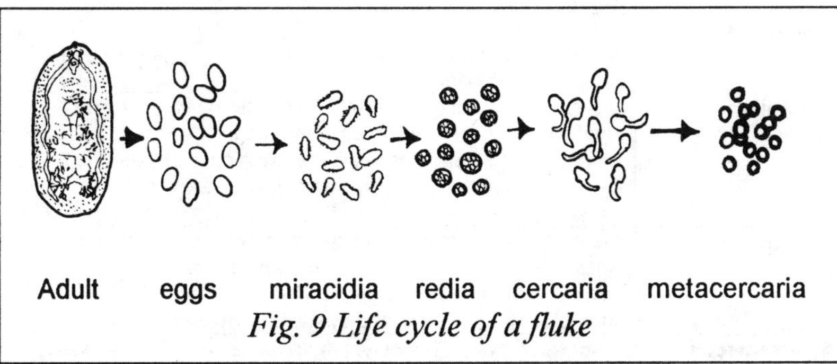

Fig. 9 Life cycle of a fluke

---

[5] Perhaps it is the changed electrical charge or magnetic force of these damaged organs that permits further development of the fluke stages. Perhaps it is merely low immune surveillance. Perhaps the dying cells of a damaged organ provide food for the baby stages. Only further scientific study will reveal the truth.

[6] Again, I am simplifying the Latin *cercaria* (singular) and *cercariae* (plural) to one case.

happen on a leaf growing near a pond, so the metacercaria develop an extremely thick shell around themselves to withstand the winter. Does the presence of the solvent benzene in your body dissolve this tough shell? That would remove the last barrier to the fluke completing its entire life cycle anywhere in your body!

After the shell is gone, they grow into adult flukes in your tissue. NOT IN THE INTESTINE BUT IN YOUR THYMUS! Now the cycle is complete. From egg to miracidia to redia to cercaria to metacercaria and then the adults! And all of them eating and sucking and devouring your vital body fluids.

But this is not normal for flukes. This is:

Stage	Normal Life Cycle
1 Egg	Expelled with bowel movement onto soil. Washed by rain into ponds.
2 Miracidia	Hatches from egg in water. Has cilia, can swim vigorously and must find intermediate snail host in one to two hours or may be too exhausted to invade.
3 Redia	Develop inside miracidia as little balls until expelled. Those are "mother" redia, and each one bears "daughter" redia for up to 8 months, all still inside the snail, and living on the fluids in the lymphatic spaces. Similarly, daughter redia are continually developing cercaria.
4 Cercaria	Have a tail, use it to exit from snail and swim to a plant. If the snail is feeding on a plant, cercaria can latch onto plant with sucker mouth and start to encyst (form a "cocoon") within minutes. Tail breaks off and swims away to dissolve.
5 Metacercaria	Two-walled cysts. The outer wall is very sticky. But as you eat the plant it is stuck to, the least pressure will break it, leaving the cyst in the mouth. The "almost unbreakable" inner cyst wall protects it from chewing, and the keratin-like coat prevents digestion by stomach juices. However when it reaches the duodenum, contact with intestinal juices dissolves away the cyst-wall and frees it. It then fastens itself to the intestinal lining and begins to develop into an adult.
6 Adult	Lives in your intestine and can produce 1000 eggs per bowel movement and live many years.

Fig. 10 Fasciolopsis' normal life cycle

As you can see, humans typically are the host for just the adult stage, and then only in the intestine. But can you imagine the havoc in your body if you did the snail's job, too? Suppose the host, the human, has solvent in his or her body so that the millions of eggs start hatching before they can exit with the fecal matter? They simply swim in hordes into the blood stream. They may be searching for a snail but certainly a living tissue of yours will serve as well! To survive they must avoid being eaten by your white blood cells. So a tissue where the white blood cells are filled with mercury, lead, cadmium, perfume, solvents, PCBs is the logical choice. They have found a home! In you!.

The solvents may be hexane, pentane, xylene, toluene, wood alcohol, carbon tetrachloride, propyl alcohol, as well as benzene.

Xylene and toluene accumulate in the brain so the fluke parasites choose the brain for their breeding place. Here they produce their redia and cercaria and eventually adults! Wood alcohol accumulates in the pancreas and eyes, making these organs the fluke breeding grounds. Isopropyl alcohol accumulates in the liver, making the liver the place where the stages develop into adults. And benzene accumulates in the thymus so that the intestinal fluke is raised up to adulthood in this tiny organ instead of the spacious intestine.

In this book you will learn how to kill it.

Many persons who have an adult fluke in the thymus feel a burning sensation or pain or "tightness" over the breastbone. But some persons feel nothing at all. And some persons with a "tightness" there do not have this parasite. So having a symptom here, while very suggestive of this fluke, does not prove you have it. However, it would be very wise to go on a parasite killing program such as I will describe to you later.

HIV/AIDS illness is caused by an intestinal fluke stage inhabiting the benzene-damaged thymus.

All cases of HIV seen in my office had benzene in their thymuses. It is tempting to speculate that benzene has some special role to play besides damaging the thymus.

No case of HIV was seen without benzene in the thymus.

When benzene is removed from the thymus but the fluke is not killed, does the HIV virus survive? Not enough of such cases were seen to answer this interesting question.

Purge The Parasite, Cure HIV

When the parasite is killed but benzene is still present in the thymus, does the HIV virus survive? Never! It is always gone after the last of the fluke stages has left. If you have HIV/AIDS illness...

Clearly, you must do 3 things:

1. Kill the intestinal fluke and all its stages.
2. Rid your body of benzene.
3. Clean up your thymus gland.

We have been taught to believe that every parasite is so unique that a different drug is required to kill each one. The better drugs, such as Praziquantel™ and Levamisole™ or even Flagyl™ and Piperazine™, can each kill several worm varieties.

But this is just not practical when dozens of different parasites are present. We have dozens of different parasites in us! It would be best to kill them all together even though only the intestinal fluke is bringing the HIV virus.

Look at the case histories. It is not unusual for someone to have a dozen (or more) parasites out of the 120 parasites I have samples of (they are listed in *The Tests*). You can assume that you, too, have a dozen different parasites. We are heavily parasitized beings! Our bodies are large enough to provide food and shelter for lots of these free loaders. If they were settled on the outside where we could see them, like lice or ticks, we would rid ourselves in a flash. Nothing is more distasteful to the imagination than hordes of biting, chewing, crawling, sucking creatures on our flesh. But what about IN our flesh? We cannot see inside ourselves, so we mistakenly assume that nothing is there.

Parasite Remedies

The Native American peoples knew that humans are parasitized. Other native peoples from the Arctic to Antarctic knew that we are parasitized like other animals. They had frequent purgings that included diarrhea or vomiting to rid themselves of their slimy invaders. Many cultures continued such practices right up to my own childhood. I remember being forced to swallow a spoonful of sulfur and molasses and raw onion! How dreadful it seemed. But it reduced the body's burden of worms and other parasites that we all have. **Where have we gone astray? Why have we forsaken these wise practices?** I have seen that eczema is due to round worms. Seizures are caused by the roundworm, *Ascaris*, getting into the brain. Schizophrenia and depression are caused by parasites in the brain. Asthma is caused by *Ascaris* in the lungs. Diabetes is caused by the pancreatic fluke of cattle, *Eurytrema.* Migraines are caused by the threadworm, *Strongyloides* Acne rosacea is caused by a *Leishmania.* Much human heart disease is caused by dog heartworm, *Dirofilaria.* And the list goes on.

Getting rid of all these parasites would be absolutely impossible using clinical medicines that can kill only one or two varieties each. Such medicines also tend to make you quite ill. Flagyl™ is used for amoebas and *Giardia*; when the correct dosage is used, it can cause extreme nausea and vomiting. Quinine for malaria is quite toxic. Imagine taking 10 such drugs to kill a dozen of your parasites! Good news, perhaps, for the drug makers but not for you.

Yet three herbs can rid you of over 100 types of parasites! And without so much as a headache! Without nausea! Without any interference with any drug that you are already on! Does this sound too fantastic? Just too good to be true? They are nature's gift to us. The herbs are:

- **Black Walnut Hulls** (from the black walnut tree)
- **Wormwood** (from the *Artemesia* shrub)
- **Common Cloves** (from the clove tree)

These three herbs must be used together. Black walnut hull and wormwood kill adults and developmental stages of at least 100 parasites. Cloves kill the eggs. Only if you use them together will you rid yourself of parasites. If you kill only the adults, the tiny stages and eggs will soon grow into new adults. If you kill only the eggs, the million stages already loose in your body will soon grow into adults and make more eggs. They must be used together as a single treatment.

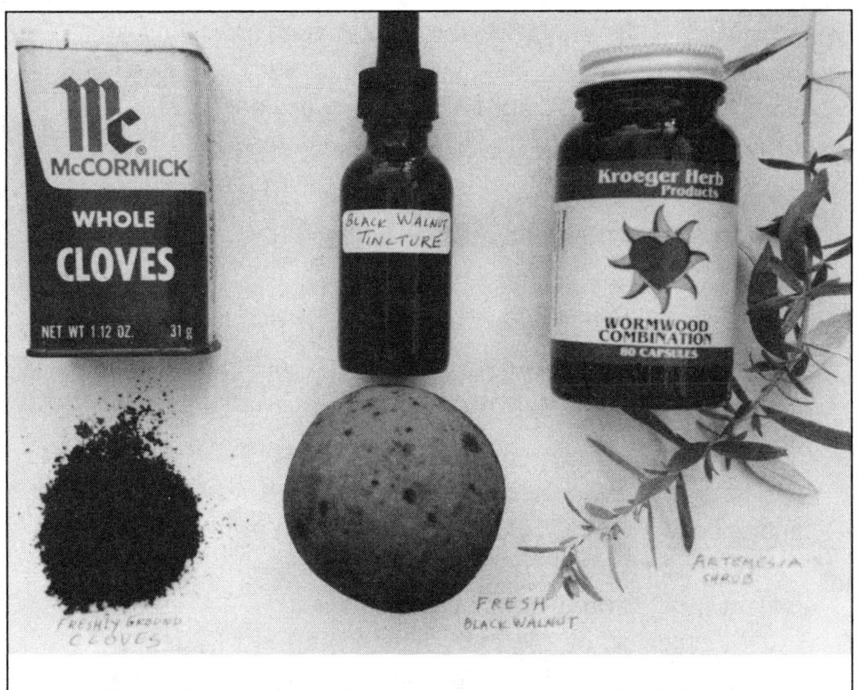

These three herbs, taken together, can cure HIV infection.

Fig. 11 Cloves, black walnut, and wormwood

It is the green hull surrounding the nut of the black walnut tree that has this miraculous parasiticide. After it has turned black, it is useless. The large green balls fall to the ground early in the fall. In a week or two they will be black and decaying. Therefore, anyone wishing to make parasiticide must be careful not to let the critical time for harvesting pass.

I encourage everyone to make their own parasiticides and to take back the responsibility for keeping themselves and their families free of these tiny monsters. The recipe for Black Walnut Hull Tincture is given in *Recipes*.

Note that it is a <u>tincture</u> (extracted using grain alcohol), not an ordinary extract (which uses water). The black walnut extract that is available from herb companies is <u>not</u> <u>potent</u> as a parasiticide. It is black, not pale green, indicating that the critical harvesting time had passed. Of course there is no time to make your own if you are HIV positive or have AIDS. See the chapter on *Sources*.

You will only need one 1 oz. bottle. While you are waiting for it to arrive, get your other 2 herbs ready: wormwood and cloves.

Wormwood consists of the leaves of the *Artemesia* shrub. My recommendation is that you grow it yourself if you have any space to do so. Wormwood seed is available from seed catalogs, see *Sources*.

The amount you need to eliminate HIV is very small, yet you cannot do without it. But the FDA (Food And Drug Administration) has regulated it as toxic! It is therefore unavailable in concentrated form from herb companies. The evidence for toxicity accepted by the FDA must have been hearsay. I have never seen a case of toxicity, not so much as a headache or nausea[7]. The toxic level must be much higher than is needed to kill these parasites.

This shrub is called wormwood for good reason: it kills worms! There is quite a bit of confusion over which *Artemesia* is the true wormwood. Books and nurseries can be wrong, even though they assure you they are correct! Buy *Artemesia absynthium* for your garden. Wormwood goes back to antiquity and is mentioned in the Bible.

If you grow your own, dry the leaves when they are in their prime. The leaves are greenish silvery gray and quite bitter. Nobody would accidentally eat too much of them. For a child,

---

[7] Of course, the FDA cannot be expected to accept experiences such as mine. We should find out what evidence they did accept.

roll up a single leaf and put it into a capsule or shred it and stir into honey.

Wormwood capsules are available as a combination of *Artemesia*, male fern, quassia, black walnut leaves and cloves (see *Sources*). This small amount of *Artemesia* is legal.

You will need one bottle of 80 Wormwood Combination capsules to cure your HIV and another bottle to kill your remaining parasites.

The third herb necessary to eliminate HIV is cloves. This is the common spice used in baking. It needs to be ground up in order to release its parasite killing properties. You can buy a can of whole cloves and grind them in a blender or grinder. Store-bought "ground cloves" do not work! Their parasite killing properties have evaporated long ago. Ground cloves from a health food store or herb shop may not work either! They may have been ground years ago. Don't take a chance, grind your own. Remember, the responsibility of the cloves is to kill eggs. Nothing else known can kill eggs of parasites within the body! If an herb company were to grind cloves and fill capsules with them right away and store the capsules in closed bottles, the potency of the herb would be protected. Don't take these details for granted. You must question your source and get a satisfactory answer or grind your own (see *Sources*).

You will need about 100 capsules of cloves. To make your own, purchase size 00 (double-zero) capsules at a health food store. (Don't try to mix cloves straight in water! It is much too strong; you may try mixing with apple sauce or buttermilk.) Size 0 capsules will also be acceptable.

You now have:

- One 30 cc bottle of pale green Black Walnut Hull Tincture. This is 1 ounce.

- 2 bottles of 80 Wormwood Combination capsules or ½ cup of *Artemesia* leaves gathered from a friendly neighbor's shrub.
- One bottle of 100 capsules of freshly ground cloves or ¼ cup bulk.

These are the only essential items that you will need to eliminate HIV from your body.

But there is another essential herbal product you will need to get completely well. I have found all HIV/AIDS sufferers also have "tapeworm disease". It is normal for us to have tapeworm stages in our bodies, probably going back to our childhood when we ate dirt. It is not normal for these stages to hatch in us. But they do hatch in HIV/AIDS sufferers because of the large amounts of solvents, especially benzene, in their bodies. Hatching tapeworm cysts spew unfertilized eggs plus bacteria and viruses all over the body, making you feel sick. To kill these emerging tapeworm stages you need Rascal™ (see *Sources*).

Two additional items, *ornithine* and *arginine*, improve this recipe. Parasites produce a great deal of ammonia as their waste product. Ammonia is their equivalent of urine and it is set free in our bodies by parasites in large amounts. Ammonia is very toxic, especially to the brain.[8] I believe this causes insomnia and other sleep problems at night and anxiety by day. By taking ornithine at bedtime, you will sleep better.[9] Arginine has similar

---

[8] The brain lacks the enzyme ornithine carbamyltransferase which is essential for making ammonia harmless by changing it into urea.

[9] I published this discovery in *Townsend Letter For Doctors*, July 1991, p554.

ammonia reduction effects but must be taken in the morning because it gives alertness and energy.

Do not try to substitute drugs for herbs. **Drug parasiticides can be extremely toxic, even in the small doses needed. Nor do they kill all the stages.** Here is a clipping I saw recently:

Common Drugs For Parasitic Infections

Infection	Drug	Adult Dosage	Pediatric Dosage
Amebiasis			
Asymptomatic	Iodoquinol	650 mg tid x 20d	30-40 mg/kg/d, 3 doses x 20d
Symptomatic	Metronidazole	750 mg tid x 10d	35-50 mg/kg/d, 3 doses x 10 d
	followed by Iodoquinol	650 mg tid x 20d	30-40 mg/kg/d, 3 doses x 20d
Blastocystis	Metronidazole	750 mg tid x 10d	
	or Iodoquinol	650 mg tid x 20d	
Dientamoeba	Iodoquinol	650 mg tid x 20d	40 mg/kg/d, 3 doses x 20d
Giardia	Quinacrine HCl	100 mg tid p.c.x5d	6 mg/kg/d, 3 doses p.c.x5d
	or Metronidazole	250 mg tid x 5d	15 mg/kg/d, 3 doses x 5 d

Names & Adverse Effects of Common Drugs

Drug: **Iodoquinol** Trade Name: **Yodoxin.** Adverse Effects: Occ: rash, acne, slight enlargement of thyroid gland, nausea, diarrhea, cramps, anal pruritus. Rare: optic atrophy, loss of vision, peripheral neuropathy after prolonged use in high dosage (months), Iodine sensitivity.

Drug: **Metronidazole** Trade Name: **Flagyl** Adverse Effects: Freq: nausea, headache, dry mouth, metallic taste. Occ: vomiting, diarrhea, insomnia, weakness, stomatitis, vertigo, aparesthesia, rash, dark urine, urethral burning. Rare: seizures, encephalopathy, pseudo-membranous colitis, ataxia, leukopenia, peripheral neuropathy, pancreatitis.

Drug: **Quinacrine HCl** Trade Name: **Atabrine** Adverse Effects: Freq: dizziness, headache, vomiting, diarrhea. Occ: yellow staining of skin, toxic psychosis, insomnia, bizarre dreams, blood dyscrasias, urticaria, blue and black nail pigmentation, psoriasis-like rash. Rare: acute hepatic necrosis, convulsions, severe exfoliative dermatitis, ocular effects similar to those caused by chloroquine.

Fig. 12 Some clinical parasiticides

Procedure For Cure

Start by taking ornithine, 2 at bedtime on the first night you get it. You don't need to wait for the rest of the program to start on ornithine. Take 4 ornithines on the second night. Take 6 ornithines at bedtime on the third night. After this take 4 or 6 ornithines at bedtime every night till you are sleeping soundly. Then go off ornithine and see whether your sleep is as good without it. Use as needed. It is not habit forming.

Taking ornithine at bedtime may give you so much energy the next day that you don't need to take arginine in the morning. But if going off caffeine (recommended) has you dragging yourself through the morning, take one arginine upon rising and another one before lunch and supper. It can make you a bit irritable. Cut back if this happens.

Ornithine and arginine, each about 500mg, are available in capsules, in separate bottles (see *Sources*).

There are no side-effects as you can see from the case histories.

There is no interference with any other medication. There is no need to stop any treatment that a clinical doctor or alternative therapist has started you on.

To summarize:

What you'll need for killing the intestinal fluke which brings with it the HIV virus, in the first five days, followed by the remaining parasites in another two weeks, are:

1. Black walnut tincture, an alcohol extract of the green hull (for alcoholics, a water recipe is given)
2. Wormwood combination, in capsules
3. Cloves, fresh ground, together with size 00 empty capsules
4. Ornithine, 500mg
5. Arginine, 500mg
6. Rascal™ (start this after three weeks). Take as directed on label.

Don't wait to begin until you have all 6 items! Start as soon as you get each item! Consider your body like a flower garden. Tiny insects are eating your leaves and petals. They are laying eggs that hatch into hungry caterpillars, spinning cocoons and emerging into new adults continually. You can't wait for anything! You must kill whatever you can as soon as you can in order to save as many petals and leaves as possible!

Are there any substitutes for the Black Walnut Hull Tincture and Wormwood Combination? The answer to this question is NOT YET. I have not worked out any substitutes, although they must exist. I believe there **must be dozens** of plant products that could kill the intestinal fluke. What is just as important is not picking them up again. But we will come to this point soon.

HIV Curing Recipe

Parasite Program Detailed Instructions

1. Black Walnut Hull Tincture:

Day 1: (this is the day you begin; start the same day you receive it)

Take one drop four times. Put it in a beverage like warm juice, milk or water. A warm liquid evaporates the alcohol. The timing does not matter. The drops can be 1 hour apart if you start at 6:00 p.m. They can be 4 hours apart if you start in the morning. Take them before meals or on an empty stomach.

Day 2: Take 2 drops four times as above.

Day 3: Take 3 drops four times.

Day 4: Take 4 drops four times.

Continue increasing in this way till you have taken 20 drops four times. After this, continue taking 20 drops once a day for 3 months. If you get interrupted, don't start over, just continue. The flukes will be dead by day 5! Don't get interrupted before day 6. After 3 months switch to the Maintenance Parasite Program

2. Wormwood Combination capsules:

Day 1: Take 1 capsule before supper (with water).

Day 2: Take 2 capsules before supper.

Day 3: Take 3 capsules before supper.

Continue increasing in this way to day 14. You take the capsules all in a single dose (you may take a few at a time until they are all gone). Then you do 2 more days of 14 capsules each. After this, you take 14 capsules twice a week, such as on Monday and Thursday forever, as it states in the Maintenance Parasite Program. Try not to get interrupted before the 6th day, so you know the intestinal flukes are dead. After this, you may proceed more slowly if you wish. Many persons with sensitive stomachs prefer to stay 2 days on each dose instead of increasing every day. You may choose the pace after the sixth day.

3. Cloves. Fill size 00 capsules with ground cloves; if these are not available, use size 0 or 000. In a pinch, buy gelatin capsules and empty them or empty other vitamin capsules.

Day 1: Take one capsule 3 times a day before meals.

Day 2: Take two capsules 3 times a day.

Days 3, 4, 5, 6, 7, 8, 9, 10: Take three capsules 3 times a day. After day 10, take 3 capsules once a day for 3 months. Then take 3 capsules twice a week forever, as in the Maintenance Parasite Program

Prevent Reinfection

It only takes five days on the three herbs together to kill the intestinal fluke adults, eggs, miracidia, redia, cercaria and metacercaria. The parasite killing program continues, though, to a peak at three weeks, followed by a tapeworm treatment, in order to rid your body of most other parasites. After this, a maintenance program is followed in order to kill any new parasite that you pick up.

YOU ARE ALWAYS PICKING UP PARASITES! PARASITES ARE EVERYWHERE AROUND YOU! YOU GET THEM FROM OTHER PEOPLE, YOUR FAMILY, YOURSELF, YOUR HOME, YOUR PETS, AND UNDERCOOKED MEAT.

I believe the main source of the intestinal fluke is undercooked meat. After we are infected with it this way, we can give it to each other through blood, saliva, semen, and breast milk, which means kissing on the mouth, sex, nursing, and childbearing.

Stay on a maintenance program of killing parasites. Give yourself a high-dose program twice a year; more often if it makes you feel better. Family members nearly always have the same parasites. If one person develops HIV (or cancer), the others probably have the intestinal fluke also. These diseases are caused by the same parasite. They should give themselves the same de-parasitizing program.

Maintenance Parasite Program

Twice a week (any 2 days will do) take:

1. Black Walnut Hull Tincture: 30 drops once a day on an empty stomach, like before a meal.
2. Wormwood Combination capsules: 14 capsules once a day on an empty stomach.
3. Cloves: 3 capsules once a day on an empty stomach.
4. Rascal capsules: 4 capsules three times a day.
5. Take ornithine and arginine as needed.

You may take these at different times in the day or together.

The only after-effects you may feel are due to dead parasites! If this maintenance treatment gives you any noticeable after-effects on the same or next day, it means you have indeed killed something, and you shouldn't wait 3 more days to resume killing it. Go after it immediately with the high dose program for three days in a row. You will know it is gone when there are no after-effects from the high dose program.

High Dose Parasite Program

Do this at least twice a year while on the maintenance parasite program. Take for three to five days in a row:

1. Black Walnut Hull Tincture: 30 drops twice a day on an empty stomach.
2. Wormwood Combination capsules: 14 capsules once a day on an empty stomach.
3. Cloves: 3 capsules three times a day on an empty stomach.
4. Rascal: 4 capsules three times a day.
5. Ornithine and arginine (500 mg each) as desired.

You may take these at different times in the day or together.

There are NO side-effects to these herbs at these dosages.

Cleanse Pets Too

Pets have many of the same parasites that we get, including *Ascaris* (common roundworm), hookworm, *Trichinella, Strongyloides,* heartworm and a variety of tapeworms. Every pet living in your home should be deparasitized (cleared of parasites) and maintained on a parasite program. Monthly trips to your vet are not sufficient.

You do not need to get rid of your pet to keep yourself free of parasites.

Your pet is part of your family and should be kept as sweet and clean and healthy as yourself. This is not difficult to achieve. Here is the recipe.

Pet Parasite Program

1. Parsley water: cook a big bunch of fresh parsley in a quart of water for 3 minutes. Throw away the parsley. After cooling, you may freeze most of it in several 1 cup containers. This is a month's supply. Put 1 tsp. parsley water on the cat's food. Put 1 tbs. parsley water on the dog's food. You don't have to watch it go down. Whatever amount is eaten is satisfactory.

Pets are so full of parasites, you must be quite careful not to deparasitize too quickly. The purpose of the parsley water is to keep the kidneys flowing well so dead parasite refuse is eliminated promptly. They get quite fond of their parsley water. Perhaps they can sense the benefit it brings them. Do this for a week before starting the Black Walnut Hull Tincture.

2. Black Walnut Hull Tincture: 1 drop on the food for a cat. For a dog that weighs twice as much as a cat you work up to 2 drops on the food. Start with 1 drop, then 2. Don't force them to eat it. Count carefully. Very young or old cats should get half a drop. Treat cats only twice a week. Treat dogs daily.

For a dog that weighs ten times as much as a cat, work up to 10 drops a day. If your pet vomits or has diarrhea, you may expect to see worms. This is extremely infectious and hazardous. Never let a child clean up a pet mess. Begin by pouring salt and iodine[10] on the mess and letting it stand for 5 minutes before cleaning it up. Clean up outdoor messes the same way. Finally, clean your hands with diluted grain alcohol (dilute 1 part alcohol with 4 parts water) or vodka. Be careful to keep all alcohol out of sight of children; don't rely on discipline for this. Be careful not to buy isopropyl rubbing alcohol for this purpose (it is the cancer related solvent).

Start the wormwood a week later.

3. Wormwood Combination: open a capsule and put the smallest pinch possible on their dry food. Do this for a week before starting the cloves.

4. Cloves: put the smallest pinch possible on their dry food.

Keep all of this up as a routine so that you need not fear your pets. Also, notice how peppy and happy they become.

Go slowly so the pet can learn to eat all of it. To repeat:

- Week 1: parsley water.
- Week 2: parsley water and black walnut.
- Week 3: parsley water, black walnut, and wormwood.
- Week 4: parsley water, black walnut, wormwood, and cloves.

Pets should not stroll on counters or table. They should eat out of their own dishes, not yours. They should not sleep on

[10] "Povidone" iodine, topical antiseptic, is available in most drug stores.

your bed. The bedroom should be off limits to pets. Don't kiss your pets. Wash your hands after playing with your pet. NEVER, NEVER share food with your pet. Don't keep a cat box in the house; install a cat door. Wear a dust-mask when you change the cat box. If you have a sandbox for the children, buy new sand from a lumber yard and keep it covered. Don't eat in a restaurant where they sweep the carpet while you are eating (the dust has parasite eggs tracked in from outside). Never let a child crawl on the sidewalk or the floor of a public building. Wash children's hands before eating. If feasible, leave shoes at the door. Eat "finger" foods with a fork.

Solvents are just as bad for your pet as for you. Most flavored pet foods are polluted with solvents such as carbon tetrachloride, benzene, propyl alcohol, wood alcohol, etc. Don't buy flavored pet food.

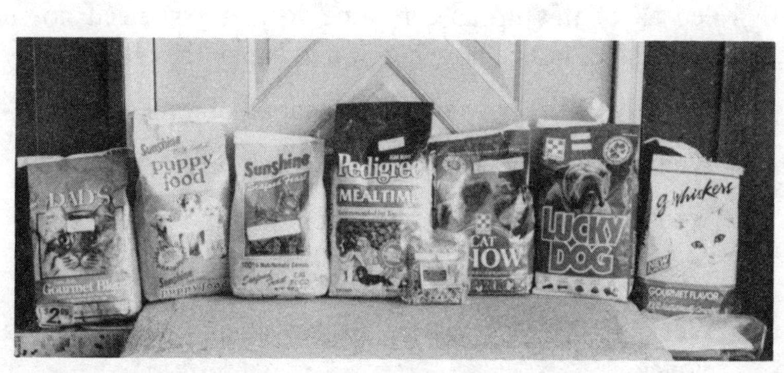

Of the collection of pet foods shown, only two were NOT polluted.
Fig. 13 Polluted and safe pet foods

Pets add a great deal to human lives. **Get rid of the parasites, not the pets.**

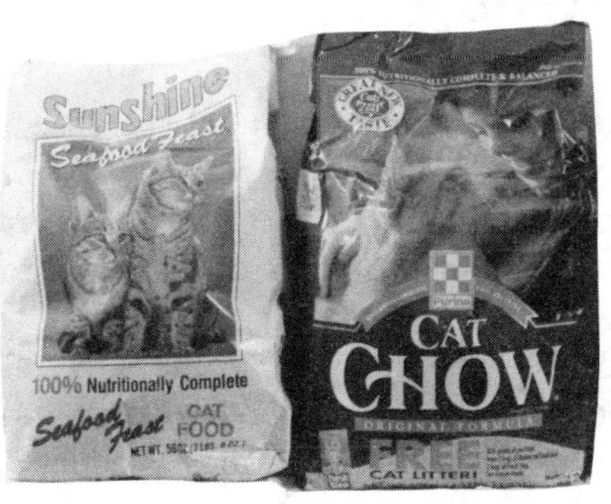

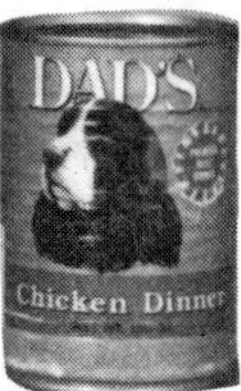

The two safe dry foods, and one safe canned food.
Fig. 14 Safe pet foods

Parasites Gone, Benzene Next

Now that you have killed the intestinal fluke and cured your HIV virus, what's next? Two tasks remain:

1. Stop getting benzene into your body.
2. Get rid of the heavy metals and common toxins in your body, diet and home. (This is covered in *Part Two: Getting Well Again*). This will heal the damaged thymus.

Banish Benzene

Benzene deserves special attention not only because it is the AIDS-related solvent, but because it is presumed to be absent from our consumer environment. Yet I have found traces in everything from bottled water to toothpaste! It is so toxic its concentration is even regulated and tested in gasoline and dry cleaning fluid to reduce exposure to it in the air. Can you imagine eating it or putting it on our bodies, even in minute quantities? Benzene is not put in our foods intentionally, we probably get it accidentally from countries where it is not illegal as an extraction or cleaning agent.

It is present in foods and products that have flavor added. This suggests that benzene was used to extract the flavor, for example, mint from mint leaves. It is not legal in the United States to use benzene to make food extracts. Our regulatory agencies have been vigilant in checking beverages, body products, and gasoline for benzene. Occasionally, benzene pollution is found and the product is quickly taken off the market. Nevertheless, the present extent of benzene pollution is unthinkable and unexpected.

These are the foods and products which I have found to be polluted with benzene STOP USING THEM IMMEDIATELY. DO NOT FINISH UP ANY ONE OF THEM. THROW THEM OUT NOW! Throw them into the garbage and take the garbage out of your house. Benzene is very volatile and will fill your air-space. Just because you can not smell it does not mean you are not inhaling it.

Benzene Polluted Products

THROW THESE OUT

Your health is worth more than the fortune you spent on them!

- **Flavored food** (yogurt, Jello™, candies, throat lozenges, store-bought cookies and cakes)
- **Hand cream**, skin cream, moisturizers
- **Toothpaste** including health brands
- **Tea Tree** oil products (Melaluca™)
- **Beverages** including bottled water, and store-bought fruit juice
- **Vaseline products** (Noxzema™, Vick's™, Lip Therapy™), Chapstick, hand cleaners
- **Cold cereal**
- **Cooking oil** and shortening (use only olive oil, butter and lard)
- **Ice cream** and frozen yogurt
- **Chewing gum**
- **Personal lubricant**
- Amyl nitrate, butyl nitrite, and similar products, commonly called "**Rush**"
- **Marijuana**
- Flavored pet food, both for cats and dogs
- Bird food made into cakes
- Cattle and poultry feeds, except simple grains

Your Substitutes:

All persons with HIV or AIDS associated illness have benzene accumulated in them. But what about the rest of us? We, too, have been using benzene polluted items. Why does it not accumulate in everybody? The answer, of course, lies in how much benzene you get. But is that all? Is there some special toxin that only some of us get, and that specifically causes benzene buildup? Indeed there is. People with a benzene buildup have been eating a lot of grilled food, toast, wieners, and open flame heated food. Such foods have benzopyrenes in them. Benzopyrenes use up the liver's detoxifying ability for benzene and leave benzene to accumulate. Stop eating these foods.

Another tip for reducing benzene buildup: vitamin B_2 is known to help detoxify benzopyrenes. Make sure you are taking at least 50 mg of vitamin B_2 (riboflavin) with each meal, and don't visit tanning booths! Ultraviolet light destroys the B_2 already in your body. But don't rely on vitamin B_2 alone. Stick to all the rules carefully.

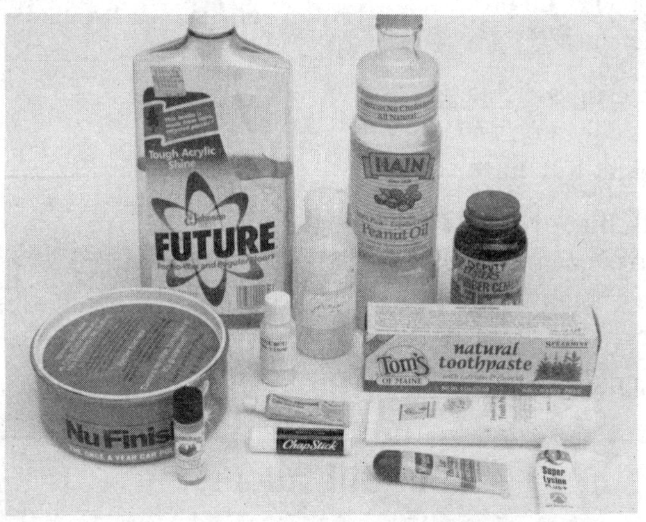

BEWARE! Our household products, body products and even foods have benzene pollution in them.

Fig. 15 Some benzene-polluted products

Stop using benzene-polluted products as soon as you read this. **This includes health brands!** Don't wait until you have low immunity. Don't wait until you have killed parasites. If you can't believe this extensive pollution with benzene and wish to have this verified by our government agencies first, set the items aside, in a twist-tied plastic bag, outside your living space. Use other products while you are waiting!

Make your own replacements from our recipes!

The body rids itself of benzene in three to five days after stopping the use of polluted products.

It is impossible for me to have tested every batch of every food and product, but so many test positive you simply can not risk any of the foods and products on the list.

You have now accomplished two goals:

1. You have killed the intestinal fluke and all its stages and are on the way to killing all of your parasites. YOU NO LONGER HAVE THE HIV VIRUS.
2. Your body has eliminated benzene. It is out of the thymus where T cells are made. Will your T cell count go up? Will you recover from AIDS?

YOU CAN RECOVER FROM AIDS BY CLEARING YOUR THYMUS OF ALL PARASITES AND HARMFUL CHEMICALS.

Review

The intestinal fluke can reproduce itself from beginning to end inside your body (not needing a snail) if you have solvent in your body. There are many solvents around us. If the solvent is benzene, which accumulates in the thymus, the human intestinal fluke colonizes there and brings you HIV. The damage to your thymus reduces your immunity, allowing other parasites and pathogens to multiply. This is AIDS.

Because benzene is a solvent, I think it dissolves the shells of the eggs and lets them all hatch! Right inside you! The tiny baby stages (miracidia) then get into your blood and travel everywhere in your body! They land, become redia, and reproduce into thousands more! They finally turn into cercaria, metacercaria, and then adults.

- Adults in your liver, if you have propyl alcohol in it, causing cancer!
- Adults in your thymus, if you have benzene in it causing HIV disease!
- Adults in your brain, if you have toluene or xylene in it, causing Alzheimer's disease!
- Adults in your kidneys (Hodgkin's disease), uterus (endometriosis) or prostate (chronic prostatitis) if you have other solvents there!
- Adults in your skin if you have Kaposi's sarcoma.

I had to mention these diseases even though this book is just about HIV/AIDS because you should know what a scourge this parasite is, and how deadly it is to have both the intestinal fluke and solvents. In every case (100%) of these diseases that I have seen, <u>both</u> have been present.

In addition to avoiding the benzene hidden in the foods and products listed, do not buy products that list propyl alcohol, propanol, isopropyl alcohol, isopropanol, and so forth, in their contents. Propyl alcohol is the second most dangerous solvent to avoid and is discussed in more detail later. Solvents will leave your body by themselves. You only need to stop using them. Tear out the benzene list and stick it to your refrigerator so the whole family can help you eliminate those products.

Part Two: Getting Well Again

You are not transformed magically into a healthy person on the day the HIV is gone. However, when both HIV and benzene are gone, you will feel noticeably better each day. In 100 days you can feel 100% better. But will you ever get your health back completely? Will your body ever be able to detoxify small amounts of solvents without developing AIDS again? You need a complete set of T cells to be healthy again. You need *helpers, suppressors, natural killers* and the whole range of specialized white blood cells that you once had, and in the right proportions. How long your recovery takes depends on how damaged your thymus is today, and <u>how well you treat it from now on</u>.

Your thymus has been assaulted by benzene, other solvents, parasites, pathogens, (bacteria and viruses), heavy metals, and regular pollutants (such as radon, asbestos, and so forth). These must all come out, to let the thymus heal.

The principle is the same as wound-healing anywhere else in your body. **The wound must be clean.** Recall a wound you once had in your skin. It had to be scrubbed clean of glass or wood splinters or dirt; only then could it be bandaged. What happened under the bandage? **It healed.** Healing is not understood. It is still in the realm of mystery. Your body knows how to heal you and, best of all, it always does. Even if you are terminally ill, your body can still turn around and be healed. **Don't delay for a minute.** You must clean up your thymus gland. This will be a marvelous adventure.

Getting well will be the most exciting part of your recovery. You will feel yourself getting stronger, more clear-headed, breathing freer, more like your old self. How does this happen? Because when you remove all obstacles from your body, you can count on it, **it will heal**!

Getting well from AIDS depends on cleaning foreign things out of your thymus so it can heal. You have already removed all the parasites from your body and the benzene. That was critical, but keep going if you want to get your immunity back.

You can clean your thymus by removing unnatural chemicals.

- Remove all unnatural chemicals from your mouth
- Remove all unnatural chemicals from your diet.
- Remove all unnatural chemicals from your body.
- Remove all unnatural chemicals from your home.

A bit of every one of these is in your thymus!

That is all there is to it. Let us look at each step, the mouth, the diet, the body, the home. The changes you need to make could cost up to $5000.00. Decide, first of all, that you are worth it. Of course you are worth it! What a fine example you will be setting for your friends and family. By getting well, you are rewarding them for helping you. And you are teaching them a valuable lesson about the toxic pollution of our environment. Your recovery will be an inspiration to everybody. You may be saving lives!

Cleaning up your thymus will bring your former health back to you. These changes will herald a new era in your life. Don't delay for a single day. Begin now—with your mouth.

Clean Up Your Dentalware

(This section on dentistry was contributed by Dr. Frank Jerome, D.D.S.)

Dr. Jerome: The philosophy of dental treatment taught in America is that teeth are to be saved by whatever means available, using the strongest, most long lasting materials. Long-term toxic effects are of little concern. The attitude of the majority of dentists is: whatever the A.D.A. (American Dental Association) says is OK, they will do.

A more reasonable philosophy is that there is no tooth worth saving if it damages your immune system. Use this as your guideline.

The reason dentists do not see toxic results is that they do not look or ask. If a patient has three mercury fillings placed in the mouth and a week later has a kidney problem, will she call the dentist—or the doctor? Will they ever tell the dentist about the kidney problem or tell the doctor about the three fillings? A connection will never be made.

It is common for patients who have had their metal fillings removed to have various symptoms go away but, again, they do not tell the dentist. The patient has to be asked! Once the patient begins to feel well they take it for granted, and don't make the connection, either. If everybody's results were instantaneous, there would be no controversy.

Find an alternative dentist. They have been leading the movement to ban mercury from dental supplies. Not only mercury, but all metal needs to be banned. If your dentist will not follow the necessary procedures, then you must find one that will. The questions to ask when you phone a new dental office are:

1. Do you place mercury fillings? (The correct answer is NO. If they do, they don't have enough experience in the use of non-metal composites.)
2. Do you do root canals? (The correct answer is NO. If they do, they do not understand good alternative dentistry)
3. Do you remove amalgam tattoos? (The correct answer is YES. Tattoos are pieces of mercury left in the gum tissue.)
4. Do you treat cavitations? (The correct answer is YES. By cleaning them.)

The complete name of *cavitations* is *alveolar cavitational osteopathosis*. They are holes (cavities) left in the jawbone by an incompletely extracted tooth. A properly cleaned socket which is left after an extraction will heal and fill with bone. Dentists routinely do NOT clean the socket of tissue remnants or infected bone. A dry socket (really an infected socket) is a common result. These sockets never fully heal. Thirty years after an extraction, a cavitation will still be there. It is a form of *osteomyelitis*, which means bone infection.

Ninety percent or more of dental offices will not be able to answer <u>any</u> of the above questions correctly. If you allow the work to be done by a dentist who does not understand the importance of the above list, you could end up with new problems. Find the right dentist first even if you must travel hundreds of miles. Dentists are not equal. You can find a dentist in your area by calling the Huggins Diagnostic Clinic (800-331-2303).

There are 6,000 to 10,000 dentists who should be able to help. Some can do part of the work and refer you to a specialist for the rest. Five hundred to one thousand of these dentists can do it all.

Normal treatment cost is about $1,000 for replacement of 6 to 8 metal fillings, including the examination and X-rays. For people with a metal filling in every tooth, or for the extraction of all teeth (plus dentures), it may be up to $3,000 (or more in some places).

Remember, the simpler the treatment, the better. If the dentist says that he or she can change your metal fillings to plastic but it would be better to CROWN them, say "NO!"

Guidelines For A Healthy Mouth

If you have	*they must*
Metal fillings	change to plastic fillings
Inlays and onlays	change to plastic fillings
Crowns (all types)	change to plastic crowns
Bridges	change to plastic crowns, partials
Metal partials	change to plastic partials(Flexite™)
Pink dentures	change to clear plastic
Porcelain denture teeth	change to plastic denture teeth
Badly damaged teeth	become extractions
Root canals	become extractions
Braces and implants	avoid
Cavitations	need to be surgically cleaned
Temporary crowns	use plastic
Temporary fillings	use Duralon™

The guidelines can be summarized as:

1. Remove all metal from the mouth.
2. Remove all infected teeth and clean cavitations.

Dr. Clark: *Removing all metal means removing all root canals, metal fillings and crowns. Take out all bridge work or partials made of metal and never put them back in. But you may feel quite attached to the gold, so ask the dentist to give you everything she or he removes. Look at the underside. You will be glad you switched.*

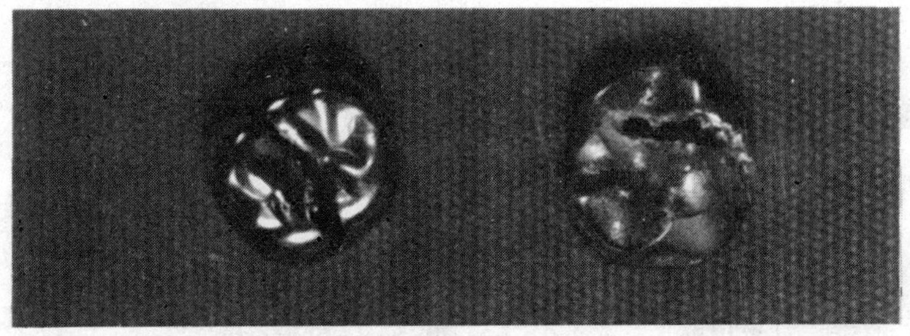

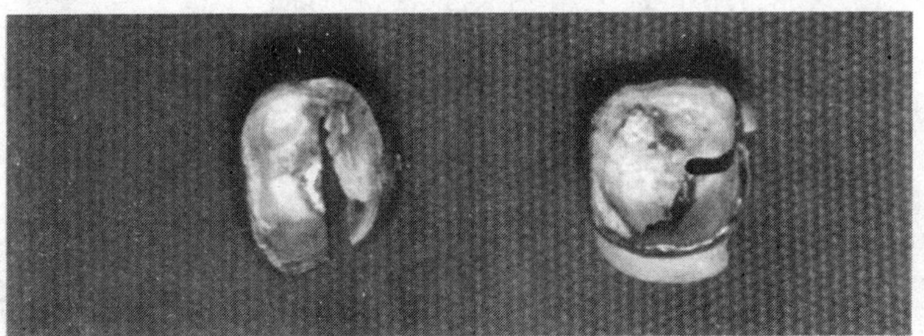

The top surfaces of tooth fillings are kept glossy by brushing (you swallow some of what is removed). Underneath is tarnish and foulness. Ask to see your crowns when they are removed.

Fig. 16 Tops and bottoms of some metal crowns

The stench of the infection under some teeth may be overwhelming as they are pulled. Bad breath in the morning is due to such hidden tooth infections, not a deficiency of mouthwash!

All metal must come out, no matter how glossy it looks on the surface. Metal does not belong in your body. It is an unnatural chemical. Do this as soon as you have found a dentist able to do it. Find a dentist with experience and knowledge about this subject. It is more than replacing acknowledged culprits like mercury-amalgam fillings. This is metal-free dentistry. *ONLY METAL-FREE PLASTIC SHOULD BE PUT BACK IN YOUR MOUTH.*

Dr. Jerome: If your dentist tells you that mercury and other metals will not cause any problems, you will not be able to change his or her mind. Seek treatment elsewhere!

Your dentist should do a complete X-ray examination of your mouth. Ask for the *panoramic* X-ray rather than the usual series of 14 small X-rays (called full mouth series). The panoramic X-ray shows the whole mouth including the jaws and the sinuses. This lets the dentist see impacted teeth, root fragments, bits of mercury buried in the bone and deep infections. Cavitations are visible in a panoramic X-ray that may not be seen in a full mouth series.

The cost of removing metals should be viewed in the proper light. It took years or decades to get into your present condition. When you do a lot of dental repair in a short time, it can seem to be costly. Unfortunately, many people are in a tight financial position because of the cost of years of ineffective treatment, trying to get well.

Your dentist may recommend crowning teeth to "protect" or strengthen them. Unfortunately, the very concept of crowning teeth is flawed. First, the enamel is removed from a tooth to prepare for the crown. This is permanent and serious damage!

Many teeth, up to 20%, may die after being crowned and will need to be extracted at a later time. For this reason, you should only get replacement crowns and no new crowns. Your metal crowns can be changed to plastic. (Remember, no metal must be left under the crown.)

If you have many crowns, you should have them all removed as quickly as possible. But you should not spend more than two hours in the dentist's chair at any one time. That is too much stress for your body. It is quite all right to have a temporary (plastic) crown placed on all teeth that need them in the first visit. You may then go back and complete treatment over the next 6 to 12 months. It is common to find a crowned tooth to be very weak and not worth replacing the crown, particularly if you are already having a partial made and could include this tooth in it.

Dr. Clark: *We are accustomed to thinking that plastic is metal-free. This is wrong. The original dental plastic, methyl methacrylate was metal-free. But modern plastic contains metal. The metal is ground up very finely and added to the plastic in order to make it harder, give it sheen, color, etc.*

Dr. Jerome: Dentists are not given information on these plastic-metals. The information that comes with dental supplies does not list them either. The A.D.A., however, has a library full of such information.[11]

Dr. Clark: *There are many lanthanide (Rare Earth) metals used in dental plastic. Their effects on the body from dental ware have NOT been studied. Only metal-free plastic is safe.*

---

[11] Call the American Dental Association at (800) 621-8099 (Illinois (800) 572-8309, Alaska or Hawaii (800) 621-3291). Members can ask for the Bureau of Library Services, non-members ask for Public Information.

Dr. Jerome: these are the acceptable plastics; they can be procured at any dental lab.

- Plastic for dentures: *Methyl Methacrylate*. Available in clear and pink. Do not use pink.[12]
- Plastic for partial dentures: *Flexite™* Available in clear and pink. Do not use pink.
- Plastic for fillings: *Composite Materials*. This is the material that has been used in front teeth for 30 years. It has been used in back teeth for 10 years. There are many brands and there are new ones being marketed constantly. The new ones are very much superior to those used 10 years ago and they will continue to improve. They do, however, contain enough barium to make them visible on X-rays. There are no alternatives available without barium.

Dr. Clark: *Composites with barium are not good, but I haven't seen enough barium toxicity from fillings at this time to merit advising extraction instead. Hopefully, a barium-free variety will become available soon to remove this health risk.*

Dr. Jerome: Many people (and dentists too) believe that porcelain is a good substitute for plastic. Porcelain is aluminum oxide with other metals added to get different colors (shades). The metal does come out of the porcelain! It has many technical drawbacks as well. Porcelain is not recommended. Sometimes the white composite fillings are called porcelain fillings but they are not.

---

[12] The pink color is from mercury or cadmium which is added to the plastic.

If you have a large bridge, it cannot be replaced with a plastic bridge because it isn't strong enough. A large bridge must be replaced with a removable partial (Flexite™).

The methods used to remove metals and infections are technical and complicated. See *Sources* for more information. And read Dr. Huggins' book *It's All In Your Head.*[13]

Dr. Clark: *I'd like to thank Dr. Jerome for his contributions to this section, and his pioneering work in metal-free dentistry. I hope more dentists acquire his techniques.*

Horrors Of Metal Dentistry

Why are highly toxic metals put in materials for our mouths? Because not everyone agrees on what is toxic at what level. Just decades ago lead was commonly found in paint, and until recently in gasoline. Lead was not less toxic then, we were just less informed! The government sets standards of toxicity, but those "standards" change as more research is done (and more people speak out). You can do better than the government by dropping your standard for toxic metals to zero! Simply remove them.

The debate still rages over mercury amalgam fillings. No one disputes the extreme toxicity of mercury compounds and mercury vapor. The A.D.A. feels that mercury amalgam fillings are safe because they do not vaporize or form toxic compounds to a significant degree. Opponents cite scientific studies that implicate mercury amalgams as disease causing. Many dentists advocate mercury amalgam fillings simply because they are

[13] Available through the Huggins' Diagnostic Clinic (800) 331-2303.

accepted by the A.D.A., which they believe protects them from malpractice litigation. Why risk your health and life on their opinions? Remember everything corrodes and everything seeps, so amalgams must too.

Older fillings may not only contain lead, but cadmium, too. Cadmium is five times as toxic as lead, and is strongly linked to high blood pressure. Cadmium is also used to make the pink color in dentures!

Occasionally, thallium and germanium are found together in mercury amalgam tooth fillings. Thallium causes leg pain, leg weakness, and paraplegia. If you are in a wheelchair without a very reliable diagnosis, have all the metal removed from your mouth. Ask the dentist to give you the grindings. Try to have them analyzed for thallium using the most sensitive methods available, possibly at a research institute or university.

I was astonished to find thallium in mercury amalgams! It couldn't be put there intentionally, look how toxic it is:

TEJ500 ***HR: 3***

THALLIUM COMPOUNDS

Thallium and its compounds are on the Community Right To Know List.

THR: Extremely toxic. The lethal dose for a man by ingestion is 0.5-1.0 gram. Effects are cumulative and with continuous exposure toxicity occurs at much lower levels. Major effects are on the nervous system, skin and cardiovascular tract. The peripheral nervous system can be severely affected with dying-back of the longest sensory and motor fibers. Reproductive organs and the fetus are highly susceptible. Acute poisoning has followed the ingestion of toxic quantities of a thallium-bearing depilatory and accidental or suicidal ingestion of rat poison. Acute poisoning results in swelling of the feet and legs, arthralgia, vomiting, insomnia, hyperesthesia and paresthesia

> [numbness] of the hands and feet, mental confusion, polyneuritis with severe pains in the legs and loins, partial paralysis of the legs with reaction of degeneration, angina-like pains, nephritis, wasting and weakness, and lymphocytosis and eosinophilia. About the 18th day, complete loss of the hair on the body and head may occur. Fatal poisoning has been known to occur. Recovery requires months and may be incomplete. Industrial poisoning is reported to have caused discoloration of the hair (which later falls out), joint pain, loss of appetite, fatigue, severe pain in the calves of the legs, albuminuria, eosinophilia, lymphocytosis and optic neuritis followed by atrophy. Cases of industrial poisoning are rare, however. Thallium is an experimental teratogen [used to induce birth defects for study]. When heated to decomposition they [sic] emit highly toxic fumes of Tl [thallium]. See also THALLIUM and specific compounds.[14]

Fig. 17 Thallium excerpt

Even if you do not have HIV/AIDS, it would make sense to have all of your metal fillings out if you have several of the listed symptoms.

Thallium pollution frightens me more than lead, cadmium and mercury combined, because it is completely unsuspected. Its last major use, rat poison, was banned in the 1970s. One current use for thallium is in Arctic/Antarctic thermostats. When added to mercury the mercury will stay liquid at lower temperatures. Are mercury suppliers then providing the dental industry with tainted amalgam?

---

14 *Dangerous Properties of Industrial Materials* 7th ed. by N. Irving Sax and Richard J. Lewis Sr. Van NOSTRAND Reinhold N.Y. 1989.

Dental Rewards

After your mouth is metal and infection-free, notice whether your sinus condition, ear-ringing, enlarged neck glands, headache, enlarged spleen, bloated condition, knee pain, foot pain, hip pain, dizziness, aching bones and joints improve.

Keep a small notebook to write down these improvements. It will show you which symptoms came originally from your teeth. Symptoms often come back! So go back to your dentist, to search for a hidden infection under one or more of your teeth, or where your teeth once were! That infection can be the cause of tinnitus, TMJ (Temporal Mandibular Joint), arthritis, neck pain, loss of balance, and heart attacks! Most importantly, these tooth bacteria easily find their way to your thymus. After cavitations are cleaned, the bacteria in the thymus will leave in a few days.

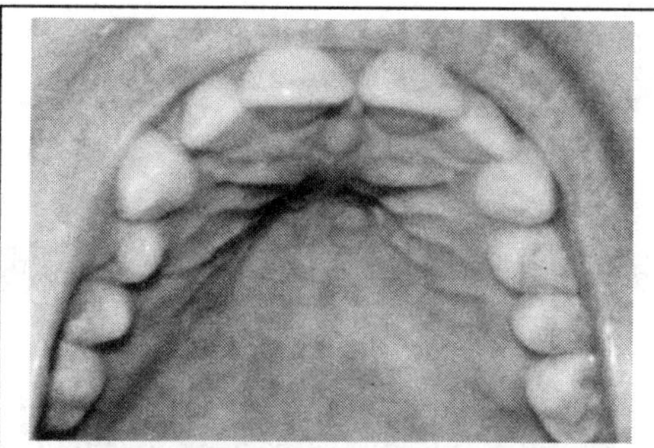
Fig. 18 Beautiful plastic mouth

Dentures can be beautiful. Of course, plastic isn't natural, but it is the best compromise that can be made to restore your mouth. At least it isn't positively charged like metals; it can't set up an electric current nor a magnetic field in your mouth, all of which may be harmful.

Do not be swayed by arguments that plastic is not as strong as metal. You see dentures everywhere and they seem strong enough to eat with. You will be told that "noble" metals like gold and platinum and silver are OK, that they are "inert" and do not corrode or seep. Nothing could be more untrue. You may be keeping them glossy by the constant polishing action of your toothpaste. But if you look at the underside, the view is frightful. Your mouth is quite corrosive! You wouldn't expect a handful of metal, even noble metal, that was dropped in a well 50 years ago, to be intact. As it corrodes your body absorbs it!

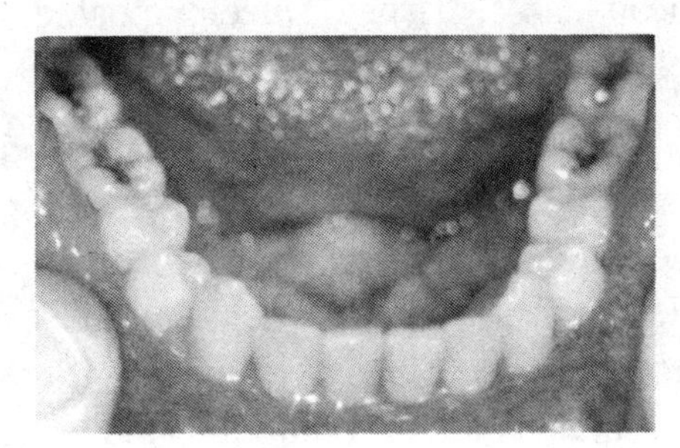

Fig. 19 Ugly metal in mouth

Getting well is the magic you can expect from removing unnatural chemicals To do this for your mouth, get started immediately, since your dentist may need more than one day to complete it. Get started the day you read this book! Don't wait till the parasite program is completed.

You now have accomplished 4 things:

1. You have killed the intestinal fluke, and all of its stages, and eliminated HIV.
2. You have killed all your other parasites and have yourself and your pet on a maintenance program to keep killing parasites.
3. You have gotten rid of all benzene sources.
4. You have started getting well by cleaning up your dentalware. You are measuring your progress against a list of all of your symptoms.

Clean Up Your Diet

This is the easiest part of your get-well program since YOU are completely in charge.

There is really only one rule:

EAT CHEMICAL-FREE FOOD.

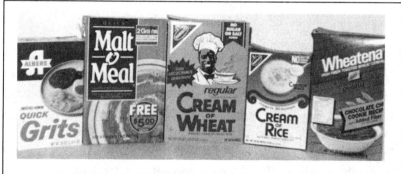

Fig. 20 Unpolluted breakfast cereals

Breakfast

Cook your cereal from scratch. Don't eat cold cereal; it has numerous solvents and added chemicals. Buy hot cereals that say "no salt added," like Cream of Wheat, steel cut oats or old fashioned oats,[15] millet, corn meal, cream of rice, or Wheatena.™ Cook it with milk to add nutritive value. Add your own (non-aluminum) salt. Make granola from a recipe (there are two in this book). Use honey, not sugar (honey is less processed). Add raisins that aren't sulfited. Don't use nuts; they carry aflatoxins. Use whipping cream or half-n-half if you need to gain weight. Isn't this a delicious way to start your day! Use ground cinnamon to flavor, or frozen fruit and honey (see *recipes*).

> The biggest obstacle to eating natural food is time. Find a friend who has the time to cook for you, if you are not up to it.

Or start your day with fried potatoes and an egg and glass of milk. Don't worry about cholesterol while you are recovering.

Eat the simplest dairy products you can find, not cheese, not ice cream, not cream cheese, not kefir. Choose milk, buttermilk and yogurt (homemade). **Always sterilize the milk yourself, first** (page 91). It should be 2% or more butterfat because the calcium in milk cannot be absorbed without at least this much fat. Eat homemade yogurt and add honey or homemade preserves yourself. You need 3 cups of a milk product each day. If you don't tolerate milk, and get diarrhea from it, try a milk digestant tablet to go with it. Start with only ¼ cup at a time. Do not choose chocolate milk. There is no substitute for milk; calcium tablets are not satisfactory. Vegetable matter, although

---

[15] Rolled oats have 235 mcg nickel per serving of 4 ounces, picked up from the rollers, according to *Food Values* 14th ed. by Pennington and Church 1985. I have only found nickel in the "one-minute" or "instant" variety of oats, however.

high in calcium, does not give you *available* calcium either, unless you buy a juicer and make vegetable juice out of it. Eating fish can give you a lot of calcium, but it is in the tiny bones hidden in the fish. Don't try to remove them. Canned salmon has a lot of calcium; tuna does not. On a day that you eat fish, you would not need milk. Goat milk is probably better than cows' milk, but more difficult to get used to and needs to be boiled, too.

No food is perfect.

You don't have to be perfect in your food selection to get well.

It can be difficult to know which chemicals are unnatural. This book can't go into a long discussion of different definitions of "natural" and "unnatural." What counts for an AIDS patient is whether the immune system will be called upon to remove something from the food you eat. Your immune system is precious. You have (or had) 5000 white blood cells in every little dot of blood.[16] They have the job of keeping you clear of parasites, bacteria, viruses and unnatural chemicals. Even if the unnatural chemicals you eat do not do great harm, they must still be removed. White blood cells that are busy removing aluminum, nickel, mercury, copper, fragrance, or even soap are not free to fight bacteria and viruses and parasites.

Give your immune system a chance to heal your body by removing the burden on it: the burden of countless, frivolous

[16] 5000 white blood cells per cubic millimeter.

cleaning-up jobs. Clean yourself up so your immune system does not have to.

Lunch

Cook your food from scratch. Don't start with cans or packages or frozen items to make some recipe. In fact, don't bother with <u>any</u> fancy recipes. Just cook two or three vegetables for lunch and eat them with butter[17] and salt. Bread and milk rounds it out, plus fruit (not canned or frozen). Soup is a nice change. Cook it with all the vegetables you can find. Don't start with a can or packet or cube. Use a bit of onion and genuine herbs to give it zest.

If all this is too much work, make fresh vegetable juice once a week and freeze enough so that you can have a daily nutritious meal just by pouring a glass of it, together with bread and yogurt or milk.

Never try to lower your cholesterol while regaining your health from HIV/AIDS.

This is a rule based on common sense. Synthetic eggs, margarine and cholesterol reduced products are extremely "chemical" foods.

[17] Butter is our only source of butyric acid in the intestine. There is some evidence that butyric acid favors beneficial bacteria in the intestine and kills parasites!

Bake your own bread! I found aflatoxins in commercial bread after just four days in my breadbox, but none in homemade bread even after two weeks! Aflatoxin is a most potent carcinogen. Aflatoxin may be the toxin in your diet that keeps the liver from clearing solvents from your body! Aflatoxin is a substance made by mold; bread goes moldy easily. Don't ever eat moldy food, whether it is fruit, breads or leftovers in the refrigerator. Throw them out. Buy a bread maker. It can do everything, including baking the bread. Use unbleached (unbrominated) flour and add ½ tsp. vitamin C powder per loaf to help retard mold further.

Do not toast your bread! This makes 4,5 benzopyrene which inhibits benzene detoxification so that it accumulates in the first place.

Supper

Cook your supper from scratch. Emphasize fish for animal food, not beef, pork, turkey or chicken. Do not grill, broil or barbecue (it makes benzopyrene); instead, fry, bake, poach or boil. Don't buy bread crumbs, use your own. Don't buy batter, make your own. Use genuine eggs, not substitutes. Wash your hands after handling raw eggs or meat. Cook real potatoes, not instant varieties. Make your own salad and salad dressing out of olive oil, lemon juice, white distilled vinegar(not apple cider vinegar which has aflatoxins) honey, salt and herbs to flavor. If your digestion isn't strong enough for raw vegetables or fruit, make juice. Get a sturdy juicer and make your juice about half carrot juice and half from vegetables like celery, squash, lettuce, and broccoli. Make your own tomato sauce with pure herb seasoning, not from a jar or can (home canned foods are fine, of course, as long as they are not made in a big aluminum pot with aluminum-containing salt).

Make mashed potatoes from scratch – not box potatoes, nor chips nor French fries. Box potatoes have added chemicals. Chips and fries were made in chemical grease called "hydrogenated vegetable (or other) oil." There is a large amount of nickel in hydrogenated fats.[18] Fry your potatoes in butter, lard or olive oil. Find butter that is not wrapped in foil and is not salted.[19] Salt your own butter, using aluminum-free salt.

Eat no meat that hasn't been cooked as thoroughly as if it were pork.

Other animals are as parasitized as we, full of flukes and worms and *schistosomes* in every imaginable stage, and if the blood carries many of these, would we not be eating these live parasites if we eat these animals in the raw state? We have been taught to cook thoroughly any pork, fish or seafood. Now we must cook thoroughly any beef, chicken or turkey. It must be at cooking temperature (212°F or 100°C) for 20 minutes. Freezing is not adequate. Canned meats are safe from living parasites, but are not recommended due to added chemicals.

If you have been very ill, the best advice is to be a vegetarian for three months, then start back on some fish or seafood only.

---

[18] 114 mcg/100 g. Taken from *Food Values* 14ed by Pennington and Church 1985.

[19] Salt has aluminum in it to keep it from caking. Buy Hain Sea Salt, which uses magnesium carbonate as an anti-caking agent, but bake it first to kill mold (3 minutes at 400°F).

Of course, you are protecting yourself with a parasite killing maintenance program. But killing a parasite AFTER it is IN your tissues will not keep you healthy; you must avoid parasites.

Beverages

Drink 6 kinds of beverages:

- milk
- water
- fruit juices
- vegetable juices
- herb teas
- homemade (see recipes)

This means getting off caffeine. And if you are already fatigued, this means you might be even more fatigued for a short time. You might have headaches from withdrawal, too. But they will only last 10 days. Mark your calendar and count off the days. Take headache medicine, if necessary, but make sure it does not contain caffeine. For energy, to replace caffeine, take one arginine (500 mg) upon rising in the morning and before lunch. Soon you won't need it.

Cutting down on coffee, decaf, soda pop and powdered drinks won't do. You must be completely off. They contain very toxic solvents due to careless, unregulated production methods. Much is imported and can't be sufficiently regulated.

Even though grain (drinking) alcohol is the recommended antiseptic, that doesn't mean you may safely drink it. It is inadvisable to drink any form of alcohol at least until you are fully recovered (two years). This is why Black Walnut Hull Tincture, which is 25% grain alcohol, is taken in a warm beverage, to evaporate the alcohol.

Researchers have found even small amounts of alcohol, like three beers over a two day period, cause a ten-fold increase in the rate of HIV multiplication.[20] Alcohol also slows down the detoxification of benzene, allowing your levels to go higher.

1. Milk: 2% or higher, drink three 8 oz. glasses a day. Homemade yogurt is fine. Goat milk is also fine. Start with ¼ cup and increase gradually, if you are not used to it. If you do not drink milk because it gives you more mucous, try to drink milk anyway. If you have other reactions, like diarrhea, try milk digestant tablets (available at health food stores). Milk is too valuable to avoid: there are many unwanted chemicals in most brands of milk, but it is solvent-free and very nutritious. The only exception should be for serious symptoms, like colitis, bloating, flu, or chronic diarrhea. All milk should be sterilized, then cooled and refrigerated (page 91).

2. Water: 2 pints. Drink one pint upon rising in the morning, the other pint in the afternoon sometime. The cold water faucet may be bringing you cadmium, copper or lead, but it is safer than purchased water, which may have solvents in it. Let it run before using it. Filters are rather useless because water pollution comes in surges. A single surge of PCB contaminates your filter. All the water you use after this surge is now polluted, so you will be getting it chronically, whereas the unfiltered water cleans up again after the surge passes. Until you can test your own water for solvents, PCBs and metals, no expensive filter is worth the investment. An inexpensive carbon filter that is replaced <u>every month</u> may improve your tap water, though. Plastic pitchers fitted with a carbon filter pack are

---

[20] *Journal Of Infectious Diseases*, 167:789, 1993.

available. Never buy filters with silver or other chemicals, even if they are "just added to the carbon." If you have copper or galvanized pipes, switch to PVC to be safe from cadmium, copper and lead.

3. Fruit juice: fresh squeezed only. Some stores make it while you wait. If they freeze some of it, you could purchase the frozen containers. Bottled fruitjuices have traces of numerous solvents, as do the frozen concentrates, as do the refrigerated ones, don't buy them. You have to see it being made, but watch carefully: I recently went to a juice bar where they made everything fresh, before your very eyes. And I saw them take the fruit right from the refrigerator and spray it with a special wash "to get rid of any pesticides", then put a special detergent on it to clean off the wash! So instead of getting traces of pesticide, I got traces of propyl alcohol![21] Another grocery store had a machine that squeezed the oranges while you watched. But if you did not watch them filling the jugs, you missed seeing them add a tablespoon of concentrate, from a bottle out of sight, to give it better flavor. It still qualifies as "Fresh squeezed 100% orange juice," but thanks to that concentrate it now has toluene and xylene in it! Best of all, buy a juicer, wash fruit with plain water, and make your own juice (enough for a week—freeze it in half-pint plastic bottles). For stronger flavor, leave some of the peel in the juice.

4. Vegetable juice: fresh or frozen only. If you or a friend would be willing to make fresh juice, this would be much better than purchased juice. Start with carrot juice. Peel carrots (don't scrape them, it's too easy to miss small dirt spots) and remove all blemishes carefully, then rinse. Drink ½ glass a day. After you are accustomed to this, add other vegetables and greens to the juice to make up half of it. Use celery, lettuce, cabbage,

---

[21] Yes, I took a sample of the wash to test.

cucumber, beet, squash, tomato, everything raw that you normally have in your refrigerator. But never anything with soft spots! Then drink one glass a day.

5. Herb tea: fresh or bulk packaged if available. If only tea bags are available, cut them open and dump out the tea. Throw away the bag, it is full of antiseptic. Buy a non-metal (bamboo is common) tea strainer. Sweeten with honey. Be careful not to buy foil packs of tea or tea blends. Tea blends are mixtures of herb teas; these have solvents in them from the extracts used.

6. Homemade beverage. If you will miss your coffee or decaf, try just plain hot water with whipping cream. Sweeten with honey. Please see *Recipes* for many more suggestions.

Horrors In Commercial Beverages

Commercial beverages are especially toxic due to traces of solvents left over from the manufacturing process. There are solvents found in decaffeinated beverages, herb tea blends, carbonated drinks, beverages with Nutrasweet™, flavored coffee, diet and health mixes, and fruit juices, even when the label states "not from concentrate" or "fresh from the orchard," or "100% pure."

Some of the solvents I have found are just too toxic to be believed! Yet you can build the test apparatus yourself (*How To Test Yourself*), buy foods at your grocery store, and tabulate your own results. I hope you do, and I hope you find that the food in your area is cleaner than mine! Remember that the equipment described later can only determine the presence or absence of something, not the concentration. There may only be a few parts per billion, but an AIDS patient trying to get well cannot afford any solvent intake. For that matter, none of us should tolerate any of these pollutants:

- **Acetone** – in carbonated drinks
- **Benzene** – in store-bought drinking water, store-bought "fresh squeezed" fruit juice
- **Carbon tetrachloride** – in store-bought drinking water
- **Decane** – in health foods and beverages
- **Hexanes** – in decafs
- **Hexane dione** – in flavored foods

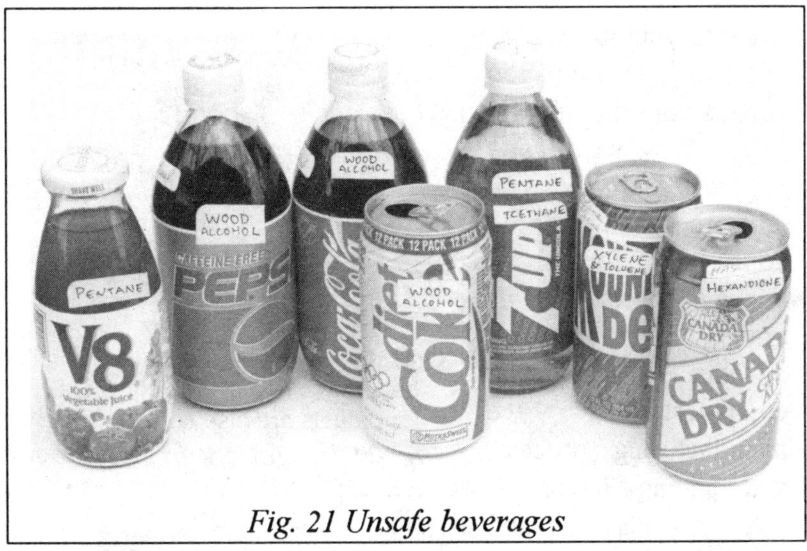

Fig. 21 Unsafe beverages

- **Isophorone** – in flavored foods
- **Methyl butyl ketone** and **Methyl ethyl ketone** – in flavored foods
- **Methylene chloride** – in fruit juice
- **Pentane**– in decafs

- **Propyl alcohol** – bottled water, commercial fruit juices, commercial beverages.
- **Toluene** and **xylene** – in carbonated drinks
- **Trichloroethane**(TCE), **TCEthylene**– in flavored foods
- **Wood alcohol** (methanol) – in carbonated drinks, diet drinks, herb tea blends, store-bought water, infant formula

If you allowed a tiny drop of kerosene or carpet cleaning fluid to get into your pet's food every day, wouldn't you expect your pet to get sick? Why would <u>you</u> not expect to be sick with these solvents in your daily food? I imagine these solvents are just tiny amounts, introduced by sterilizing equipment, the manufacturing process, and adding flavor or color. Flavors and colors for food must be extracted somehow from the leaves or bark or beans from which they come. But until safe methods are invented, such food should be considered unsafe for human consumption (or pets or livestock!).

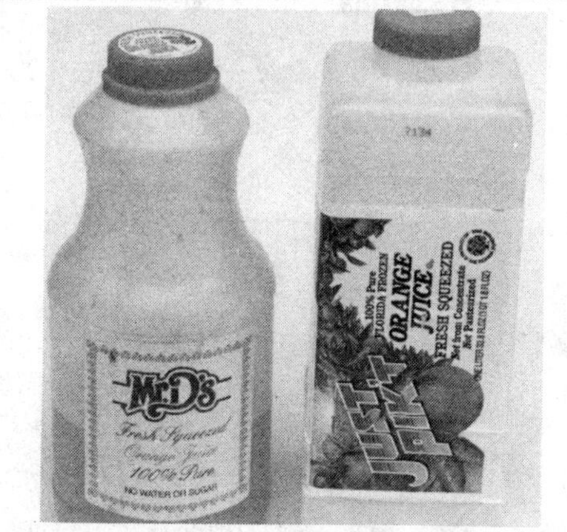

Only these two commercially available beverages had no solvents. Dairy products are also solvent-free.

Fig. 22 Two solvent-free beverages

Sore Mouth Remedy

Thrush (*Candida*) or *Herpes* in your mouth is especially hard to get rid of. Here is how to treat it:

a) While your mouth is bleeding, treat with one drop Lugol's Iodine Solution (see *Recipes*) in one tbs. water, enough to swish in your mouth, and swallow. Do this at bedtime.

b) If your mouth is not bleeding, put one drop of Lugol's Iodine Solution right on your tongue, directly, at bedtime.

This will kill surface fungus. But *Candida* grows right into your living cells, which of course you can't kill. The fungus will gradually die out as it rises to the surface due to stopping its growth. It takes a month! During this time follow these special dietary rules:

1. Drink and eat nothing very hot or ice cold.
2. Drink no fruit juice; it feeds yeast. Even though the sugar is natural, yeast thrives on it, preventing you from clearing up a thrush.
3. Don't eat ice cream or suck on candy for the same reason. If you have thrush stay off sweets until it is gone. Then test yourself on fresh sliced fruit (not juice) with cream and honey to see if you notice a recurrence.
4. Use no alcohol. Even Black Walnut Hull Tincture should be put in a warm beverage to evaporate the alcohol.
5. Don't eat nuts, sunflower seeds, pumpkin seeds, popcorn or even toast if your mouth is bleeding. Also avoid tomatoes (too acidic) and highly salted foods. As a mouthwash use milk or baking soda water or crushed lysine tablets in water.

6. Don't brush your teeth more often when your mouth is sore or bleeding. Use monofilament nylon fish line, two to four pound test, to floss once a day, followed immediately by brushing with food grade hydrogen peroxide. Use three or four drops on your toothbrush. It is very important to kill amoebas and all bacteria because they invade under the gum line and cause terrible tooth and bone loss. In serious situations use several drops of white iodine (see *Recipes*) on a wet toothbrush.

Food Preparation

Cook your food in glass, enamel, ceramic or microwavable pots and pans. Throw away all metal ware, foil wrap, and metal-capped salt shakers since you will never use them again. If you don't plan to fry much (only once a week), you might keep the Teflon™ or Silverstone™ coated fry-pan, otherwise get an enamel coated metal pan. Stir and serve food with wood or plastic, not metal utensils. If you have recurring urinary tract infections, you should reduce your metal contact even further; eat with plastic cutlery. Sturdy decorative plastic ware can be found in hardware and camping stores. Don't drink out of styrofoam cups (styrene is toxic). Don't eat toast (many toasters spit tungsten all over your bread besides making benzopyrenes). Don't buy things made with baking powder (it has aluminum) or baked in aluminum pans. Choose goods made with baking soda and sold in paper or microwavable pans. Don't run your drinking water through the freezer or fountain or refrigerator. Don't heat your water in a coffee maker or tea kettle. Don't use a plastic thermos jug (the plastic liner has lanthanides) the inside must be glass.

Why are we still using stainless steel cookware when it contains 18% chromium and 8% nickel? Because it is rustproof and shiny and we can't see any deterioration. **But all metal seeps!** Throw those metal pots away.

Nearly all bacteria have a requirement for nickel so that their enzyme urease will work for them. Urease attacks urea, present in all our body juices, and makes ammonia from it. Ammonia is a utilizable nitrogen source for bacteria, urea isn't. If our bodies weren't polluted with nickel, many of our bacterial invaders couldn't grow! Why do we take in nickel and supply our bacteria? Nickel is in the soil, where bacteria belong, too. But if we insist on keeping plenty of it in our tissues, we have only ourselves to blame for bacterial invasion.

It is hard to believe that metals we handle every day in our coinage, food and beverage containers, body products, and home and garden products could be hazardous. Yet this has been well studied. The real question is how are most people able to handle these toxins without succumbing sooner?

Again, I want to emphasize that the amount and the form of the metal is very important. For instance, plain zinc is carcinogenic (cancer producing). However an appropriate dose of zinc sulfate is anti-carcinogenic.[22] **Get your essential minerals from foods, not cookware.**

Never, never drink or cook with the water from your hot water faucet. If you have an electric hot water heater the heating element releases metal. Even if you have a gas hot water heater, the heated water leaches metals or glues from your pipes. If your kitchen tap is the single lever type, make sure it is fully on cold.

---

[22] *Inhibition of Carcinogenesis by Dietary Zinc*, Nature, Vol. 231, No. 5303, pp. 447-448, June 18, 1971.

Food Guidelines

It is impossible to remember everything about every food, but in general do not buy foods that are highly processed. Here are a few foods; see if you can guess whether they should be in your diet or not.

breads	Yes, but not fancy varieties that have flavor listed in the ingredients, nor "day-old", or "cholesterol-reduced" bread.
cheese	Yes in baked or cooked dishes only. It must have no mold (throw it out if you see any). Rotate brands.
chicken	Only if cooked for 20 minutes at boiling point, as in soup, or canned (never prepare raw chicken yourself).
wine with dinner	No.
peanut butter	Yes if all natural, but very thoroughly stir in ¼ tsp. vitamin C powder to remove aflatoxins.
cottage cheese	Yes if sterilized by baking or cooking.
desserts	Yes, but again, only if not flavored with extracts (maple and vanilla are OK).
rice	Yes. Add vitamin C after cooking.
pasta	Yes, with homemade sauce.
jello	No, it has artificial flavor and color.
egg dishes	Yes, but not "imitation", cholesterol-free or cholesterol-reduced varieties.
pop corn	Yes, with butter or olive oil, and aluminum free salt.
fish, seafood	Yes!
soy foods (tofu)	No. It's the extensive processing that taints it.
soup	Yes, if seasoned only with herbs (no bouillon cube).

Fig. 23 Some good foods

Choose brands with the shortest list of ingredients. Alternate brands every time you shop. If friends are cooking for

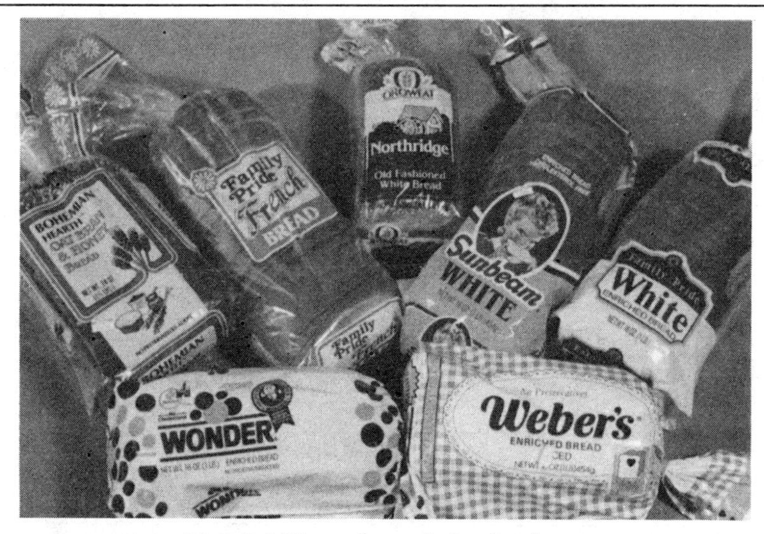

Fig. 24 These breads had solvents

you, give them a copy of these pages about the diet. Carry your own aluminum-free salt with you. The support of your family and friends is very valuable to you, but don't eat with their dishes (dish detergent is on them).

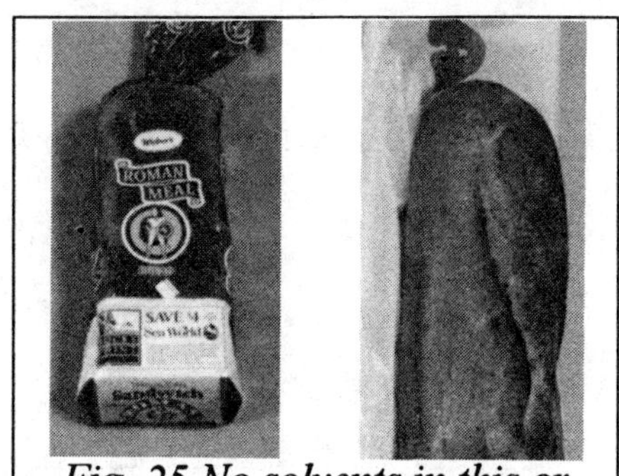

Fig. 25 No solvents in this or bakery bread

You can always eat off paper plates, use plastic cutlery and a plastic cup you wash yourself under the tap. Keep a set of everything handy to take out with you. Your friends are not made ill by these pollutants—YOU ARE. They can excrete them efficiently—YOU CAN'T.

Because you cannot supervise restaurant chefs, many normally safe foods should not be ordered. Here is a list of things that are generally safe to order:

pancakes, french toast, waffles	But add vitamin C to any natural syrup.
eggs	Not scrambled—the added milk or cheese does not get sterilized, and not soft boiled—the white should be solid.
hash browns	If lightly fried, not deep fried.
soup	Only if nothing else is available. (It probably came in a can and was cooked in an aluminum pot and is full of aluminized salt.)
vegetarian sandwiches	But no soy products (too processed).
baked or boiled potatoes	Use only real butter, bring your own salt, don't eat the skin if it was wrapped in foil or has black spots..
cooked vegetables	Broccoli, brussel sprouts, beets, corn, squash, and so forth.
vegetable salads	Don't eat the croutons, bacon bits, and anything that doesn't look fresh.
vegetarian dishes	Especially chinese food, but no soy ingredients.
bread and biscuits	But not "cholesterol-free" varieties.
fish and seafood	Anything but deep fried (the oil may have benzene) is fine: baked, steamed, fish cakes, seafood cocktails, etc.
fruit cup	With whipped cream if not from a pressurized can.
fruit pies, cobblers	But not with ice cream (every flavor has benzene).
lemon or lime meringue pie	Indulge yourself.

Fig. 26 Good restaurant foods

The only beverages you should order in a restaurant are water and boiled milk. Herb teas are all right if you bring your own and make sure the hot water comes from a non-metal pot. Bring your own brown sugar and salt.

If you order food "to go", ask the chef to line the metal or styrofoam containers or cups with plastic wrap. Clear plastic containers are OK, but do not store leftovers in them.

Diet Review

You now have accomplished 5 things:

- You have killed the intestinal fluke and cured HIV.
- You have killed all your other parasites and have yourself and your pet on a maintenance program to keep killing parasites.
- You have removed all products with benzene in them from your house and are eating no foods with benzene pollution.
- You have taken out all the metal from your mouth and are waiting (patiently?) for metal-free plastic teeth or fillings or dentures.
- You have switched from eating food concoctions to eating simple foods, free from solvents and metal, and have eliminated most meats. You are starting to strike symptoms off your list.

As you see your symptoms disappear, one after another, you will feel the magic of healing. Most HIV patients have a few symptoms, but AIDS sufferers can fill a page. It can be quite shocking to see a list of all your symptoms.

Sometimes a new symptom appears as fast as an old one disappears. The coincidence makes it tempting to believe that one symptom turns into a different one. But it is not so. If a new symptom appears, it is because another pathogen has become activated due to a new toxin Try to identify the new item. Stop using any new food, supplement, or body product, even if it is a health variety, and see if it goes away.

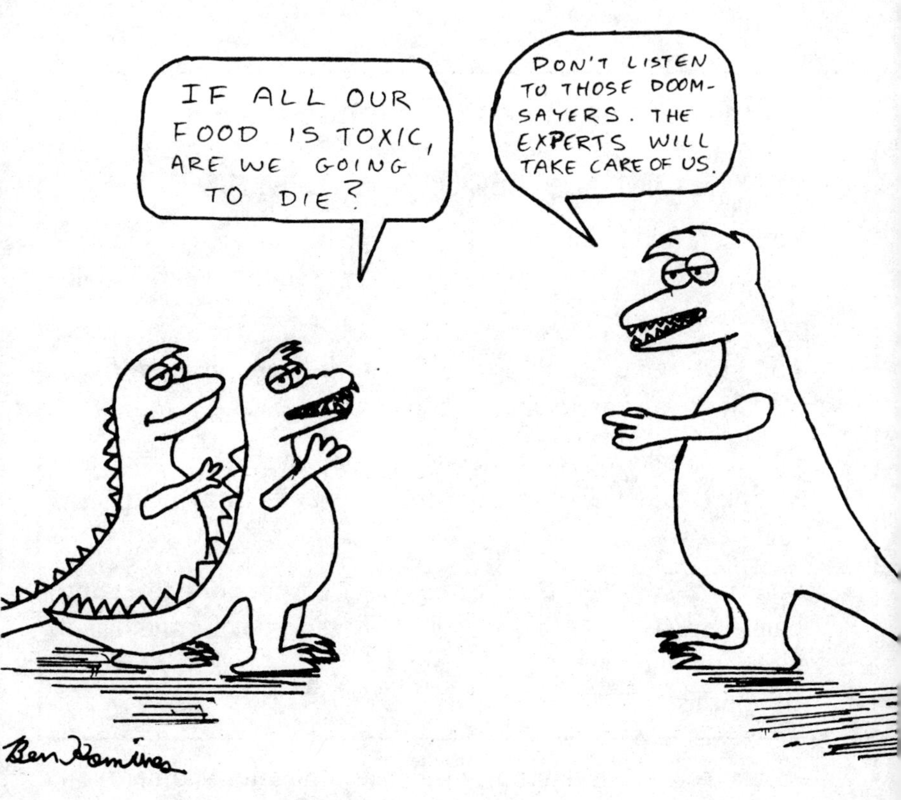
IF ALL OUR FOOD IS TOXIC, ARE WE GOING TO DIE?
DON'T LISTEN TO THOSE DOOM-SAYERS. THE EXPERTS WILL TAKE CARE OF US.
Ben Ramirez

Fig. 27 Our future, unless we act

Clean Up Your Body

We are living in a very fortunate time. We are not expected to all look alike! The 60's brought us this wonderful freedom. Freedom to dress in a variety of styles, use make-up or no make-up, jewelry or no jewelry, any kind of hair style, any kind of shoes.

You will need to go off every cosmetic and body product that you are now using. Not a single one can be continued. They are full of titanium, zirconium, benzalkonium, bismuth, antimony, barium[23], strontium[24], aluminum, tin, chromium, not to mention pollution solvents such as benzene and PCBs.

Do not use any commercial salves, ointments, lotions, colognes, perfumes, massage oils, deodorant, mouthwash, toothpaste, even when touted as "herbal" and health-food-type. See *Recipes* for homemade substitutes.

People are trying desperately to use less toxic products. They seek health for themselves. So they reach for products that just list herbs and other natural ingredients. Unfortunately, the buyers are being duped. The F.D.A. (Food and Drug Administration) requires all body products to have sufficient antiseptic in them. Some of these antiseptics are substances you must avoid! But you won't see them on the label because manufacturers prefer to use quantities below the levels they must disclose. And by using a variety of antiseptics in these small amounts they can still meet sterility requirements. The only ingredient you might see is "grapefruit seed" or similar healthy-

---

23 Barium is described in the *Merck Index* as "Caution: All water or acid soluble barium compounds are POISONOUS." 10th ed. p. 139 1983.

24 This element goes to bones.

sounding natural antiseptic. This is sad for the consumer of health food varieties.

- I have seen rocks sold as "Aluminum-Free Natural Deodorant". You rub the rock under your arms. It works because the rock is made of magnesium-aluminum silicate.
- Men's hair color has lead in it.
- Lipstick has barium, aluminum, titanium.
- Eye pencil and shadow have chromium.
- Toothpaste has benzene, tin, and strontium.
- Hair spray has propyl alcohol and PCBs.
- Shampoo has propyl alcohol!
- Cigarettes have lead, mercury, nickel and Tobacco Mosaic Virus
- Chewing tobacco has ytterbium
- Marijuana has benzene

Some of the unnatural chemicals listed are present because of residues in the manufacturing process, but others you will actually see listed on the label!

See *Recipes* for easy-to-make, natural substitutes. But you might consider just stopping them all. Especially if you're going on vacation.

Use nothing that you wouldn't use on a new-born baby. This is a permissive age. You will be the only one feeling "naked." Others won't even notice. Don't forget advertising is aimed at you, even if other people's eyes are not!

Don't even use soap unless it is homemade soap (see *Recipes*) or borax[25] straight from the box. Borax was the traditional pioneer soap. It is antibacterial and can be made into a concentrate. It is also a water softener and is the main ingredient in non-chlorine bleaches. Borax has excellent solvent power for grease. But even borax is not natural to your body and it is therefore wise to use as little as necessary. See *Recipes* for antibacterial natural borax soap.

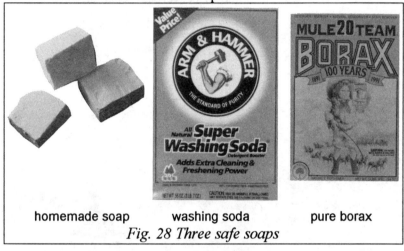

homemade soap washing soda pure borax

Fig. 28 Three safe soaps

Don't use toothpaste, not even health-food varieties. To clean teeth, use baking soda straight from the box – but dissolve it in water first, otherwise it is too abrasive. Or brush with hydrogen peroxide food grade, not the regular variety; it is available at health food stores, not pharmacies or grocery stores. To floss before brushing, use monofilament nylon fish line (two to four pound test). Throw away your old toothbrush—solvents don't wash away.

---

[25] 20 Mule Team Borax™ works well for soap and is free of metals and other pollutants. Borax inhibits the bacterial enzyme *urease*. Urease is used by bacteria that live in us to utilize our urea as a source of nitrogen for themselves.

Don't use mouthwash. Use saltwater (aluminum-free salt) or food grade hydrogen peroxide (just a few drops in water).

Don't use hair spray.

Don't use massage oils of any kind. Use olive oil.

Don't use bath oil. Take showers, not baths, if you are strong enough to stand. Showers are cleaner.

Don't use perfumes or colognes.

Don't use lotions or personal lubricants except homemade.

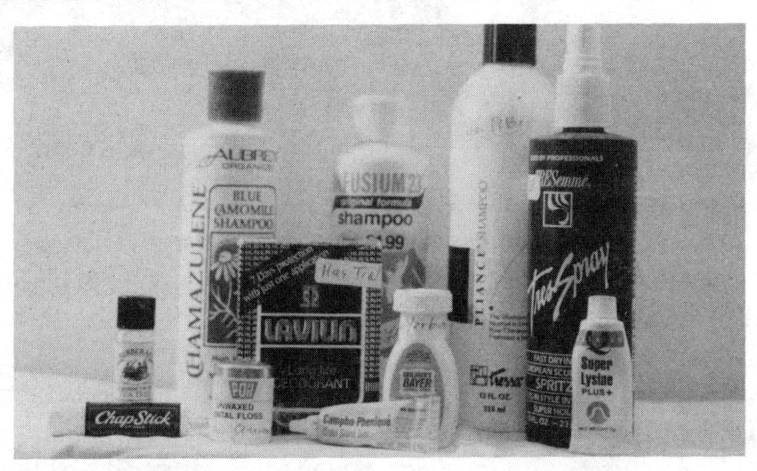

Our household, health, and body products, and drugs are polluted with solvents, heavy metals, PCBs and lanthanides.

Fig. 29 Some polluted body care products

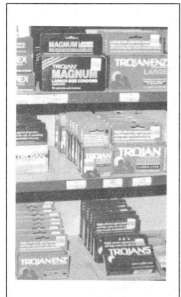

Fig. 30 Lubricated condoms have benzene.

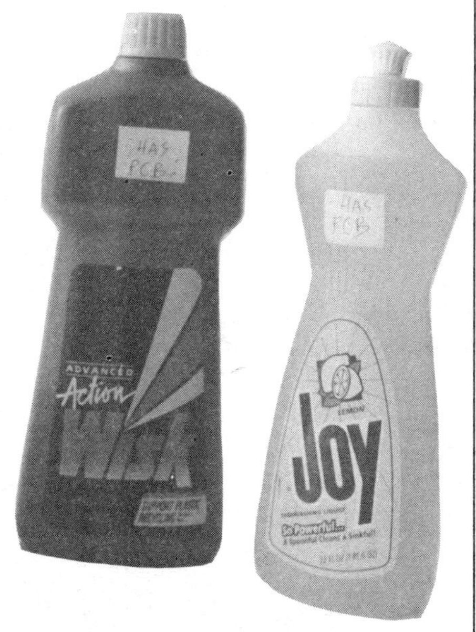

Our dishes and clothing are our primary source of PCBs.

Fig. 31 Detergents with PCBs.

Prohibit Propyl Alcohol

> **CANCER is caused**
>
> in part by propyl alcohol. The other part is the same human intestinal fluke that you had! You are at <u>much</u> greater risk of developing cancer for this reason. You must be especially careful to avoid propyl alcohol.

Propyl alcohol is the antiseptic commonly used in cosmetics. Check all your cosmetics for the word "propanol" or

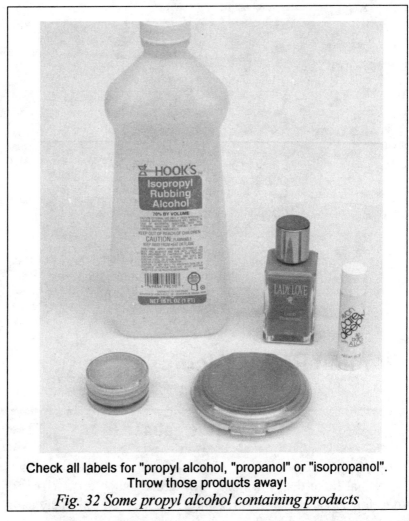

Check all labels for "propyl alcohol, "propanol" or "isopropanol".
Throw those products away!

Fig. 32 Some propyl alcohol containing products

"isopropanol" on the label. It is usually put on the label, since it is not currently suspected of causing cancer.[26] I don't know if propyl compounds like propamide, propacetamide, propyl gallate, or calcium propionate could be converted by the body to propyl alcohol, so don't take chances. Do not use anything that has "prop" in the list of ingredients. Don't give your discarded cosmetics to anybody. Don't save them. Don't have them in the house anywhere. Throw them out.

Here is a list of common body products that may have propyl alcohol in them: cosmetics, shampoo, hair spray, mouthwash, mousse, body lotions, shaving supplies, and, of course, rubbing alcohol. **If in doubt, throw it out!**

Propyl alcohol is a pollutant in cold cereals. Stop buying all cold cereals. I suspect the manufacturers of these cereals add flavors to them. Flavors are extracted using very toxic solvents, including propyl alcohol, benzene, wood alcohol and many others. Of course, these solvents are then reduced to a minimum (but can never be eliminated). You must have NONE. Even the most natural cold cereals are polluted, and I don't know why. Perhaps manufacturers sterilize their equipment with propyl alcohol. I haven't tested every cereal on the market, but I have tested so many that you should not take a chance on a single one. See *Recipes* to make your own.

THE GOOD NEWS IS THAT PROPANOL, LIKE BENZENE, LEAVES YOUR BODY, BY ITSELF, IN FIVE DAYS AFTER YOU STOP GETTING IT.

---

[26] Many people use cosmetics with propanol in them and do not develop cancer. The propanol is detoxified for them by their livers. Eating moldy food with aflatoxins in it poisons the liver's ability to detoxify propanol.

Read all labels on the body products you buy. Keep a lighted magnifying glass with you for this purpose while shopping. Tear out the next page and stick it to your refrigerator so the whole family can help you eliminate them.

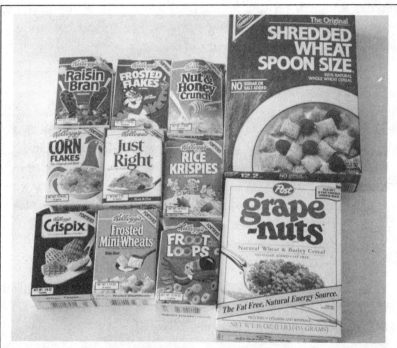

All cold cereals I tested, including health-food varieties, are polluted with solvents such as benzene, carbon tetrachloride and propyl alcohol. DON'T EAT THEM.

Fig. 33 Some polluted cold cereals

Propyl Alcohol Polluted Products

THROW THESE OUT

even if propyl alcohol is not listed on the label!

- **shampoo**, even health brands
- **hair spray** and **mousse**
- **rubbing alcohol**
- **cold cereals**, including granolas and health food varieties
- **cosmetics** (unless the label does not have any "prop" ingredients)
- store-bought and **bottled water**, including distilled, mineral, health store varieties
- store-bought **fruit juice**, including 100% natural and health store varieties
- **white sugar** (use any kind of brown sugar)
- **mouthwash**
- all **shaving supplies** including aftershave
- **carbonated beverages**
- **decaffeinated coffee**, Postum™, herb tea blends (single herb teas are OK)

Remember propyl alcohol is also called propanol, isopropanol, isopropyl alcohol and rubbing alcohol.

Your Substitutes:

Stop Using Supplements

Stop using your vitamin supplements. They, too, are heavily polluted. This is the saddest, most tragic part of your instructions. I haven't found solvents or xenobiotics (unbiological chemicals that require special liver detoxifying processes) in supplements, but I see heavy metals and lanthanides in 90% or more of the popular vitamin and mineral capsules and tablets I test. These substances will do more harm in the long run than the supplement can make up for in benefits.

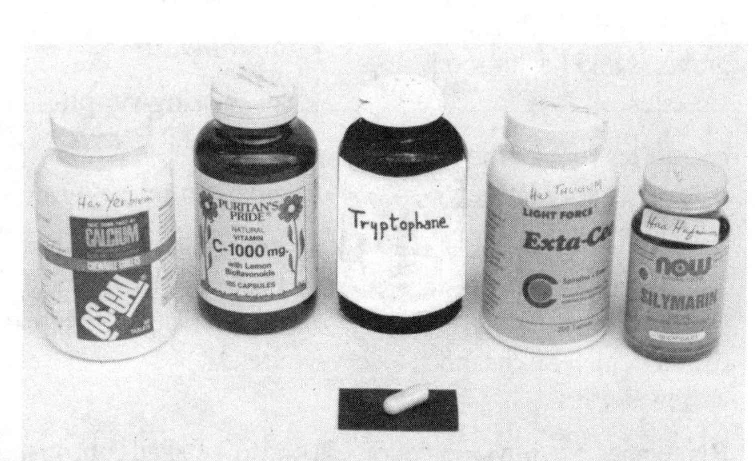

The capsule in the foreground is a notorious tryptophane capsule. It had the following pollutants: PCBs, mercury, ruthenium, thulium, strontium, praseodymium, aluminum, benzalkonium.

Fig. 34 Some polluted supplements

Until all vitamins and minerals and other food supplements have been analyzed for pollutants, <u>after they are encapsulated or tableted</u>, they are not safe. We need more disclosure on our products. No manufactured product is pure. We can't expect that. But at least we should be able to tell what impurities we are getting, and how much.

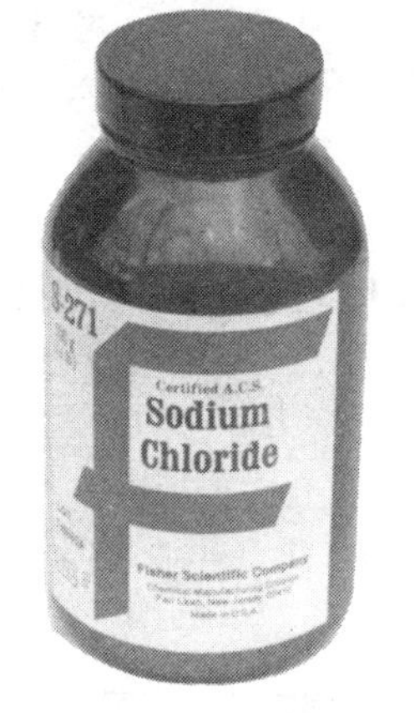

Fig. 35 Pure salt

It is possible to do detailed analysis of foods or products at a reasonable price. Look at the bottle of common table salt, sodium chloride, that is used by beginning chemistry students to do experiments. It must be thoroughly analyzed for them because minute impurities affect their results. (Those minute impurities, like lead, affect you, too.) Look at the label on the bottle in the picture. Even after all of these tests, the cost of laboratory salt is only \$2.80 per pound.[27]

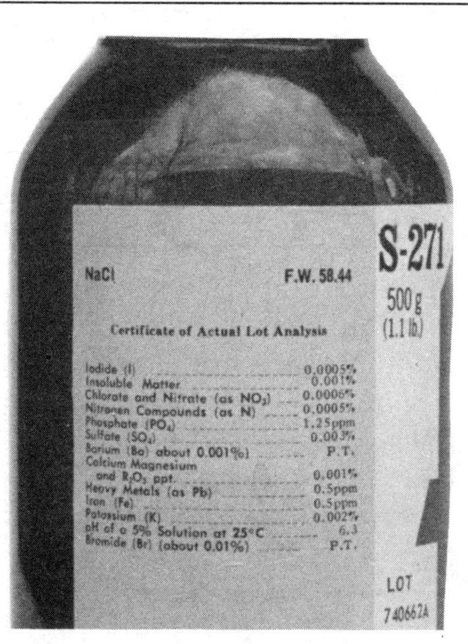

Common table salt for student use is thoroughly analyzed for pollution. The label gives you the final "Actual Lot Analysis" of the product. It is not expensive.

Fig. 36 Laboratory salt label

---

27 You will pay about \$8.00 per pound (Spectrum Chemical Co.) for USP (United States Pharmaceutical) grade. But the same anaylsis is done on the cheaper grades, and my point is that the analysis is cost effective enough that it should be done on our daily foods.

It is most important not to be fooled by ingredient claims, like "made from organically grown vegetables". Sure that's great, but the analysis *I* trust would be done on the final, cleaned, cooked and packaged product on the shelf. The package is a major unlisted ingredient.

Toxic solvents like decane, hexane, carbon tetrachloride and benzene will get more flavor or fat or cholesterol out of things than metabolizable grain alcohol. Of course, the extraction process calls for washing out the solvent later. But it can't all be washed out, and a detailed analysis on the final product would give the public the information they need to make informed choices.

If your supplements

are from Bronson Pharmaceuticals, you do not have to throw them all out. As of this writing only their 1 gram ascorbic acid, children's chewable vitamin C, and flax seed mixture were polluted. Other companies all have numerous polluted products. Unless specifically recommended in this book, it is safer to just throw them out.

Safe Supplements

There are, no doubt, lots of safe supplements to be had. The problem is knowing which are polluted. The nature of pollution is such that one bottle might be safe, while another of the same brand is not. In view of this, as I found a polluted bottle, I stopped using any more of that brand. That is why I am reduced to recommending just one brand, Bronson's, at this time, with the execeptions noted.

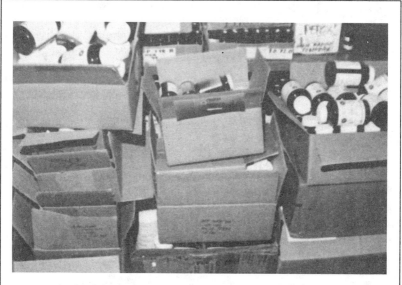

Fig. 37 Boxes of vitamins I discarded

Vitamin C, in powdered form, is a must in your lifestyle. It helps the liver, and possibly other organs, detoxify things. It also helps retard mold. Keep some next to your refrigerator so it is handy when you put away groceries. Add 1/8 tsp. to maple syrup, ketchup, vinegar, popcorn, cooked cereal, fruit juice, leftovers. I have not seen it help to detoxify benzene, though. Have ¼ tsp. (1 gram) with each meal. This much can be stirred into milk without changing the flavor.

Vitamin B_2, 50 mg to 125 mg per meal. Is essential for HIV sufferers. This vitamin helps to detoxify the benzopyrene in food. Can be part of a B-complex. (If you get 250 mg tablets, take ½ tablet with each meal.) Another substance, *ellagic acid*, found in brazil nuts, has also been reported to detoxify benzopyrenes.[28] Benzopyrenes may be responsible for your tendency to accumulate benzene. During an acute illness, increase it to 300 mg three times a day.

Vitamin B_6, 250 mg. Undoubtedly helps the liver and kidneys in many ways. One per day.

Magnesium oxide, 300 mg, is another must. Take one or two a day. It is a major mineral; all of our cells need lots of it. Only leafy vegetables provide it.

L-G stands for "lysine-glutamic acid". This is a supplement you can make yourself (see *Recipes*). It seems to go directly to the thymus and helps greatly. We have used it for four or five years for persons with EBV, CMV and chronic *Herpes*. Perhaps it would be good for other viral diseases, too. We use it for all HIV or AIDS cases even when it isn't mentioned in the case histories. See *The Story Of L-G* to learn more about it.

Hydrogen peroxide, food grade. It is advantageous to kill bacteria and viruses to some extent every day. Hydrogen peroxide lets you do this. It should never come in contact with metal, including its container or metal tooth fillings. If you get a few drops on your skin it may turn white and sting, but does no harm, so simply wash it off. HIV/AIDS sufferers should use 10 or more drops at each meal, in a beverage. Chlorine dioxide("07") is another bactericide and virus killer. It comes under various brand names. Because I have not tested it for many pollutants, I have a preference for hydrogen peroxide.

Herbs. These are excellent supplements, both in bulk and capsules, <u>but not extracts or concentrates</u>. There are many books that describe their uses.

---

[28] *Merck Index*, 10th ed. p. 512 1983.

Thioctic acid or lipoic acid. Presumably this chelates (traps and prepares for elimination) heavy metals, and helps the liver in detoxifying obscure and deadly poisons. Everyone would benefit from 100 mg per day. We find it outstanding, and give it to most HIV clients, even when not mentioned in the case histories. It comes as a 100 mg capsule (see *Sources*). We use it at doses from one capsule, 3 times a day, to 2 capsules, 5 times a day. We have seen no side effects at these dosages, even in very sick persons.

Lugol's Iodine Solution (see *Recipes*) is made of potassium iodide and plain, pure iodine. It is made this way because plain iodine does not dissolve well in water; it dissolves much better in potassium iodide. Potassium iodide dissolves well in water and stays clear; for this reason it is also called "white iodine." By mixing the two, we can get stronger concentrations of iodine than either can provide by itself. Commercially available Lugol's is polluted with propyl alcohol. Make it yourself from scratch.

DO NOT TAKE LUGOL'S IODINE IF YOU ARE ALLERGIC TO IODINE. IT COULD BE FATAL.

Iodine has a distinctive trait: it hangs up on anything and everything. In fact, it attaches itself so quickly we consider everything it touches as "stained." This is just the property we want to make it safe for use. The amount you use is immediately hung up, or attached, to your mucous and can not be quickly absorbed into the blood or other organs. It stays in the stomach. And for this reason it is so useful for killing vicious bacteria like *Salmonella* and *Shigella*.

Salmonella and *Shigella* are two stomach and digestive tract bacteria. They can give you terrible bloating and gas which is often misdiagnosed as *lactose intolerance*. Younger persons often have a fever when *Salmonella* attacks. Summer "flu" or

"24-hour flu" is really *Salmonella* getting you. It comes into you with deli food, chicken, past-dated dairy food, not to mention picnic food that has stood around for a while. Hands carry these two bacteria, so always wash hands before eating and after shaking someone's hand. People can have chronic *Salmonella* and *Shigella* infections. Every new strain they eat or drink forms hybrids with the old strain they already had in their stomachs. This results in much more vicious strains that actually make you feel sick. *Shigella*, especially, makes you feel angry, irritable, and short-tempered as a mule. *Shigella* goes to your nervous system. All cases of multiple sclerosis I have seen had rampant *Shigella*!

Six drops of Lugol's solution can end it all for *Salmonella*. If you have gas and bloating, pour yourself ½ glass of water. Add 6 drops of Lugol's (not more, not less), stir with wood or plastic, and drink all at once. The action is noticeable in an hour. Take this dose 4 times a day, after meals and at bedtime, for 3 days in a row, then daily at bedtime. This eradicates even a stubborn case of *Salmonella*.

Notice how calming 6 drops of Lugol's can be, soothing a manic stage and bringing a peaceful state where anxiety ruled before.

Lugol's is perfectly safe (if not allergic) to take day after day, when needed, because of its peculiar attaching property. It arrives in the stomach, reattaches to everything in proximity. Doomed are *Salmonella* and *Shigella*; doomed also are eggs (cysts) of parasites that might be in the stomach.

Naturally, one would not leave such medicine within the reach of children. Also, one would not use anything medicinal, including Lugol's unless there were a need, like digestive distress. Store it in a perfectly secure place. In the past, 2/3 of a teaspoon (60 drops) of Lugol's was the standard dose of iodine given to persons with disease.

Shigella is not killed by Lugol's after it leaves the stomach to reside in the bowel. Nothing but frequent bowel movements (3 to 4 a day) plus *Acidophilus* liquid can expel them, even after a week. Both bacteria come to us in dairy foods.

Sterilize Dairy Foods. All dairy products should be sterilized before consuming.

Pasteurization is not sterilization.

Milk goes sour after the expiration date on the carton even when refrigerated and unopened. (Sour milk isn't caused by *Salmonella* or *Shigella*, my point is that it is obvious that milk isn't sterile.)

Boil milk for 10 seconds to kill *Salmonellas* and *Shigellas*. Then cool and refrigerate. Make yogurt and buttermilk with this milk.

If you simply cannot tolerate dairy products, try cooking buttermilk. Separate the curds (sterile cottage cheese) and whey. Whey is a traditional, delicious beverage with all the calcium of milk in it. Dairy products are <u>too important</u> to your recovery to abandon.

Other supplements. The concept of supplementing the diet is excellent, but the pollution problem makes it prohibitive. In *How To Test Yourself* you learn how you can test any product, including supplements to make sure they are safe.

Clean Up Your Home

There is only one job left. Clean up your environment. This is the easiest task because it mostly involves throwing things out, so it was left to the last. But don't delay for a minute to get this done. Hopefully your family and friends will jump to your assistance.

- The basement gets cleaned.
- The garage gets cleaned.
- Every room in the house gets cleaned.

Clean Basement

To clean your basement, remove all paint, varnish, thinners, brush cleaners, and related supplies. Remove all cleaners such as carpet cleaner, leather cleaner, rust remover. Remove all chemicals that are in cans, bottles or buckets.

You may keep your laundry supplies: borax, baking soda, washing soda, white distilled vinegar, chlorine bleach and homemade soap. You may keep canned goods, tools, items that are not chemicals. You may move your chemicals into your garage. Also move any car tires and automotive supplies like waxes, oil, transmission fluid, and the spare gas can (even if it is empty) into your garage or discard them.

Seal cracks in the basement and around pipes where they come through the wall with black plastic roofing cement. In a few days it will be hard enough to caulk with a prettier color. Spread a sheet of plastic over the sewer or sump pump.

Clean Garage

Do you have a garage that is a separate building from your home? This is the best arrangement. You can move all the basement chemicals into this garage. Things that will freeze, such as latex paint, you may as well discard. But if your garage is attached, you have a problem. Never, never use your door between the garage and house. Walk around the outside. Don't allow this door to be used. Tack a sheet of plastic over it to slow down the rate of fume entrance into the house. Your house acts like a chimney for the garage. Your house is taller and warmer than the garage so garage-air is pulled in and up as the warm air in the house rises. See the drawing.

In medieval days, the barn for the animals was attached to the house. We think such an arrangement with its penetrating odors is unsavory. But what of the gasoline and motor fumes we are getting now due to parked vehicles? These are toxic besides! This is even more medieval.

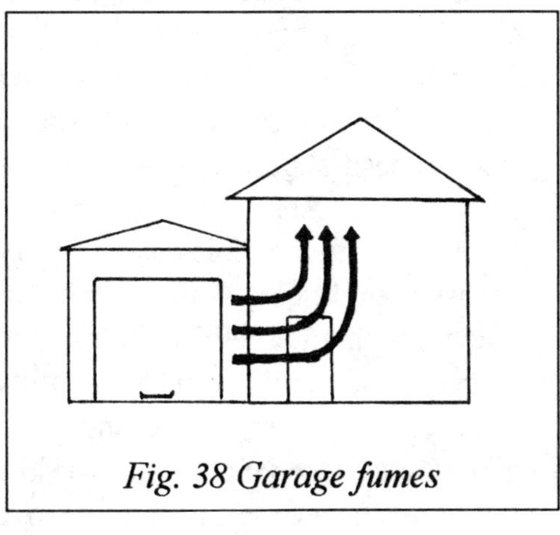

Fig. 38 Garage fumes

If your garage is under your house, you cannot keep the pollution from entering your home. In this case, leave the cars and lawnmower outside. Remove cans of gasoline, solvents, etc. Put up a separate shed for these items.

Clean House

To clean the house, start with the bedroom. Remove everything that has any smell to it whatever: candles, potpourri, soaps, mending glue, cleaners, repair chemicals, felt markers, colognes, perfumes, and especially plug-in air "fresheners". Store them in the garage, not the basement. Since all vapor rises, they would come back up if you put them in a downstairs garage or basement.

Next clean the kitchen. Take all cans and bottles of chemicals out from under the sink or in a closet. Remove them to the garage. Keep only the borax, baking soda, washing soda, white distilled vinegar and bottles of concentrated borax and 50% vinegar you have made. You may also use homemade soap. Use these for all purposes. For exact amounts to use for dishwasher, dishes, windows, dusting, see *Recipes*. Remove all cans, bottles, roach and ant killer, mothballs, and chemicals that kill insects or mice. These should not be stored anywhere. They should be thrown out. Remember to check the crawl space, attic and closets for hidden poisons also. To keep out mice, walk all around your house, stuffing holes and cracks with steel wool. Use old-fashioned mouse traps. For cockroaches and other insects (except ants) sprinkle handfuls of boric acid[29] (not borax) under your shelf paper, behind sink, stove, refrigerator, under carpets, etc. Use vinegar on your kitchen wipe-up cloth to leave a residue that keeps out ants. Do this regularly. To wax the floor, get the wax from the garage and put it back there. An HIV/AIDS patient should not be in the house while house cleaning or floor waxing is being done.

---

[29] Boric acid is available by the pound from farm supply stores and from Now Foods. Because it looks like sugar keep it in the garage to prevent accidental poisoning.

Remove all cans and bottles of "stuff" from the bathroom, to the garage. The chlorine bleach is stored in the garage. Someone else can bring it in to clean the toilet (only). Leave only the borax-soap, homemade soap, and grain alcohol antiseptic. Toilet paper and tissues should be unfragranced, uncolored. All colognes, after shave, anything you can smell must be removed. Family members should buy unfragranced products which must not contain propyl alcohol. They should smoke outdoors, blow-dry their hair outdoors or in the garage, use nail polish and polish remover outdoors or in the garage.

Do not sleep in a bedroom that is paneled or has wallpaper. They give off arsenic fumes and formaldehyde. Either remove them or move your bed to a different room. Leave the house while this is being done. If other rooms have paneling or wallpaper, close their doors and spend no time in them.

Do not keep new foam furniture in the house. If it is less than one year old, move it into the garage until you are well. It gives off formaldehyde. Wash new clothing for the same reason.

Turn off radiators and cover them with big plastic garbage bags, or paint them, or remove them. They give off asbestos from the old paint.

Do not use the hot water from an electric hot water heater for cooking or drinking. It has tungsten. Do not drink water that sits in glazed crock ware (the glaze seeps toxic elements like cadmium) like some water dispensers have. Do not buy water from your health food store that runs through a long plastic hose from their bulk tank (I always see cesium picked up from flexible clear plastic).

If your house is more than 10 years old, change all the galvanized pipe to PVC plastic. Although PVC is a toxic substance, amazingly, the water is free of PVC in three weeks! If your house is more than 15 years old, change all the copper pipe to PVC plastic. If you have a water softener, by-pass it immediately and replace the metal pipe on the user side of the softener tank. Softener salts are polluted with strontium and chromate; they are also full of aluminum. The salts corrode the pipes so the pipes begin to seep cadmium into the water. After changing your pipes to plastic, there will be so little iron and hardness left, you may not need a softener. If the water comes from a well, consider changing the well-pipe to PVC to get rid of iron. While the well is open, have the pump checked for PCBs. Call the Health Department to arrange the testing. If you must have softening after all this, check into the new magnetic varieties of water softener (although they only work well when used with plastic plumbing).

The cleanest heat is electric. Go total electric if possible. If you must stay with gas, have a furnace repair person check your furnace and look for gas leaks before the heating season starts. Don't call the gas company even though it is free. The gas company misses 4 out of 5 leaks! The Health Department does not miss any; call them!

Don't stop because you are already feeling better. Illness can return with a vengeance. Get every clean-up job completed so you can feel secure for your next doctor's checkup and for your future.

It is possible to get most of this house cleaning done in one day. Do all you possibly can. The more difficult jobs may take a week. This is a week of lost time if you are scheduled for a biopsy.

Persons with AIDS should not have a pet. The pets pick up parasites daily and are continually infectious. This is too much of a challenge for your weakened immune system.

Finally, search the whole house for holes in the ceiling, walls or floor that lead to insulated areas. Any fiberglass thus exposed will fill your breathing space. Even tiny holes made by pesticide companies can be deathtraps for you; the microscopic bits of glass go to your thymus gland. Merely covering holes does not work; they must be airtight—fill and paint them. Use duct tape to seal attic entrance ways. Check furnace and air conditioner fans; pull out any fiberglass stuffed around them or used as filters. Vacuum afterwards. Best of all, find a contractor willing to remove your fiberglass insulation, vacuum, and replace it with paper or vermiculite insulation.

Suppose you have nobody who is willing to clean up the house, basement, garage for you, or take on your pets for a month while you find them a new home. Don't delay for a minute if you should be invited to stay with a friend or relative who is willing to clean up their place for you and take you to the dentist. If there are no invitations, go on vacation or put yourself into a non-paneled, smoke-free motel room (bring your own soap, sheets, and pillowcases, and ask that they not "clean" your room or spray it). If you have a camper, remember to clean it up first. Foam and paneling must be out of it. Gas lines should be checked or closed off. Simply being outdoors is your safest place. A sunny beach, with shady places, where you can rest all day is ideal. Remember not to use any sunscreen or suntan lotions; make your own (see *Recipes*) or simply wear a hat.

Unnatural Chemicals

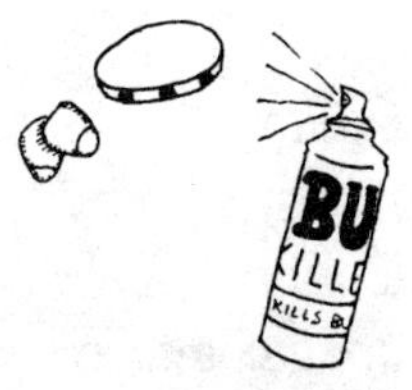

in ant & roach hives, grains of pesticide

ARSENIC

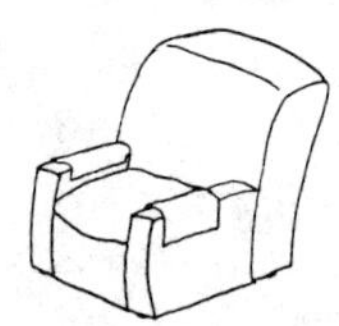

in carpet & furniture treated for stain resistance

in wallpaper

BARIUM

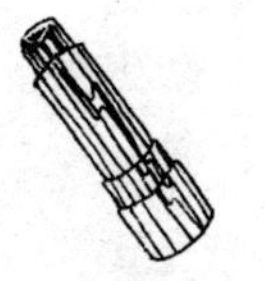

in lipstick

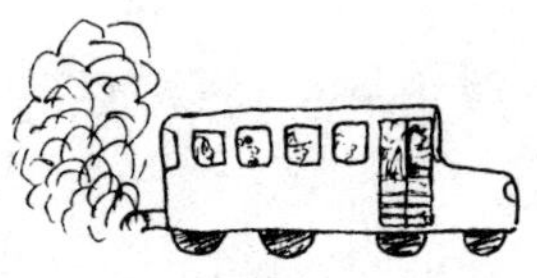

in bus exhaust

MOLYBDENUM

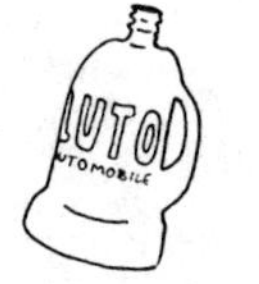

in "molys"

COBALT

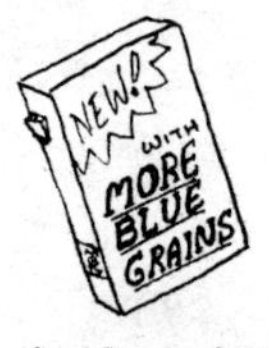

in laundry detergent

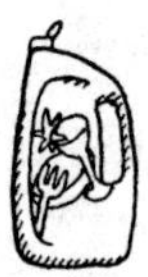

in dishwasher detergent

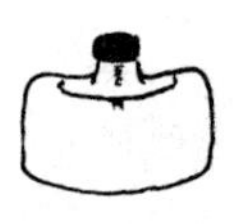

in skin bracer

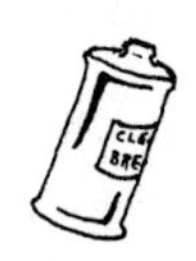

in mouthwash

ANTIMONY

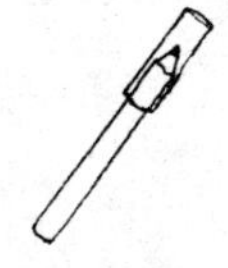

in eye liner

CADMIUM and COPPER

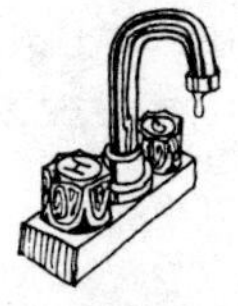

in water running through old metal pipes

TITANIUM

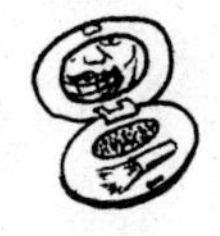

in face powder & other powders, an in metal dental wa

PCB's

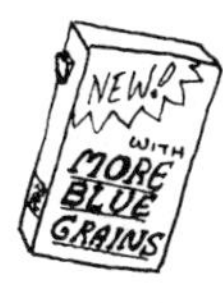

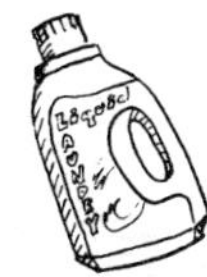
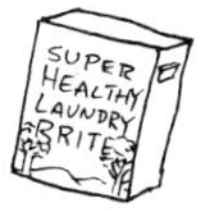

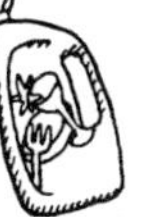

in regular & health store detergents and soaps

CHROMIUM

VANADIUM

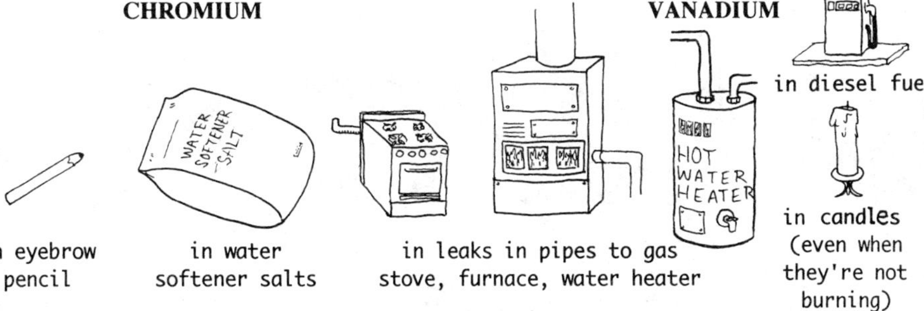

in diesel fue

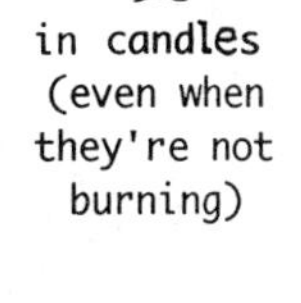

in candles (even when they're not burning)

n eyebrow pencil

in water softener salts

in leaks in pipes to gas stove, furnace, water heater

NICKEL

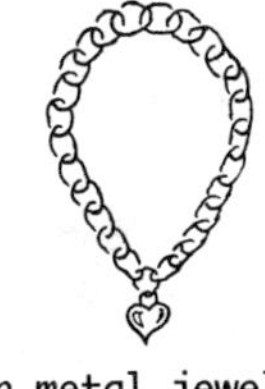

in metal jewelry worn on the skin

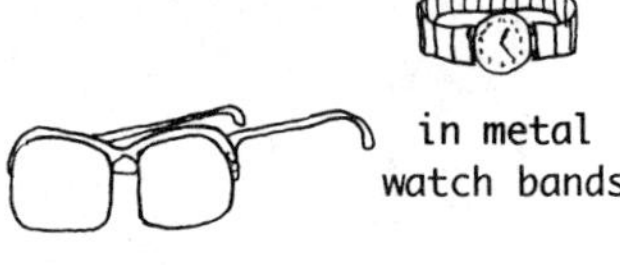

in metal watch bands

in metal glasses frames

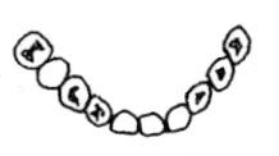

in metal tooth fillings and retainers

LEAD

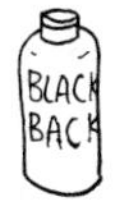

in men's hair color restorer

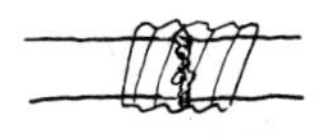

in solder at joints of copper pipes

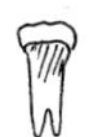

in old root canals

THULIUM

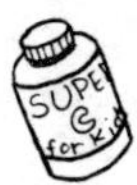
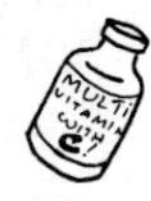
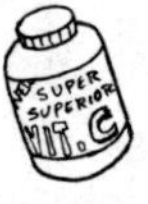

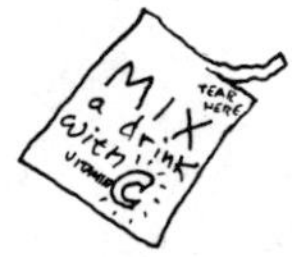

in all new varieties of Vitamin C

DYSPROSIUM and LUTETIUM

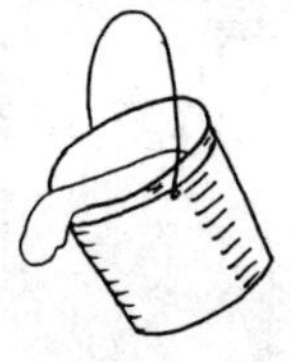

in paint, varnish, shellac

HOLMIUM

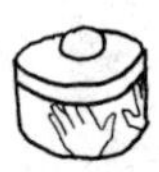

in hand cleaners

HAFNIUM

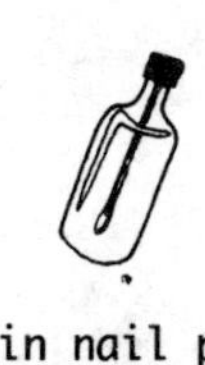
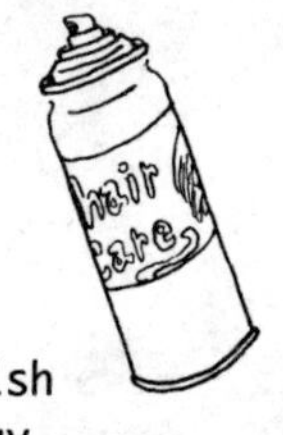

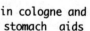

in nail polish & hair spray

RHENIUM

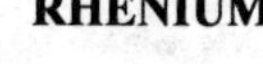
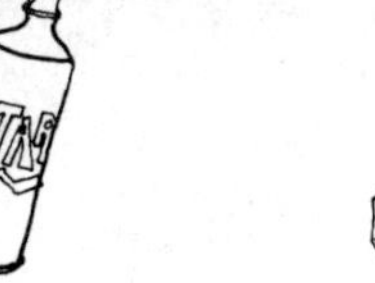

in spray starch

BISMUTH

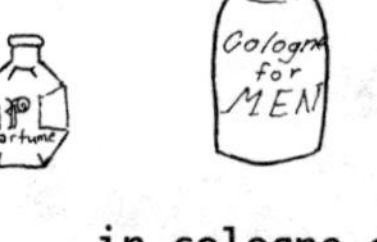

in cologne and stomach aids

CESIUM

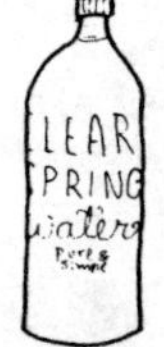

in clear-as-glass plastic

TIN and STRONTIUM

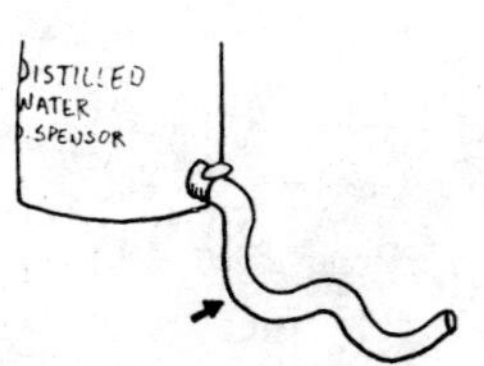

after running through long plastic hose

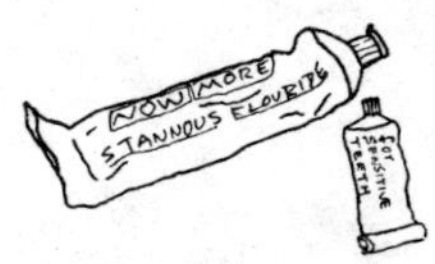

in toothpaste

YTTERBIUM, ERBIUM TERBIUM

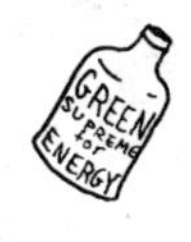

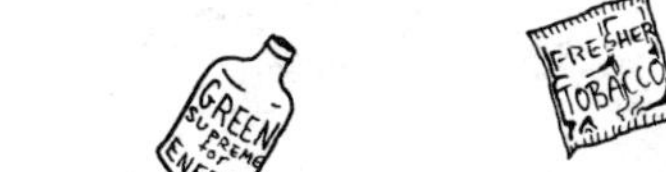

in foil packaging

in plastic tooth fillings

in vitamins and supplements

PRASEODYMIUM, NIOBIUM, NEODYMIUM, YTTRIUM

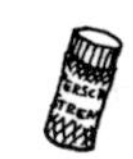

in over the counter drugs

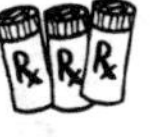

in prescription drugs

RADON, URANIUM, THORIUM

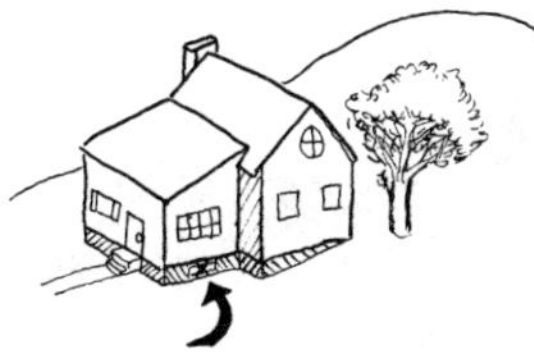

in crawlspace without open vents

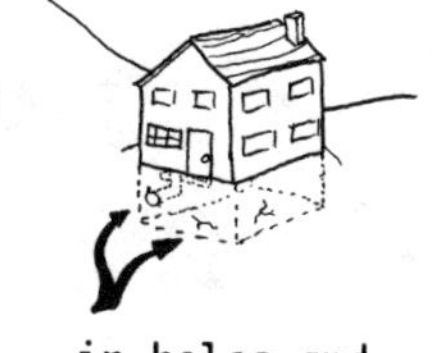

in holes and cracks in basement

LANTHANUM

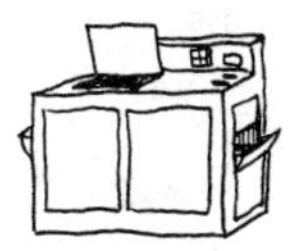

in duplicator and copier ink

BENZALKONIUM and ZIRCONIUM

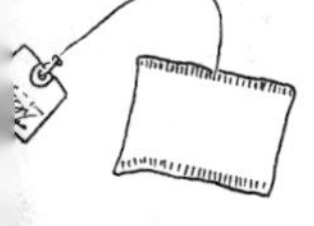

in tea bags

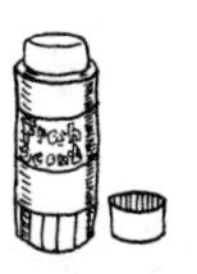

in deodorant

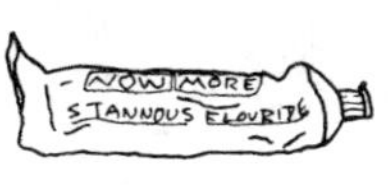

in toothpaste

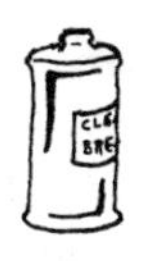

in mouthwash

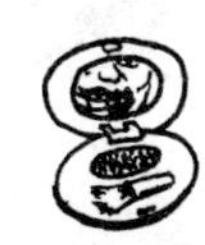

in cosmetics

ALUMINUM

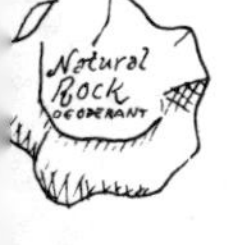

"natural"
deodorant
vertised as
uminum-free

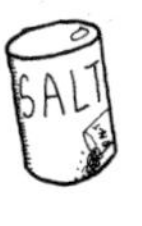

in salt

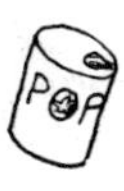

in cans

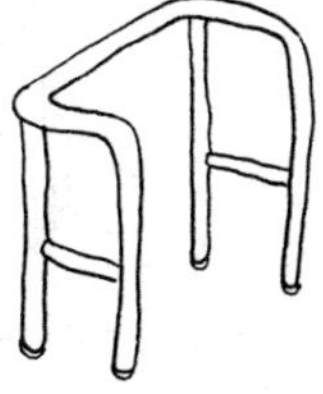

in walkers for the elderly

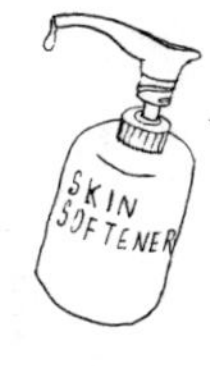

in lotions

TUNGSTEN

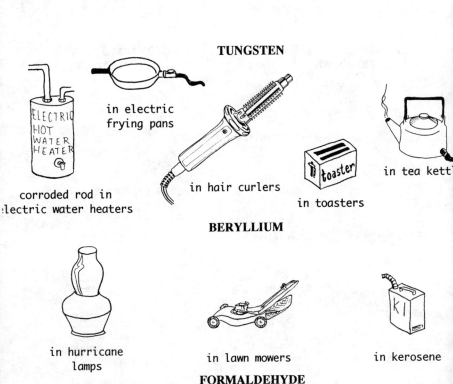

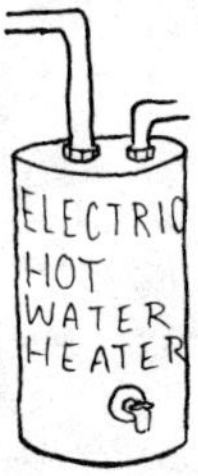

corroded rod in
lectric water heaters

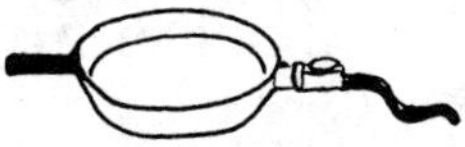

in electric
frying pans

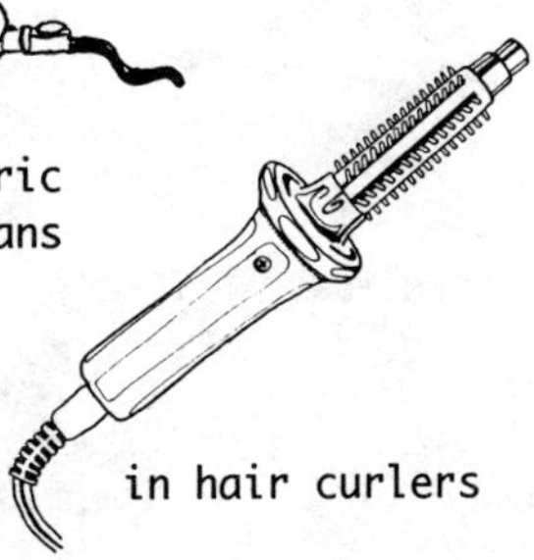

in hair curlers

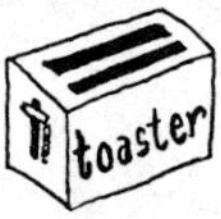

in toasters

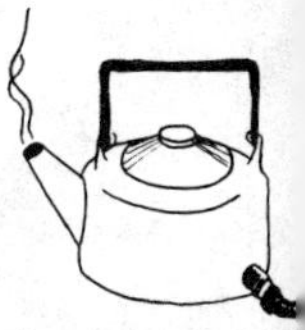

in tea kett

BERYLLIUM

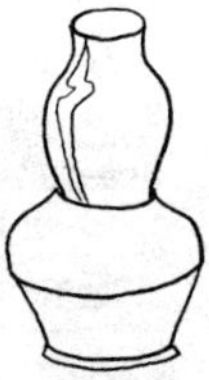

in hurricane
lamps

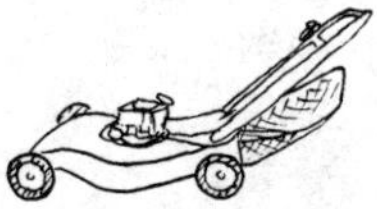

in lawn mowers

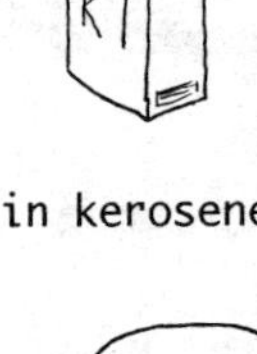

in kerosene

FORMALDEHYDE

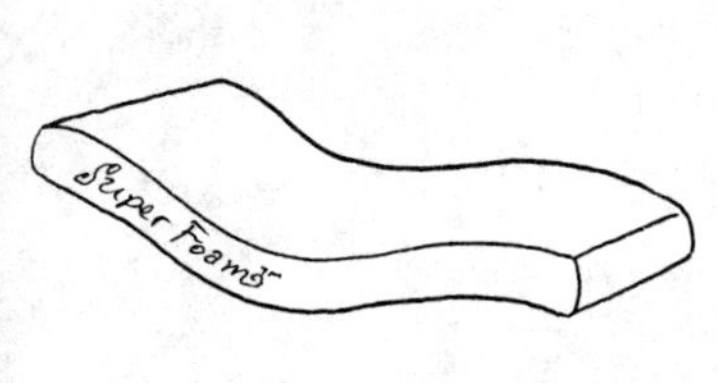

in foam mattresses

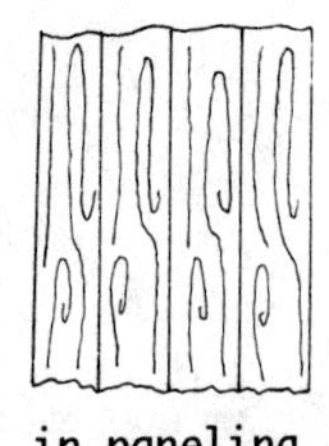

in paneling

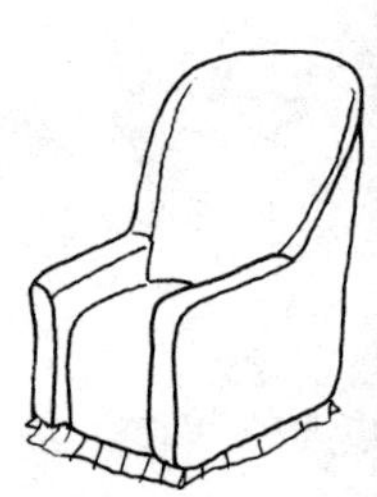

in foam chairs

ASBESTOS

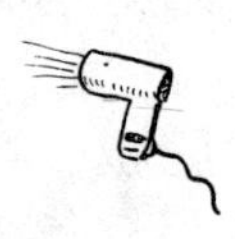

in hair blowers

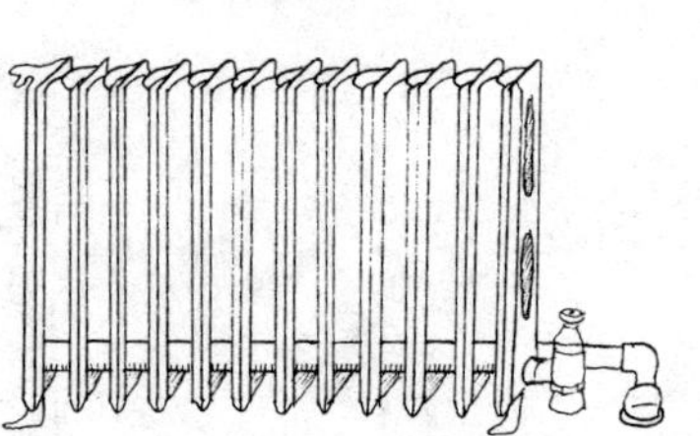

in radiator paint

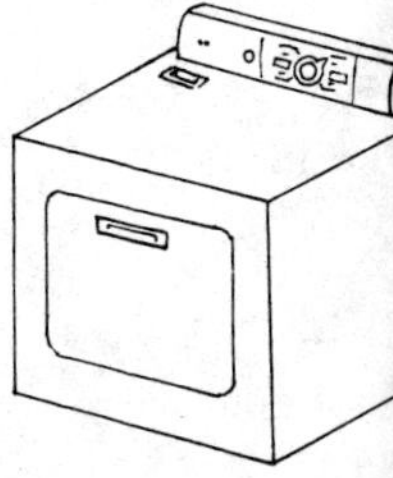

in clothes dryer bel

Watch Your Health Improve

NOW YOU HAVE DONE IT ALL!

Look forward to your next blood test.

- Your parasites are gone. Without the intestinal fluke you can not have HIV.
- You have cleaned out the benzene from your body and surroundings. Without this solvent you can't get AIDS Notice from the case histories how benzene disappears from the body simply by removing the sources.
- You have removed the metal from your mouth and cleaned up hidden infections under old pulled teeth in the jaw bone.
- You have switched to foods that are not moldy or processed. This means foods that are fresh and have not been chopped, ground, extracted and mixed with other chopped, ground, extracted foods to create concoctions. This includes health foods and supplements except a few as indicated.
- You have stopped putting chemicals on your skin, in your mouth, on your hair, in your armpits, on your eyelids, on your teeth, on your scalp, on your nails, or in your nose, lungs or genital tract.
- You have cleaned the house of all the chemicals that your body considers toxic.

Congratulations, this is a big accomplishment!

I hope you did all this in the first week after you bought this book and started on the parasite killing program. You stand an excellent chance of turning your future around!

Will your next blood test say HIV positive or negative? How could your HIV test say positive if you no longer have the virus? It can't. But you must select the test that searches for the virus. It is called the HIV antigen test. Your original test may have been the antibody test; it measures your antibodies to the virus. It will always stay positive. Your body will always remember to make antibodies to the HIV virus, just as your body remembers to make antibodies to chicken pox and measles. YOUR TEST MUST NOW BE THE HIV ANTIGEN TEST, such as the P24 test.

Ask your doctor to schedule the P24 antigen test for you. If it comes back NEGATIVE be especially cautious! The virus may be gone but you could reinfect yourself in a single day. And you have no way of knowing whether you are free of benzene. Only this can protect you from AIDS. Repeat the test every two months.

How long does it take to recover from AIDS after cleaning up the thymus? About 3 weeks. Your body is exceedingly swift. And it is age-related. The younger you are, the faster you recover.

How do you know you are recovering?

1. Your fatigue lessens.
2. Your mind is clearer.
3. Your temperature goes toward normal.
4. Your skin lesions fade.

5. Your breathing is deeper.
6. Your night sweats stop.

These improvements should encourage you to leave no stone unturned; that is, leave no pollutant in your thymus. Don't be satisfied with half measures. Your life is important to all of society; and your life affects all of humanity.

You need not only to recover from AIDS, but to be well, not fatigued. Only you have a profound understanding of the destructive course our so-called "civilization" is taking. Only you understand pollution as nobody else understands it. Only you may foresee the end of the planet's biosphere, or major branches thereof, as you were destined. You have an important mission to this planet's creatures. Your suffering must not be in vain. Heal yourself *completely* so that the rigors of politics, business, education and entertainment are not overwhelming to you.

Stay Clean

Here are a few more facts on where we are getting the human intestinal fluke stages,and other parasites. Since the infective stage in nature is the metacercarial[30] stage, are we eating metacercaria from vegetation like lettuce? I have not seen evidence for this but it must be researched, thoroughly, as a possibility.

You will see in the case histories how some people test YES (positive) for parasites in spite of having completed the parasite

---

[30] Remember, in nature, the cercaria swim to a plant and attach themselves to a leaf. There they lose their tails and are called *metacercaria*. It is the overwintering stage.

killing program and being on the maintenance program (twice a week treatments). This is possible because a reinfection can occur in as little as one hour! In every case of persistent re-infection the patient had indulged in fast foods or delicatessen meats consistently. Parasites can make good progress in two days (eating you up and reproducing in you) if given the chance.

Unfortunately for fast food lovers, the solution is not to make a daily routine out of the maintenance program. Herbs powerful enough to kill parasites probably are not advisable on a daily basis.

You must avoid parasites in daily life!

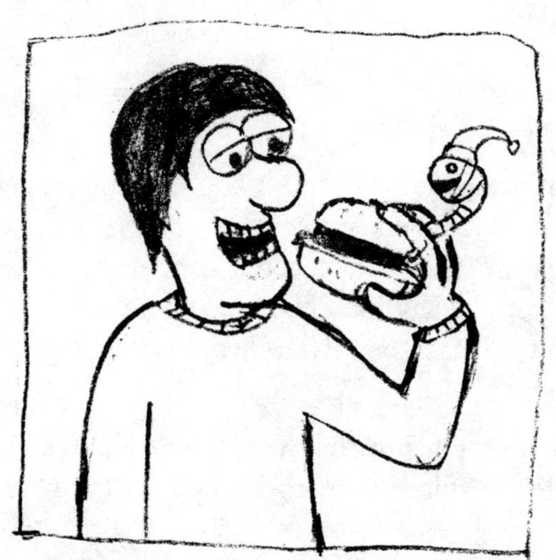

THIS MEAL REALLY GROWS ON YOU! Ben Hamines

Meat Could Be A Source

Are we getting metacercaria from eating animals that have the parasite[31]? Suppose we eat the raw blood of an animal that has this parasite. The animal's blood has eggs, miracidia, redia, cercaria and metacercaria in it. We swallow those live eggs, miracidia, redia, cercaria and metacercaria.

The metacercaria are meant to attach themselves to our intestine and grow larger, into adults that lay more eggs. But could the eggs, miracidia and redia that we eat also survive and develop in us? The miracidia and cercaria with their tails could simply swim away into our bodies. The eggs could hatch into more miracidia. Benzene will invite the stages into the thymus and the time clock for AIDS begins to tick.

When would we eat raw blood? In raw beef such as rare hamburger or steak! In raw turkey as in turkey burgers! And in raw chicken as in chicken burgers! Just handling these raw meats would put the infective stages on your hands! What a terrifying risk this gives us!

Some flukes are large enough to be seen with the naked eye, although their various stages usually need a low powered microscope. Therefore it should be possible to examine any meat sample from the grocery store to verify this source.

[31] Nobody has checked beef herds in the U.S.A. or the imported sources for the presence of *Fasciolopsis buskii.* It is urgent to find out whether cattle, fowl and pets have become a biological reservoir and are transmitting it to some of us. *Fasciola hepatica, Eurytrema* and *Clonorchis* should also be searched for because I find them so frequently.

Look at the photos of ground meats. There are objects that look identical to the stages of flukes. Research needs to be done to culture them in order to classify them accurately.

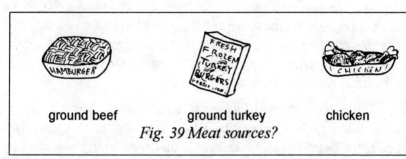

Fig. 39 Meat sources?

This raises the possibility, in fact, the <u>probability</u>, that our meat animals are the "biological reservoir," namely <u>source of infection</u>, by the HIV causing parasite! The human intestinal fluke was first studied in certain snails in ponds in China. Are our farm ponds similarly infested? If so, our animals have an obvious source of metacercaria.

The best advice is to become vegetarian immediately.

The second best advice is to cook all meats for at least 20 minutes at the boiling point, as in baking. Roast it until the meat falls off the bone. Don't eat any meat except fish and seafood in a restaurant. Restaurants cannot be entrusted with so important a cooking rule. Don't eat delicatessen meat. Are there other sources of this parasite? We need to search our food supply for other possible sources.

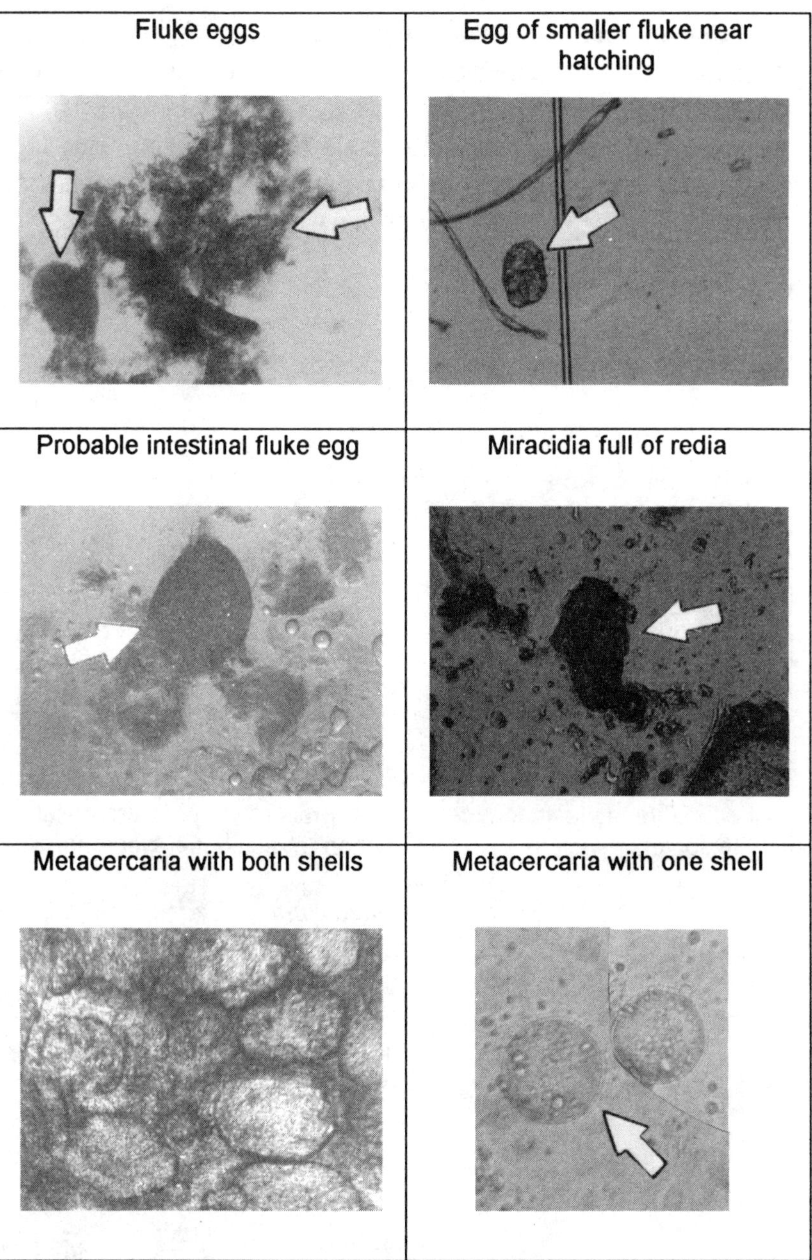

Fig. 40 Likely fluke stages in meat (100x)

Animals could not always have been infested with these fluke parasites. Cows, chickens and turkeys are not the natural hosts of the *human intestinal fluke* (although pigs are). And parasite stages, should never be found inside these animals. But their feeds are now full of solvents, which promotes abnormal parasitism in them, just as it does in us.

All animal feeds tested, except simple grain mixtures, were polluted with solvents such as benzene, carbon tetrachloride, isopropanol, wood alcohol, etc.

Fig. 41 Some polluted animal feed

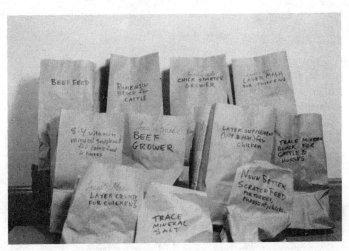

Fig. 42 Solvent free

Even bird feed was found to have benzene and other solvents in it. Buy seed only.

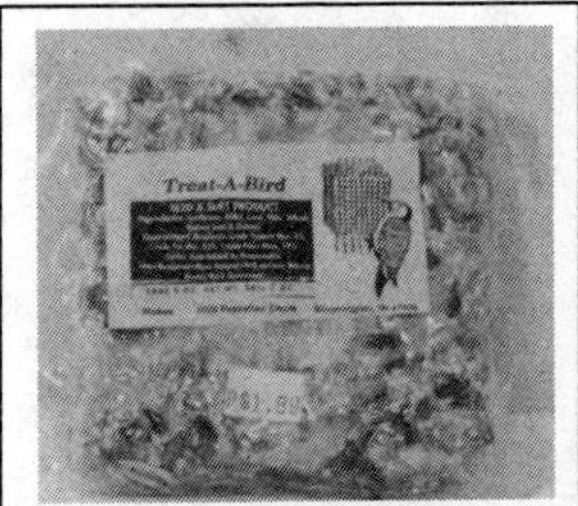

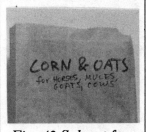

Fig. 43 Bad bird feed

Sex Could Be A Source

Since the infective stages of the intestinal fluke are microscopically tiny and can travel throughout the body in the blood, it is possible that some may get into the genital tract and genital fluids. It would be wise to practice protected sex. See the photos of parasite stages in urine. This is certainly evidence for sexual transmission.

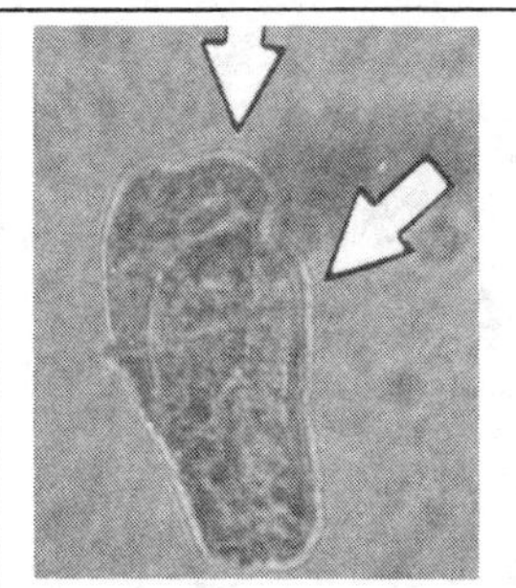

Two overlapped miracidia. (100x)

Fig. 44 Miracidia in urine

Cercaria resemble sperm, which you might expect to see in urine from a male. However the size makes them easy to distinguish.

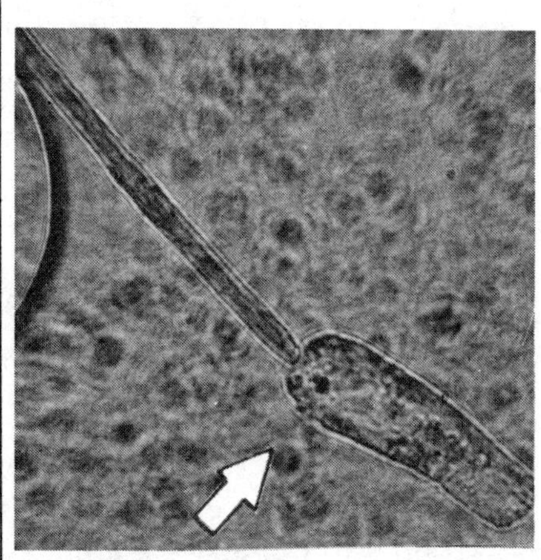

Cercaria seen in urine (400x)

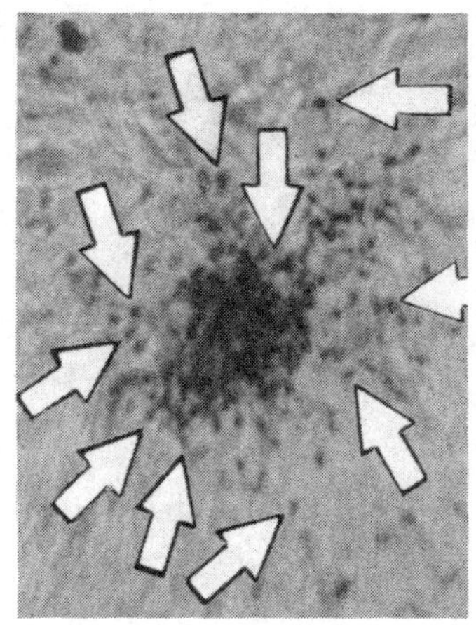

Sperm for comparison (400x)

Fig. 45 Cercaria in urine vs. sperm

Raw Milk Could Be A Source

When an animal or human is infested with the fluke stages, all the body fluids eventually have them. Milk is a body fluid. Cow's milk and goat milk should all be boiled before drinking it. Do not drink raw milk.

Mother's Milk Could Be A Source

If the body is teeming with very tiny fluke stages because of the solvent in your tissues, could they be transmitted through mother's milk? See the photograph of mother's milk. It shows a fluke egg almost ready to hatch. The mother was full of benzene. The baby was full of benzene from drinking the mother's milk. The father was full of benzene, also. The family was using a cooking oil polluted with benzene. Use only olive oil, butter or lard.

If you are nursing a baby and have HIV/AIDS illness, your milk could have infective stages in it. You can stop infecting your baby by:

1. Going on the parasite killing program yourself. The ingredients will come through the milk and kill the baby's parasites at the same time.
2. Stopping the use of any food or product that has benzene pollution in it. This will clear your baby of it, as well as you, in five days.
3. Stopping eating beef, chicken and turkey. Eat fish and seafood for protein. Don't broil or flame cook your foods. Don't eat toast or hot dogs. Strictly following the dietary guidelines in this book will prevent your baby from getting parasites and benzene buildup back.

4. Taking vitamin C and B-complex with each meal.
5. Stopping exchanging body fluids (through kissing on the mouth and sex) with persons who may be infected. You will be non-infective as soon as you have completed the parasite program.

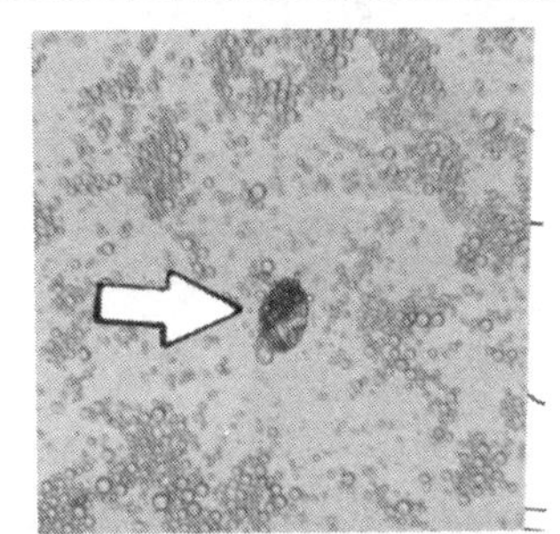
Egg (100x)

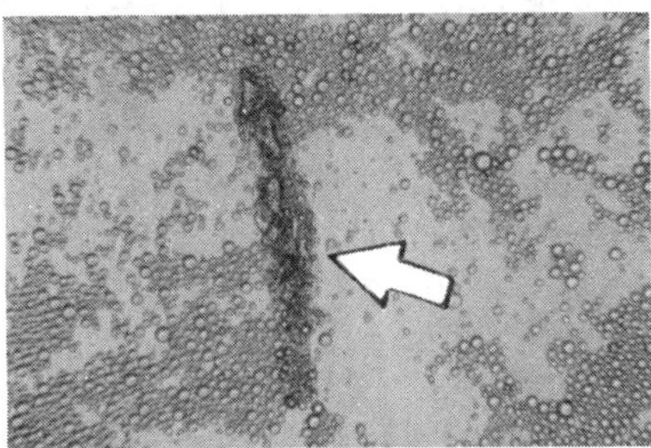
Miracidia developing redia (100x)

Fig. 46 Parasites in human milk

Until your intestinal flukes are dead (five days), you may be giving the baby parasites in your milk, but <u>don't stop</u> breast feeding, since this will become the baby's cure, too. Also, switching to canned formula would worsen the situation with solvent pollution. If your baby is very ill with AIDS, express your milk with a breast pump. Heat it to steaming in order to pasteurize it. Cool and refrigerate. Don't use metal pans for this, use enamelware that is used for nothing else. Store in glass jars. After five days of parasite killing, using the recipe given earlier, your milk will be safe from the human intestinal fluke and the HIV virus it brings.

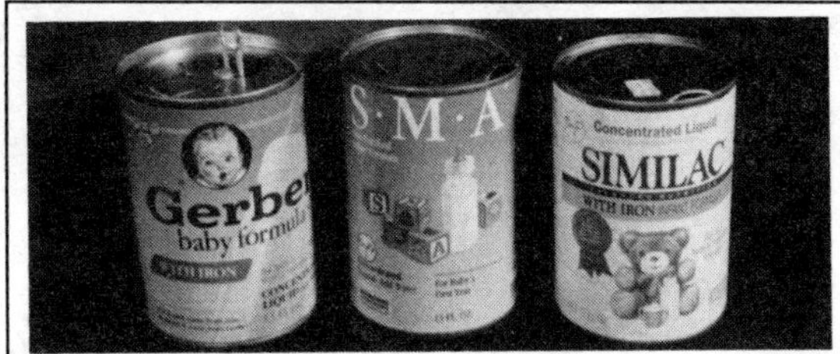

Fig. 47 Infant formulas with wood alcohol

Saliva Could Be A Source

Saliva is another body fluid that carries the tiny developmental stages of the fluke parasites. This means that kissing on the mouthcould transmit the HIV/AIDS parasite. But would you eventually get HIV? Only if you had benzene in you!

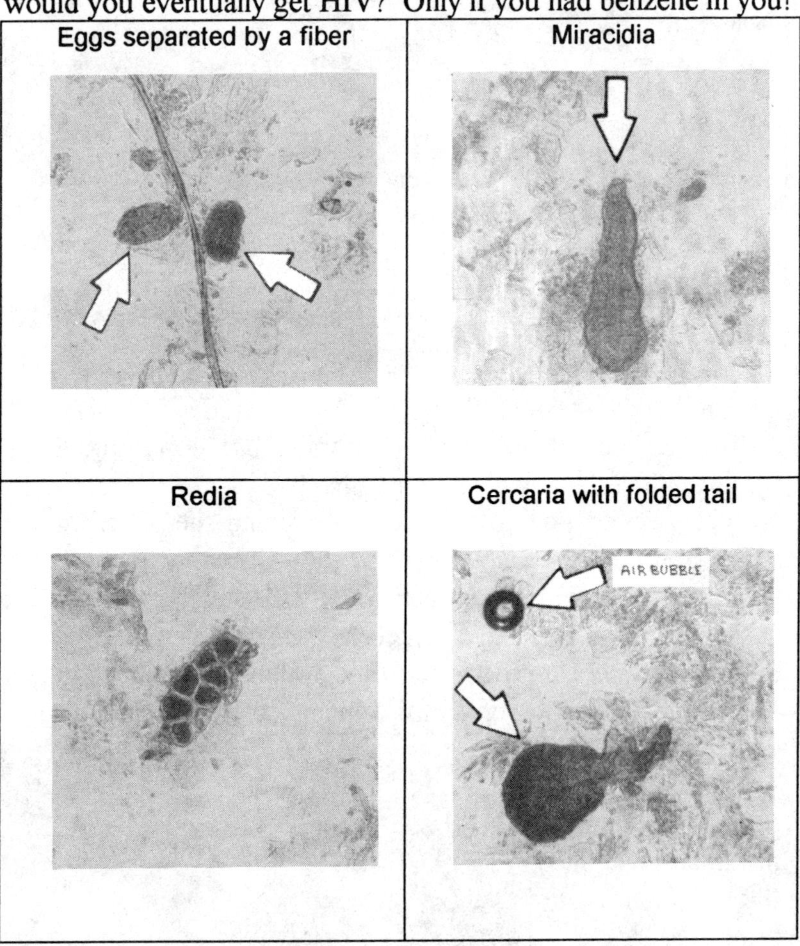

Fig. 48 Parasites in human saliva (100X)

Blood Could Be A Source

The blood carries the infective stages of the intestinal fluke. Until the public blood supply can be searched for them,[32] it is not safe. If you need surgery, use your own blood or get it from someone who has gone through the parasite-killing program. Of course, without solvents in your body, such an infection could not give you HIV/AIDS but it is still very undesirable.

Pets Could Be A Source

Because pet food is polluted with solvents, we should expect "fluke disease" to develop in our pets. This means the unnatural development of fluke stages in their bodies. Their saliva, urine and excrement become sources for transmission. We have learned to be careful with their urine and excrement. Now we must be careful with their saliva. Never let a pet lick you. Never kiss your pet.

Of course, if you fed them homemade food, in their own dishes, and kept them on the pet parasite program, there would be no danger for them or for you.

---

[32] Antibodies to the various fluke stages or antigen tests could be used to test the public blood supply for parasite stages. I know of no existing human intestinal fluke test besides my electronic method.

To summarize:

1. We are eating the infective stages of the intestinal fluke in beef, chicken and turkey
2. We then transmit it to each other by kissing on the mouth and sex.
3. Even if we pick it up in these two ways, we would not get HIV/AIDS from it unless we have benzene in our bodies.

World-wide AIDS

There are two tasks that need immediate attention:

1. Cleaning up the meat supply so that it no longer is infested with flukes. A sample of animal saliva, fixed with equal parts of 20% formaldehyde and spun down in a high speed centrifuge should provide a quick specimen for observation under the microscope. More modern methods could be devised, based on reaction of saliva or blood with antibody to fluke stages. Each animal should be tested. Animals need not be slaughtered but only deparasitized.
2. Cleaning up the feed and food supply of benzene. Even without the fluke parasites, benzene will give us AIDS. We do not need the parasites to get AIDS. As benzene spreads so will AIDS. When half the population has benzene in their bodies, half of us will also get AIDS.

Biological Questions

My tests show me the close association between parasites, solvents and HIV/AIDS. But they do not show me the detailed mechanism.

Since there is never a case of HIV without human intestinal fluke stages being present in the thymus, do the stages bring in the HIV virus? Evidently the virus originates with them. Perhaps the virus is even a snail virus, hitching a ride on the parasite stage.

Why must there be benzene in the thymus? Are the eggs and cercaria attracting the benzene or is the benzene damaged tissue attracting the parasite stages? Or is benzene simply force-hatching the eggs or metacercaria?

Why do some people have benzene in their thymuses for a long time after an exposure, while others do not? Evidently, many people can detoxify it quickly so it doesn't build up. Is this a thymus problem or a liver problem? Is it caused by the fluke itself, or a toxin such as 4,5 benzopyrene, found in our daily foods? I have found 4,5 benzopyrene (but not 3,4 benzopyrene) to be present in persons with benzene buildup. Benzopyrenes are formed when food is burned as in grilling, smoking, even in common toast and wieners! We must stop eating such abnormally prepared foods.

Why does only *Fasciolopsis* bring HIV when many other flukes are also present and multiplying?

Are other flukes bringing us yet new bacteria and viruses? **Is this how we get all our new bacteria and viruses?** Namely from newcomer parasites?

What symptoms does HIV virus cause? It is not clear in a single case history which symptom might be attributed to the virus, supporting the theory that HIV is a fluke virus, dependent upon it for survival or reproduction, and that is why it goes away when the parasite is eliminated.

Fortunately, these questions don't have to be answered before you cure yourself of HIV and AIDS

Some Very Good News

- Fluke parasites are very easy to kill, much easier than many roundworms or tapeworms (tapeworms often survive the parasite herbs).
- Not everything is polluted. Only the processed foods are, and not even all of them. If we eat natural food, we will be safe.
- I have never seen a case of mercury toxicity from eating fish.
- PCB pollution is not in everything (but they are prevalent in detergents).
- I have never seen a case of lead, arsenic or pesticide toxicity from eating fruit or vegetables. Pesticides used on foods haven't penetrated them, as far as my tests show. Simply cut away the blossom and stem end, and wash thoroughly.
- Municipal water is still the safest source. I found no cases of asbestos, aluminum, fluoride or any solvent toxicity due to city water, and only a few cases of arsenic or PCBs.

- Solvents, PCBs, aflatoxins, and 4,5 benzopyrene leave the body in a few days after you stop getting them into your body, not a few years!
- Lead is not coming from paint; it is mainly coming from lead solder joints on copper water pipes.
- Asbestos is not coming from municipal water or building materials; it is mostly coming from your own clothes dryer belts (imported varieties) and hair blowers.
- Although milk (or buttermilk) is a much maligned beverage, it is still unpolluted with metals, solvents, aflatoxins or benzopyrene. But it should be ultrapasteurized, like cream, to rid it of *Salmonella*, *Shigella*, and possible fluke stages.
- Benzene and other solvents are not coming from widespread gasoline pollution; traces are in our foods and products.

Part Three: Case Histories

The case histories you are about to read are all the HIV or AIDS cases that walked or were helped into the office. None were omitted because they did not succeed, or for any other reason.

Some brought with them a clinical HIV positive test result, others were not yet identified as HIV or AIDS cases by their clinical doctors because no test had been done or the test came back negative. Because electronic testing is much more accurate, I considered them to have HIV if they tested YES (positive) to my Protein 24 antigen sample. Likewise I considered the person cured of HIV when they tested NO (negative).

*Cases marked with an asterisk are significant in that they also had clinical HIV tests repeated at the end of my program. (All were negative.)

> The names have been changed to ones of the same sex picked at random from a telephone directory. Ages have been changed by up to five years. Some personal characteristics have been changed in non-essential ways.

All of them got cured if they carried out the instructions, regardless of their degree of illness. Some did not carry out instructions or could not be followed or had special circumstances that kept them from carrying out the instructions. As you will read, the method is 100% effective. It follows that this method must work for you, too, if you are able to carry out the instructions.

Types Of Tests

HIV We test for Protein 24 antigen. As the correlation between HIV, *Fasciolopsis* (human intestinal fluke) in the thymus, and benzene became clearer, I often tested those next.

Cancer We test for ortho-phospho-tyrosine. hCG is tested occasionally as a pre-cancer indicator. Remarkably, cancer is caused (and cured) very similarly to HIV/AIDS and is the subject of another book by this author.

Parasites About 120 varieties, including intermediate stages.

Toxic elements About 70 varieties.

Solvents 27 varieties.

Pathogens (bacteria and viruses) About 80 varieties.

Kidney stones Seven varieties.

Blood (which includes urine) This testing is done by a commercial laboratory, and depending on the panels selected, could be 100 or more tests.

Obviously most of these tests are not part of eliminating parasites and curing HIV. They are essential for learning how to get well.

We have the capability of testing each of these 300 substances in any of the body's 100 tissues for which I have samples. It is unrealistic to even attempt to accomplish these 30,000 possible tests. Typically about 30 tests can be completed in an average office visit, and I select the most useful ones for the client. Only the YES (positive) results and significant NO (negative) results are shown in these case histories.

See *The Tests* chapter for more information about each test.

Not all of the cases are roaring successes, but there are lessons in all of them that can put <u>you</u> on the road to recovery.

1	**Donna Brooks**	**HIV**

Donna Brooks is 20 and came from two states South specifically for her Epstein Barre Virus diagnosis and Chronic Fatigue Syndrome. She has numerous other problems, many of them are weird, such as shaking with cold, gagging after eating, pain in the knee cap. She has pain and tightness over the mid-chest. She has a hard time breathing with shortness of breath. She has pain in the breastbone and upper chest. All this suggests HIV illness. She has severe stomach problems and is losing weight. Her mother, who did not come with her, is extremely concerned. She aches all over. She has a rash on her legs and stomach. They have a cat and a water softener. She drinks mostly Mountain Dew™.

☒ Protein 24 (HIV) YES (present in her white blood cells) and also at thymus and vagina; NO elsewhere

☐ Ortho-phospho-tyrosine (Cancer) NO (not in her white blood cells, and assumed not elsewhere)

☒ hCG (Pre-Cancer) YES at liver, thymus, vagina and at numerous other tissues!

Note: cancer marker ortho-phospho-tyrosine is NO but cancer marker hCG is YES all over her body! hCG always precedes cancer.

☒ Fasciolopsis (Parasite) YES at liver, thymus, kidney, intestine, cervix

☒ Fasciolopsis cercaria (Parasite) YES at liver, thymus, vagina only

She states that she is not sexually active and never has been; she has never had a blood transfusion. Note how heavily infested with flukes she is. The flukes in her liver are starting a cancer and the flukes in her thymus have brought her the HIV virus.

☒ Sheep liver fluke (Parasite) YES at thymus and cervix

☐ Pancreatic fluke and all stages (Parasite) NO

☐ Human liver fluke and all stages (Parasite) NO

☒ Benzene (Solvent) YES at thymus and vagina

☐ Propyl Alcohol (Solvent) NO

Double and triple checked this. She will avoid all products with "PROP" on the label anyway. Note: she did not have the cancer marker ortho-phospho-tyrosine, but she was flooded with the cancer marker hCG which is always made before ortho-phospho-tyrosine is made.

☒ Acetone (Solvent) YES

☒ Toluene (Solvent) YES high

☒ Methyl butyl ketone (Solvent) YES high

Remaining solvents: NO. She will stop all commercial beverages. She will be totally vegetarian for three months. She will go off the benzene list. She will start on the parasite killing program. She brought her latest blood test.

BLOOD TEST	Result	Comment
1. T4	10.4	slightly elevated
2. Cholesterol	very low (168)	indicating a liver problem and cancer risk
3. Triglycerides	very low (37)	cancer risk.

Very low cholesterol and triglycerides have always indicated a high cancer risk. With the emphasis on reducing these currently, this fact seems to be overlooked. Most persons are eating margarine, not butter, and therefore losing their only source of butyric acid in the diet. Butyric acid has been studied and found to have anti-parasite and anti-viral actions. This is another example where chemical food may be the true villain of human illness. Donna is extremely anxious and broke into tears. She knows her mother will not suspect her of having secret sex affairs, but she can hardly believe the whole situation herself. We reassured her that she could clear it up completely.

Five days later

She feels better, especially mentally (more alert). She can breathe easier. Her sternal pain is gone. Her stomach is the main problem now.

☐ Protein 24 (HIV) NO

☐ Ortho-phospho-tyrosine (Cancer) NO

☐ hCG (Pre-Cancer) NO

☒ Hexane dione (Solvent) YES

Has had not one sip of a commercial beverage or tea but had potato chips and cookies. She has some with her.

☒ Cookies (Food Sample) YES in her white blood cells

She will stop eating store bought cookies, crackers, and flavored things.

☒ Mineral oil (Toxic Element) YES

Stop using lotions.

☐ Propyl Alcohol (Solvent) NO

She is using make-up that has no propanol in it, but will stop all of it anyway, and make her own.

☐ Fasciolopsis and all stages (Parasite) NO

☐ Sheep liver fluke and all stages (Parasite) NO

☐ Pancreatic fluke and all stages (Parasite) NO

☐ Human liver fluke and all stages (Parasite) NO

☒ Ascaris, Ascaris megalo (Parasites) YES

These common roundworms are the probable cause of her stomach problems. She will continue the parasite program and also treat the cat . After two weeks she will begin the kidney herb recipe to make more progress in her recovery.

Summary: Donna was understandably shocked that a 20 year old person like herself, who had never had a sexual or blood contact, could have the HIV virus. And, to make matters worse, she had the begin-

nings of cancer. She could not believe it but was willing to try anything since she already had a fat file from a clinical doctor. After just five days her mother could tell she was better, and she also noticed it herself, so she began to believe our story about the true nature of HIV illness. It is tempting to believe that isopropanol is part of the chemistry that goes toward the production of ortho-phospho-tyrosine and not merely a solvent that helps to hatch eggs or break down the tissues so they will accept fluke stages.

Alyce Dean **Lung Cancer and HIV**

Alyce is a low key, sweet tempered person, age 48, brought in by her brother for a spreading numbness in her body. She has pain and numbness at the same time in her arms, legs and hands. Three years ago Alyce had a mastectomy on the right side for cancer. Now a lump is developing on the back of her neck. (I suspect this is a PCB cyst.) Her father died of liver cancer a few years ago.

☒ Ortho-phospho-tyrosine (Cancer) YES at lungs; NO at breast, etc.

☒ Fasciolopsis (Parasite) YES at liver and intestine

☒ Fasciolopsis redia (Parasite) YES in blood

She will start on parasite killing program.

Four days later

☐ Ortho-phospho-tyrosine (Cancer) NO

☐ Fasciolopsis and all stages (Parasite) NO

Her cancer is gone, but her symptoms have not improved; in fact, she is worse, and walks slowly.

☒ Terbium (Toxic Element) YES

Probably in a pill.

☒ Zirconium (Toxic Element) YES

Off deodorant. These are not enough to explain her nerve-muscle deterioration.

☒ Benzene (Solvent) YES

There are building supplies (paint thinner) in the back porch as well as insect spray and chemicals for dairy animals. She lives alone but will have one of her children remove it all and make an air sample in her home for us to test.

Fifteen days later

She is much worse. She has missed her earlier appointment It is tragic to see this young woman losing ground. If she can't find the benzene source, she may not survive.

☐ Ortho-phospho-tyrosine (Cancer) NO

Cancer has not returned.

☒ Protein 24 (HIV) YES

Now has HIV illness.

☒ Benzene (Solvent) YES and in bathroom and porch air

☐ Benzene (Solvent) NO in kitchen and bedroom air

Spray still on porch.

☐ Fasciolopsis adults (Parasite) NO

☒ Fasciolopsis cercaria (Parasite) YES at thymus, bone marrow, and blood

This is obviously from eating undercooked meat since she lives alone. Her children are cooking for her. It is impossible to say no to their cooking. Some of the chemicals have been removed from the porch. She has seen her clinical doctor who has scheduled radiation for her.

☒ Salmonella, EBV, and Coxsackie B virus (Pathogens) YES

Others not tested. She is to clear the whole house of chemicals; her highest priority is to get the benzene out of her body. Her family is sympathetic but isn't taking seriously the need to clear the house of chemicals. Alyce does not have enough immune power to combat simple infections.

Summary: This is the last time we saw Alyce. She cleared her cancer in the first four days and the future looked bright. But she was not strong enough to clean up the solvent, benzene, which was polluting the air in her house. Her family did not come with her to learn the details of cleaning up and so the job was left undone. Without immunity she was helpless against the common bacteria and viruses.

2	**Sharon Brownie**	**HIV and Liver and Lung Cancer**

Sharon Brownie came to the office for pain behind her shoulder blades, behind her ears, in both legs, and on top of her head at the scalp. These are unusual symptoms to occur together.

☒ Protein 24 (HIV) YES at thymus

Quite a surprise.

☒ Ortho-phospho-tyrosine (Cancer) YES at liver and lungs

She also has liver and lung cancer, another surprise, since there is no smoker in the house.

☒ Fasciolopsis (Parasite) YES at thymus and blood

The meaning of this result is not clear. How could an adult fluke fit into a blood vessel? She has both cancer and HIV. Yet, the adult intestinal fluke is not in the liver, only in the thymus and, apparently, blood.

☒ Fasciolopsis redia (Parasite) YES at blood, thymus, liver and lung

She will start on parasite program. She will go off items on the benzene and propanol lists.

Four days later

☐ Ortho-phospho-tyrosine (Cancer) NO

☐ Fasciolopsis and all stages (Parasite) NO

☐ Protein 24 (HIV) NO

Fifteen days later

She feels considerably better. She still gets weak spells in her arms and legs (but not pain, now).

☐ Protein 24 (HIV) NO

☒ Gallium, Gold, Ruthenium (Toxic Elements) YES

Tooth fillings. She has no tooth fillings but wears a metal partial denture. She will get a new metal-free plastic one.

Thirteen days later

- ☐ Protein 24 (HIV) NO
- ☐ Ortho-phospho-tyrosine (Cancer) NO
- ☒ Oxalate (Kidney Stones) YES
  Start on kidney herb recipe.
- ☒ Propyl Alcohol (Solvent) YES
- ☒ Pentane (Solvent) YES
- ☒ Kerosene (Solvent) YES
  Used in cook stove.
- ☒ Denatured alcohol (Solvent) YES
  Used in lamps. She will be much more careful when pouring these fuels and will stop drinking soda pop.
- ☒ Diphyllobothrium (Parasite) YES
  Dog/fish tapeworm. She will increase parasite dosage.

Eleven days later

She still has pain at left lower abdomen, upper back and lower back. This is probably still due to parasites, plus liver gallstones.

- ☐ Kidney Stones (ALL) NO
  Continue kidney herbs at half dose.
- ☐ Protein 24 (HIV) NO
- ☐ Ortho-phospho-tyrosine (Cancer) NO
- ☐ Denatured alcohol (Solvent) NO
- ☒ Pentane (Solvent) YES
  Can't give up soda pop.
- ☒ Propyl Alcohol (Solvent) YES
  Source unknown, since she uses no commercial body products.
- ☒ Gastrothylax, Trichomonas (Parasites) YES
  Continue parasite program.
- ☐ Parasites (Remainder) NO
  She will start taking peroxy and 07 in preparation for a liver gallstone cleanse. She will do a 5 day high dose parasite treatment.

Another month later

Her left arm is numb, both feet are numb. There is shoulder and shoulder blade pain. She is still putting off the dental work.

☐ Protein 24 (HIV) NO

☐ Ortho-phospho-tyrosine (Cancer) NO

☐ Diphyllobothrium, Gastrothylax, Trichomonas (Parasites) NO

☐ Solvents (ALL) NO

☒ Diplococcus pneu, Histomonas, Salmonella typh, Haemoph inf (Pathogens) YES

Two of these are teeth bacteria. She is getting a lot of headaches. Remainder of box 1 and 2: NO.

Five weeks later

She is still getting a lot of headaches, probably from tooth bacteria. She did a liver cleanse and got numerous tan-colored stones.

☐ Protein 24 (HIV) NO

☐ Ortho-phospho-tyrosine (Cancer) NO

☒ Clostridium sept. (Pathogen) YES

Probable cause of pain behind both ears. Needs to do dental work.

☒ Wood Alcohol (Solvent) YES

Is drinking Pepsi™ again.

☒ Kerosene (Solvent) YES

They are using it again; must change.

Summary: Sharon eliminated the HIV virus and her liver cancer in record time: 4 days. What was more difficult was eliminating headaches; in fact, it was not accomplished. Her isopropanol disappeared after she switched off commercial shampoo. It remains to be seen whether her arms and feet will recover. She does plan to get the dental work done.

Harriet Kader **HIV**

Harriet is a young 31 year old mother who had been seeing alternative doctors for several years because of her numerous problems that bewilder her and her husband. Mainly, she has no energy at all. She also has eczema on her hands, heart palpitation, and a history of high bilirubin.

☐ Ortho-phospho-tyrosine (Cancer) NO

☒ Protein 24 (HIV) YES at thymus and vagina; NO at liver and intestines

☐ Fasciolopsis and all stages (Parasite) NO

Note: where did the HIV virus come from if all the intestinal fluke stages are absent? Is there a stage present in an organ that did not show up in the white blood cells?

☒ Sheep liver fluke redia (Parasite) YES at thymus and vagina

☒ Pancreatic Fluke stages (Parasite) YES high at thymus

☒ Benzene (Solvent) YES at thymus and vagina

☒ Wood Alcohol (Solvent) YES at thymus and pancreas

☒ Mineral oil (Toxic Element) YES at thymus

Note: she does not have propanol in her so she has not become infested with intestinal flukes and has not developed cancer. It seems probable that she picked up the sheep liver fluke sexually, since it is in her vagina. It may have traveled to the thymus, then, to continue its cycle. The pancreatic fluke is thriving in the thymus, too, because benzene is present here. We will test her husband, Preston.

Preston Kader:

☐ Protein 24 (HIV) NO

☒ Ortho-phospho-tyrosine (Cancer) YES at intestine

The news of his cancer in the intestine was shocking.

☒ Fasciolopsis (Parasite) YES at liver

☒ Fasciolopsis eggs (Parasite) YES

☒ Fasciolopsis miracidia, redia (Parasite) YES at intestine

☒ Sheep liver fluke miracidia (Parasite) YES

If these miracidia were transplanted sexually into Harriet's vagina they could swim about, invading her blood stream and continuing their cycle in her solvent-loaded tissues.

☐ Pancreatic fluke (Parasite) NO

☒ Benzene (Solvent) YES at thymus and intestine

☒ Propyl Alcohol (Solvent) YES at thymus and liver

They will remove propanol from their home and personal use. They will stop using everything on the benzene-pollution list.

One month later

We are seeing Harriet only. They have been on a parasite program. The Protein 24 antigen test for HIV, done at the clinic the morning after her last visit here, was NO (negative). I expected it to be YES (positive) because my test was positive. Does the clinic miss early cases?

☐ Ortho-phospho-tyrosine (Cancer) NO

☒ Protein 24 (HIV) YES at thymus and vagina

☐ hCG (Pre-Cancer) NO

☒ Benzene (Solvent) YES

☐ Propyl Alcohol (Solvent) NO

The HIV virus is still there, because the benzene is still in her. But she has not used anything on the benzene list I gave her! She has been using a cooking oil I am unfamiliar with. She will stop using it and bring some in for testing. She will use olive oil only.

☒ Fasciolopsis (Parasite) YES at thymus and intestine; NO at liver and vagina

☒ Sheep liver fluke (Parasite) YES at liver, thymus, intestine and vagina

☒ Sheep liver fluke metacercaria (Parasite) YES at thymus, spleen and bladder

☒ Human liver fluke metacercaria (Parasite) YES at thymus

☒ Human liver fluke eggs (Parasite) YES at liver and thymus

Summary: It has been difficult for Harriet to get rid of the benzene because I was unable to identify the source for her. This has kept the parasites exploding their population in her. Of course, she would be infective to her husband and vice versa. They had not gone on the parasite program after the first visit because they wanted to hear the clinical test results first. This was very ill advised. Hopefully, they are committed to it now. But perhaps they are not since they have not returned.

3	John Vissers	HIV

This 35 year old man experiences numbness in his legs and arm. He was exposed to glues. He also has fatigue and poor concentration. He experiences occasional sore throats and pain in his shoulders, wrists, lower back, knees. His mood is very changeable with some depression. He only has a few good days in a month. He suffers from hay fever and chest tightness. This is a long list of ailments for a man of his youth. They have a water softener.

☒ Protein 24 (HIV) YES

☐ Ortho-phospho-tyrosine (Cancer) NO

☒ Fasciolopsis (Parasite) YES at thymus; NO at liver
Others not tested.

☒ PCB (Toxic Element) YES high
Body current was extremely low considering that 5 volts was applied to his hands during testing—alerted me to possible PCB pollution.

☒ Benzene (Solvent) YES
Others not tested. He will start on parasite program and go off all items on the benzene list. His son is with him and is not well, either. We will attend to him next.

One month later

☐ Protein 24 (HIV) NO

☐ Ortho-phospho-tyrosine (Cancer) NO

☒ TCE, TCE ethylene, Wood Alcohol (Solvents) YES

One month later

☐ Protein 24 (HIV) NO

☐ Ortho-phospho-tyrosine (Cancer) NO

☒ TCE, TCE ethylene, Wood Alcohol, Pentane (Solvents) YES
He will stop using commercial beverages and make his own.

☐ PCB (Toxic Element) NO

Went off detergents.

Summary: John is unable to come more often for follow-ups. His numbness suggests mercury toxicity but we have not even tested for toxic elements at this point. He can be commended, though, for getting rid of benzene, HIV, PCBs, and parasites.

Pete Vissers	**HIV**

This 8 year old boy has pain in his chest and cysts in the back of his neck. He also has a frequently stuffy and runny nose, dry lips, swollen glands, upset stomach after eating, leg pains, and some trouble sleeping. The chest pain is similar to his father's.

☒ Fasciolopsis (Parasite) YES at thymus; NO at liver

☒ Protein 24 (HIV) YES

☐ Ortho-phospho-tyrosine (Cancer) NO

☒ Benzene (Solvent) YES

☐ Propyl Alcohol (Solvent) NO

☒ PCB (Toxic Element) YES

Others not tested. Start on parasite program. Go off detergent and benzene products.

Summary: The chest pain drew my attention immediately to the probability of HIV virus. The cysts were immediately suggestive of PCB's. These cysts are described in the Japanese book on the PCB event that took place many years ago there. So there was little difficulty in finding it in Pete. But I did not see him for follow up. It seems likely that the child was included in the lifestyle changes made by his parents.

4	**Betty Naylor**	**HIV and Cervical Cancer**

Betty is 24 years old, arriving for Chronic Fatigue Syndrome. However, she had an impressive list of additional symptoms involving her lower back, stomach, throat, skin, ears and neck. She also had chest tightness and the need for long breaths of air and PMS. The chest problem suggested the possibility of HIV-illness. She sleeps all day and has burning over the sternum. They have a water softener. She has been sick all winter.

☒ Protein 24 (HIV) YES at thymus, vagina; NO elsewhere

☒ Ortho-phospho-tyrosine (Cancer) YES at cervix only

☒ hCG (Pre-Cancer) YES at thymus, cervix; NO at vagina

This was quite a surprise. Betty volunteered that she had never had sex in her life and had never been in the hospital except at birth. I reassured her that this could be quickly cleared up, provided she followed instructions meticulously. She was very eager to do so.

☐ Fasciolopsis adults (Parasite) NO

☒ Fasciolopsis miracidia (Parasite) YES at cervix and vagina

☒ Fasciolopsis cercaria (Parasite) YES high at cervix

☒ Fasciolopsis eggs (Parasite) YES at vagina

☒ Sheep liver fluke (Parasite) YES high at liver (one side) and intestine

☒ Sheep liver fluke eggs (Parasite) YES at liver (same side as above), cervix and vagina

☒ Human liver fluke adults (Parasite) YES at liver (same side as above)

☒ Human liver fluke eggs (Parasite) YES throughout liver

These findings suggest both benzene and isopropanol have accumulated in Betty's body. There isn't enough time to test for all solvents today.

☒ Benzene (Solvent) YES at thymus and vagina

☒ Propyl Alcohol (Solvent) YES at liver (same side as above) and thymus; NO at vagina

To avoid benzene, she is to go off all toothpaste, Vaseline products, ice cream and frozen yogurt and cooking oils, except olive oil. To avoid propanol, she is to go off all body products that have "PROP" on the label. She is to go off all commercial beverages to avoid other solvents, not yet tested. We will follow-up very soon. She is very anxious. She will start on parasite killing program. She will be strictly vegetarian for 3 months.

Five days later

She has a lot more energy and has gone off her antibiotics. She says she is very apprehensive.

☐ Protein 24 (HIV) NO

☐ Ortho-phospho-tyrosine (Cancer) NO

☐ hCG (Pre-Cancer) NO

☐ Solvents (ALL) NO

☐ Fasciolopsis and all stages (Parasite) NO

☐ Pancreatic fluke (Parasite) NO

☐ Sheep liver fluke (Parasite) NO

☐ Human liver fluke (Parasite) NO

She is elated. She will continue the parasite killing program and her other lifestyle changes.

☒ PCB (Toxic Element) YES

Off detergent; use borax and washing soda and homemade soap.

☒ Gadolinium, Tantalum (Toxic Elements) YES

Tooth fillings.

☒ Holmium (Toxic Element) YES

Probably with the PCBs.

☐ Toxic Elements (Remainder) NO

She needs metal tooth fillings replaced. After 3 months of vegetarian diet she will eat only fish and seafood in restaurants and super-well done meats at home.

Summary: This young woman fairly bounced out of the office at the good news of her second visit. The entire story of how she could have gotten the HIV virus and developed cancer of the cervix was like a revelation to her—almost unbelievable. Yet her mother, she said, was witness to her health improvement in just 5 days, and she is forced to believe it all. At any rate, she is much too scared not to believe that she had HIV virus.

Notice a peculiarity: there is no adult intestinal fluke in the liver. Not even a stage of it is in the liver! Yet there is ortho-phospho-tyrosine being produced! It is being produced at the cervix where the miracidia and cercaria are and where the sheep liver fluke eggs are.

Now, the sheep liver fluke adults are found in the liver. Could they orchestrate the production of ortho-phospho-tyrosine for the intestinal fluke? Or was there an adult intestinal fluke at some earlier time that got killed? One seldom sees both adult flukes together. Do they kill each other somehow? Notice, too, that the cancer marker, hCG, was present, along with the cancer marker, ortho-phospho-tyrosine at the cervix. But only hCG was being produced at the thymus. Is a particular stage responsible for producing hCG? I explained to Betty that she must take great care to protect her thymus for two years so that it will completely regain its health. It would be tempting to neglect the dental work but this would be a tragic mistake. Benzene leaves the thymus in a weakened condition so that other solvents and toxic substances continue to accumulate there. This would, surely, give her lowered immunity, perhaps even AIDS.

5 Kersten Mossay — HIV

Kersten is a young woman with early teenage children. We have seen her from time to time, perhaps once a year, for 5 or 6 years now. She says she does not often go to clinical doctors. Today she has a 100° temperature which she has had for a month. There is also blood in her urine. She has been to a clinical doctor who diagnosed it as *nephritis*. Her blood pressure goes from high (173/140) to extremely low. Her pulse goes to 120 in the evening. She has a sore throat and is experiencing double vision. She hurts all over, especially in her hands and feet. She has become extremely nervous, with bad memory and is very fatigued. A second clinical doctor did an anti-nuclear antibody test which was negative. He gave her a diagnosis of *fibromyalgia* and wanted to schedule her to see a psychiatrist, but she hasn't carried this out.

☒ Protein 24 (HIV) YES

☐ Ortho-phospho-tyrosine (Cancer) NO

Being positive for HIV astounded her. Neither she nor her husband have ANY risk factors. Coming from a strict religious background, there is no extra-marital sex or use of blood, nor recreational drug use. I assured her it had nothing to do with her or her husband's conduct.

☒ Fasciolopsis (Parasite) YES at thymus and kidney; NO at liver, intestine, etc.

☐ Fasciolopsis remaining stages (Parasite) NO

☒ Gardnerella vag, Salmonella, Flu A and B, Shigella, Borellia, A strep, Herpes Simplex 1, Adenovirus, Proteus, CMV, Resp Sync Virus, Chlamydia, Bacillus cereus, Strep pneu (Pathogens) YES

☐ Propionobacterium, Trichomonas, Bacteroides frag, Campylobacter pyl, Haemophillus inf, Staph aureus, Strep pneu, Coxsackie virus B4, Histoplasma cap, Human Papilloma (Plantar), Coxsackie virus B1, Nocardia, EBV, Human Papilloma 4 (Pathogens) NO

End of Box 1. She has 14 YES out of 28 tested, much too high for a regular illness; this is an immune deficiency state. Obviously, Kersten has numerous infections unleashed in her body and would soon be bedridden and terminally ill. Her generally healthy lifestyle, with avoidance of alcohol and nicotine, and ability to adapt to new personal habits, will come to her assistance now.

☒ Benzene (Solvent) YES

☐ Solvents (Remainder) NO

They will remove all solvents from their basement and house to an outdoor garage. They will lose some paint cans to damage by freezing this way. She will start on the parasite killing program and avoid eating meat altogether. She will stay off the benzene pollution list I gave her. She will bring in her husband for testing.

Three days later

Kersten's husband, Leroy, has arrived for a brief check. He is experiencing no health problems, although he works hard as a home builder.

Leroy

☐ Ortho-phospho-tyrosine (Cancer) NO

☒ Protein 24 (HIV) YES at thymus and penis; NO at liver, kidneys, brain, prostate, etc.

☐ Fasciolopsis adults (Parasite) NO

☒ Fasciolopsis cercaria (Parasite) YES at thymus and penis; NO at liver, kidney, brain, prostate

Leroy has brought a sample of the frozen beef they have been eating; it is from a special local source. It tested YES (positive) to Fasciolopsis cercaria electronically. We will examine it under the microscope also.

☒ Benzene (Solvent) YES

☐ Solvents (Remainder) NO

He will start on parasite program. He loves beef and will cook it thoroughly but is not completely convinced it is dangerous. He probably, also, does not believe his HIV POSITIVE status. However, he is willing to help Kersten get well.

Four days later (1 week after first visit)

Kersten has arrived. She is very much better. She still has a sore throat.

☐ Ortho-phospho-tyrosine (Cancer) NO

☐ Protein 24 (HIV) NO

☐ Fasciolopsis and all stages (Parasite) NO

☒ Sheep liver fluke adult (Parasite) YES at intestine

☐ Sheep liver fluke other stages (Parasite) NO

She will continue the parasite program, vegetarianism, and avoidance of benzene list. She is concerned about the children. I suggested being very careful to thoroughly cook the meat for them and avoidance of benzene polluted products and food.

Summary: It is 4 months later; evidently the family is staying well. I am especially fond of this family. Notice that they were not full of food solvents, in general, due to their habit of eating home-cooked food and beverages. Since the parasite stage could be sexually transmitted as well as eaten with meat, it was important for Kersten's husband to come in, which he did without a hostile attitude. Probably, he was not yet ill because the parasite cycle had not completed itself; he did not yet have the adult fluke. The virus can be present without an adult fluke but when all the stages are gone, it is gone, too. Note its preference for thymus and penis as a tissue site in Leroy.

6	Lenore Dale	HIV and Intestinal Cancer

This is a young 34 year old person who works for a doctor and has already tried a number of alternative health procedures. She has a long list of bizarre symptoms, such as swollen and itching lips, gagging when eating, suggesting AIDS, but the symptom of chest heaviness made it even more probable. She has a water softener.

☒ Protein 24 (HIV) YES at thymus, vagina and ovaries

☒ Ortho-phospho-tyrosine (Cancer) YES at intestine

☒ hCG (Pre-Cancer) YES everywhere
What a shocking realization this brought to her, both HIV and cancer in a single diagnosis. She could hardly bear the news in spite of my assurance that she could eliminate them both within 10 days. Perhaps she was also angry or disbelieving.

☒ Fasciolopsis (Parasite) YES at liver and intestine
Gave her cancer.

☒ Fasciolopsis eggs (Parasite) YES at intestine, adrenals, saliva

☐ Sheep liver fluke and all stages (Parasite) NO

☐ Pancreatic fluke and all stages (Parasite) NO

☐ Human liver fluke and all stages (Parasite) NO

☒ Benzene (Solvent) YES at thymus
Go off items on benzene list.

☒ Propyl Alcohol (Solvent) YES at liver
Eliminate propanol. Others not tested. She will start parasite program. Note: I failed to test for Fasciolopsis stages in the thymus. My error!

Twelve days later

☐ Protein 24 (HIV) NO

☐ Ortho-phospho-tyrosine, hCG (Cancer) NO
HIV and cancer are gone—everything was done correctly.

☒ Aluminum Silicate (Toxic Element) YES
Will disconnect water softener and switch salt.

☒ Bismuth (Toxic Element) YES
Get rid of fragranced items.

☒ Radon (Toxic Element) YES

Open the vents to the crawl space.

☒ Thallium and Germanium (Toxic Element) YES

This coincidence of thallium and germanium is only found when the tooth filling metal has these pollutants. She is very upset about this since she states that she has had weak hands (very weak) for many years already. This is a classic symptom of thallium poisoning. She had all her mercury fillings taken out by Dr. S. who is a Huggins Institute trained dentist. 5 gold crowns were put back in her mouth, and she spent $3,000 on this last fall.

☒ Gold (Toxic Element) YES

☒ Mercury (Toxic Element) YES at tooth #29 and 15

Tooth #29 has a gold crown. She says this tooth has been bothering her. I then searched for the location of the thallium and found it at teeth #29, 10, and 18. She will ask the dentist to do a fresh panoramic X-ray to search for tattoos. I shone a flashlight in her mouth and could see 2 tattoos. However, these metal pinpoint leftovers might be left from the braces she used to wear. She states she remembers seeing them after the braces were removed.

☒ PCB (Toxic Element) YES

Uses Dr. Bronner's Peppermint soap—will go off.

Summary; Lenore's case is especially tragic but nevertheless an early warning sign for all humanity. She was given 16 mercury fillings starting in early childhood, some of which were polluted with thallium. This was the probable cause of having a child with microcephaly. In an effort to improve her health she turned to health food soap only to be poisoned with PCBs. Only her good intelligence and survival instinct kept her from self-destructive anger. She will probably set herself and her family on the road to good health.

7, 8	**Brenda Stauffer & Katy**	**HIV**

This is a very pleasant but concerned mother; she has her 10 month old baby, Katy, with her. Brenda is 31 and complains of burning on her chest. (She places her hand right over her thymus, and I sincerely hope this isn't HIV disease.) She also has chronic back pains which move about, and is always sleepy. Her baby has had one illness after another, including pneumonia and has been on antibiotics all winter. She is breast feeding, and the baby appears well-grown and content.

☐ Ortho-phospho-tyrosine (Cancer) NO

☐ hCG (Pre-Cancer) NO

☒ Protein 24 (HIV) YES at thymus and vagina

This is indeed shocking. She has no risk factors. I explained the benzene problem and its link to parasites in the thymus.

☒ Fasciolopsis (Parasite) YES at thymus only; NO at liver and intestine

Other parasites not tested.

☒ Benzene (Solvent) YES

Other solvents not tested. She is not using any items on my benzene list of polluted items. She is using peanut oil in cooking. She will stop and bring it in for testing. She will switch to olive oil.

Baby, Katy, age 10 months

She was tested by surrogate technique, using her mother in the circuit.

☒ hCG (Pre-Cancer) YES throughout body

☒ Ortho-phospho-tyrosine (Cancer) YES throughout body

☒ Protein 24 (HIV) YES throughout body

The shock of seeing this apparently healthy baby riddled with cancer and HIV disease was too tragic for me to communicate to the mother. I did not tell her.

☐ Fasciolopsis adult (Parasite) NO

☒ Fasciolopsis eggs (Parasite) YES at liver, thymus, saliva

We should be able to see these eggs in the baby's saliva and have taken a sample on a cotton bud for examination under the microscope.

☐ Sheep liver fluke adults (Parasite) NO

☒ Sheep liver fluke eggs (Parasite) YES at saliva, thymus, liver

☐ Pancreatic fluke and all stages (Parasite) NO

☒ Human liver fluke adults (Parasite) YES throughout her body

☒ Benzene (Solvent) YES one of the highest levels seen

It seems likely the baby is getting the parasite stages from the mother's milk; we will get a sample of the milk and search under the microscope. The benzene must be coming through the milk too.

Summary: Since the mother will go on the parasite killing program immediately and be off benzene sources, I suspect the baby will be cleared of her problems within a week. I emphasized the importance of follow-up in one week, since the source of benzene was not proved. But the mother felt this would not be possible for various reasons. This lack of concern shocked me and irritated me. To be sure the mother returns I broke the news to her that her baby had cancer. She was overwhelmed with sadness, immediately. I hope she comes back on time.

Seven days later

Baby Katy

☐ Protein 24 (HIV) NO

☐ Ortho-phospho-tyrosine (Cancer) NO

☒ hCG (Pre-Cancer) YES at thymus

Mother, Brenda

☐ Protein 24 (HIV) NO

☐ hCG (Pre-Cancer) NO

☐ Ortho-phospho-tyrosine (Cancer) NO

☐ Benzene (Solvent) NO

☐ Propyl Alcohol (Solvent) NO

☒ Wood Alcohol (Solvent) YES at pancreas and in breast milk

☒ Regular gasoline (Solvent) YES

☐ Solvents (Remainder) NO

Father, George

☒ Benzene (Solvent) YES

☒ Propyl Alcohol (Solvent) YES

He has not observed any rules or restrictions. They will continue on parasite program and stay off benzene and propanol products.

Summary: The HIV is gone and cancer is almost gone for mother and baby. They will try to avoid commercial beverages and cold cerealls for their family. The thymus is probably somewhat damaged and care must be taken to avoid toxic substances from getting into it.

Two weeks later

The baby has not been ill since last visit. She has been kept on a sulfa drug all this time, however. The mother seems afraid to take the baby off it.

Baby, Katy

☐ Protein 24 (HIV) NO

☐ hCG (Pre-Cancer) NO

☐ Ortho-phospho-tyrosine (Cancer) NO

☐ Benzene (Solvent) NO

☐ Propyl Alcohol (Solvent) NO

Mother, Brenda

☐ Protein 24 (HIV) NO

☐ hCG (Pre-Cancer) NO

☐ Ortho-phospho-tyrosine (Cancer) NO

☒ Fasciolopsis cercaria (Parasite) YES high at thymus

This explains the burning over her chest which she still experiences.

☒ Benzene (Solvent) YES at thymus

They are using some cooking oil for baking cakes; will switch to olive oil.

☐ Propyl Alcohol (Solvent) NO

Other solvents not tested. Brenda has been drinking unpasteurized milk; she will heat it to steaming now. The baby gets heated milk. The father was not tested at this time.

Summary: Both cancer and HIV are gone but are lurking in the wings. If the parents are not very vigilant over diet and body products they will recur. Fortunately, this story has a happy ending.

Three weeks later

Baby was ill 1 week ago and got Sulfatrim from a clinical doctor. She is on the medication now.

Baby, Katy

☒ Benzene (Solvent) YES high

Don't use Baby Magic™ on baby.

☒ Propyl Alcohol (Solvent) YES high

Baby is eating Cream of Wheat™, oats, cornmeal and mashed potatoes with gravy.

Mother, Brenda

☒ Benzene (Solvent) YES

☒ Propyl Alcohol (Solvent) YES

She is eating nothing that might have benzene in it. We will test their well water. She will stop using baby shampoo.

Ten days later

They have brought a sample of their well water.

Mother, Brenda

☒ Benzene (Solvent) YES

☒ Benzene (Solvent) YES in drinking water!

Finally, the riddle of the benzene source is solved. The father, who is present, is very concerned. He will search for pollution in his well, pump and cistern.

Baby, Katy

☐ Solvents (ALL) NO

☒ Haemophilus infl, CMV, Mycoplasma, Staphylococcus aureus, B strep, EBV (Pathogens) YES

End box 1. 6 were YES (positive) out of 34. This is quite poor; suggestive of developing AIDS.

Three weeks later

Brenda says she feels better. They have switched to a different well for their drinking water.

☒ Thulium (Toxic Element) YES
Orange drink, probably from the added vitamin C; will stop.

☒ Beryllium (Toxic Element) YES
Gasoline.

☒ Fiberglass (Toxic Element) YES
Will search for a hole in the ceiling or wall, exposing insulation.

☐ Toxic Elements (Remainder) NO
I tested her other children for benzene, and one was YES (positive) for it (he is still using toothpaste; will stop).

Final Summary: Hopefully, this discovery of polluted well water will stop the nightmare these parents have experienced since the birth of their last child.

9* Mel Davison HIV

Mel is a healthy looking young man of 25. He came with a friend from a large city, five hours away. He brought with him a recent blood test, including his HIV positive test results. He was referred by a cured cancer client.

BLOOD TEST	Result	Comment
1. Creatinine	slightly high (1.1)	kidney problem
2. Uric acid	very high (9.4)	kidney problem
3. Phosphate	high (4.3)	dissolving bone
4. Calcium	very low (8.5)	he is not drinking milk
5. Total protein	very high (9.0)	probable liver problem
6. Albumin	low (3.5)	probable liver problem
7. Globulin	high (5.5)	probable liver problem
8. GGT, SGOT, SGPT	high (55, 46, 58)	liver problem
9. LDH	high (208)	check for cancer
10. Cholesterol	very low (121)	check for cancer
11. WBC	very low (3.0)	bone marrow toxin?
12. RBC	low (4.35)	parasites
13.Platelet count	low (158)	bone marrow?
14. Poly/lymph	low (47/38)	chronic virus
15. Monocytes	slightly high (8.9)	virus
16. Eos	slightly high (3.6)	parasites
17. Baso	high (2.6)	check for cancer
18. Sed rate	high (56)	inflammation somewhere
19. HIV 1	POSITIVE	antibody test by Elisa Assay
20. HIV	POSITIVE	antibody test by Western Blot

These blood test results are definitely poor; his youthful healthy appearance belies these bad results. He will start to drink milk, 2%, 3 glasses a day and later cleanse his kidneys.

☒ Protein 24 (HIV) YES at thymus and penis; NO elsewhere

☐ Ortho-phospho-tyrosine (Cancer) NO

☐ hCG (Pre-Cancer) NO

☒ Fasciolopsis (Parasite) YES in half of thymus only and at intestine

☒ Sheep liver fluke (Parasite) YES at both sides of thymus and intestine

☒ Sheep liver fluke cercaria (Parasite) YES at penis only

☐ Pancreatic fluke (Parasite) NO

☐ Human liver fluke (Parasite) NO

Note: His thymus gland is hosting both intestinal and sheep liver flukes. They tend to exclude each other in the liver. Why are they compatible in the thymus? He must have many solvents in his thymus.

☒ Benzene (Solvent) YES at thymus, intestine, penis

He will start on parasite killing program immediately. He will avoid benzene products.

Same day, 3½ hours later

He took a large dose of parasite killer, instead of beginning at day 1.

☐ Protein 24 (HIV) NO

Perhaps he killed the redia stages that carried the virus?

☒ Cobalt, PCB (Toxic Elements) YES at thymus

Off detergents.

☒ Mercury, Iridium (Toxic Element) YES at thymus

Tooth fillings.

☒ Vanadium (Toxic Element) YES

Gas leak.

☐ Toxic Elements (Remainder) NO

He is requested to get all metal out of his mouth immediately and get replacements as he is able to afford them. His only gas appliance is a stove; he will get a maintenance person to check it for leaks. After this he will do an air sampling for us to test for vanadium next time.

☒ Acetone (Solvent) YES

☒ Benzene (Solvent) YES higher than before

He brought his own water for drinking with him; he will switch to faucet water.

☒ Methyl Butyl Ketone, Wood alcohol, Carbon tetrachloride (Solvents) YES

☐ Solvents (Remainder) NO

Note: Although the parasite was killed quickly, and the HIV virus disappeared, the benzene level had not reduced. He will go off all commercial beverages and drink only milk (to which he is allergic), water (from faucet), homemade fruit and vegetable juice, single herb teas, homemade coffee substitutes. He will go off all cold cereal. This is a lot of change to put into effect rather quickly. But his friend is supportive and may help him get it accomplished.

Eighteen days later

At his last blood test he was evaluated as having AIDS with a T count of 78.

☐ Protein 24 (HIV) NO

☐ Ortho-phospho-tyrosine (Cancer) NO

☐ Solvents (ALL) NO

☒ Vanadium(Toxic Element) YES

Nothing has been done about the stove.

☒ Cobalt (Toxic Element) YES

Has not gone off detergents.

☒ Mercury and Iridium (Toxic Element) YES

Dental work not done.

☒ PCB (Toxic Element) YES

Still using detergent.

☒ CMV, EBV, Streptococcus pneumonia (Pathogens) YES

☒ Herpes 1 (Pathogen) YES everywhere in body

☒ Candida (Pathogen) YES

Obviously AIDS; others not tested at this time.

Nine days later

Mel has been well. He has bought a vegetable juicer and enjoys his new lifestyle.

☐ Ortho-phospho-tyrosine, hCG (Cancer) NO

☒ Protein 24 (HIV) YES at thymus and penis

Has the virus again.

☐ Fasciolopsis adults (Parasite) NO

☒ Fasciolopsis cercaria (Parasite) YES at thymus

But NO at white blood cells, indicating a minimal infection.

☒ Fasciolopsis redia (Parasite) YES

☒ Sheep liver fluke adults (Parasite) YES at liver, NO at thymus

☒ Sheep liver fluke miracidia (Parasite) YES

Other flukes not tested.

☐ Benzene (Solvent) NO

☐ Propyl Alcohol (Solvent) NO

Mel has probably reinfected himself by eating undercooked meat, by saliva or sexual contact very recently. Due to past injury of the thymus by benzene, the parasite stages go immediately to the thymus, interfering with T cell formation. He will increase his parasite maintenance program to daily doses instead of twice a week. This will prevent 3 days' growth opportunity for the parasites. Note that it is the cercaria or redia of the intestinal fluke that brings with it the HIV virus, not the adult. He will do a 5 day high dose parasite program, also. He will avoid eating beef, chicken, or turkey for 3 months. Also note that cercaria were not showing up in the white blood cells: if I had not also tested the thymus I would have missed them.

Ten days later

☐ Protein 24 (HIV) NO

Got rid of virus again.

☐ Ortho-phospho-tyrosine (Cancer) NO

☒ hCG (Pre-Cancer) YES throughout his body
A precancerous situation exists; it is always caused by propyl alcohol.

☒ Propyl Alcohol (Solvent) YES at thymus, one part of the liver
He has used regular commercial shampoo recently.

☒ TCEthylene, TCE, MEKetone (Solvents) YES
Flavored foods.

☒ Styrene (Solvent) YES
Off styrofoam cups.

☒ Kerosene (Solvent) YES
More careful with gasoline.

☒ Butyl Nitrite (Solvent) YES high at thymus
Commonly called "rush". Will go off. Will bring in all other body products for testing.

☐ t-Butyl Nitrite (Solvent) NO

☒ 2 Methyl propanol (Solvent) YES

☒ Grain Alcohol (Solvent) YES
Possibly from black walnut tincture. Use no alcoholic beverage. Put tincture in warm beverage.

☐ Solvents (Remainder) NO
Note: Mel has picked up a number of solvents, including propanol which is giving him the precancerous condition indicated by hCG. However these solvents, while giving him AIDS, do not bring him the HIV virus. He will need to be much more disciplined to regain his immunity. He will take charcoal capsules (3 a day) and Silymarin caps (4 a day) until his next appointment. [I have since found Silymarin to be polluted and have switched to Milk Thistle, see *Sources*.]

Seven weeks later

I fear the worst after this long absence without reinforcement and support of office visits.

☐ Protein 24 (HIV) NO

☐ Ortho-phospho-tyrosine (Cancer) NO

☐ hCG (Pre-Cancer) NO

☐ Benzene (Solvent) NO

☐ Propyl Alcohol (Solvent) NO

He has done an excellent job of changing his lifestyle and is ready for a clinical test for HIV antigen. Hopefully he will do it today, before he can reinfect himself.

☒ Balantidium troph, Babesia canis, Eimeria tenella, Fischoedrius elongatus (Parasites) YES

End of box 1.

☒ Taenia solium scolex (Parasite) YES

This is a tapeworm, he will start on Rascal for 2 bottles.

☒ Gaffkya tetragena, Klebsiella pneumoniae, Proteus vulgaris, Veillonella dispar, Staph aureus, Troglodytella, Salmonella para, Strep mitis, Sphaerotilus natans, Pseudomonas aer (Pathogens) YES

Ten positives out of forty tested. This is a good result.

Six weeks later

Although Mel's clinical test was done the same day, the results have just arrived in the mail. They are NEGATIVE for HIV. We will send him a copy.

Summary: Mel has learned the secret of HIV and AIDS illness. He is capable of steering a wise path. We wish him well.

10 Anne Burgad HIV

Anne is a 44 year old woman with shoulder pain, elbow pain, and arm pain, probably due to gallstones in her liver. She has frequent headaches. She also has lower back pain and numbness in her right hand and 2 middle fingers. Her hands seem weak. This had started about 6 years ago with a big attack of arm pain and numbness. Her foot and big toes are very painful. Her feet get numb when sitting. sometimes she can't get her breath. I discussed cleansing her kidneys and liver.

☐ Ortho-phospho-tyrosine (Cancer) NO

☐ Kidney Stones (ALL) NO

Very unusual to find a person with no kidney stones, especially when they have lower back pain and foot pain. Most strange! We will start on kidney herb recipe, in spite of no stones being present, in hopes of curing the low back pain.

Three weeks later

☒ Gallium and Mercury (Toxic Element) YES

☐ Toxic Elements (Remainder) NO
She is to get all metal fillings replaced with plastic.

BLOOD TEST	Result	Comment
1. Seg/lymphs	49/41	virus
2. T4	slightly low	
3. Phosphate	slightly high	dissolving bone. Drink: 3 glasses of 2% milk daily. Take Magnesium (300 mg) 1/day from Bronson's Pharm.
4. SGOT, SGPT	very low	Take B6 (500 mg) 1/day till problem is solved. Later take B6 (250 mg) 1/day.
5. Cholesterol	very low	liver problem, cancer risk. Eat butter, no margarine.
6. Total protein	slightly low 6.6	liver problem

One month later

She has all metal fillings out. She is experiencing worse chest "tightness."

☐ Mercury (Toxic Element) NO

☒ Babesia (Parasite) YES

☒ Echinococcus granulosus eggs (Parasite) YES

☒ Sheep liver fluke (Parasite) YES
End box 1. Start on parasite killing program.

One month later

She is coughing more, is more tired, and finds it difficult to breathe. (I will check for HIV.) She has been breaking out in Herpes.

☒ Benzene (Solvent) YES
She is using Camphophenique™. Will go off.

☐ Solvents (Remainder) NO

☒ Sheep liver fluke (Parasite) YES at thymus; NO at liver, intestine, etc.

☐ Echinococcus granulosus, Babesia (Parasites) NO

☒ Protein 24 (HIV) YES

She will go off the benzene list and continue on parasite program.

One week later

She is much improved with shoulder pain and headaches reduced.

☐ Protein 24 (HIV) NO

☐ Ortho-phospho-tyrosine (Cancer) NO

☐ Fasciolopsis and all stages (Parasite) NO

☐ Sheep liver fluke (Parasite) NO

She still has pain over her sternum.

☒ Iodamoeba, Leishmania don, Loa Loa (Parasites) YES

End of box 2. Continue parasite program. Loa loa often causes pain over heart region.

☐ Solvents (ALL) NO

One week later

The sore spot on her mid chest is finally gone.

☐ Iodamoeba, Leishmania don, Loa Loa (Parasites) NO

She will prepare to clean her liver by taking 07 and peroxy (17½%) with meals.

Six weeks later

She has done 2 liver cleanses and got hundreds of stones out. Some chest tightness persists. Finger joint pain persists.

☐ Protein 24 (HIV) NO

☐ Ortho-phospho-tyrosine (Cancer) NO

☐ Fasciolopsis and all stages (Parasite) NO

☒ Sheep liver fluke (Parasite) YES

Note: Sheep liver fluke returned, probably due to handling raw pork in a restaurant.

Two months later

Neck pain and back pain are present. There is obviously still a large source of bacteria, in spite of dental repair, liver and kidney cleansing. I will search for tapeworm heads.

☐ Protein 24 (HIV) NO

☐ Ortho-phospho-tyrosine (Cancer) NO

☐ hCG (Pre-Cancer) NO

☐ Benzene (Solvent) NO

☐ Propyl Alcohol (Solvent) NO

☒ Moniezia scolex (Parasite) YES at pancreas; NO in white blood cells

☒ Moniezia eggs (Parasite) YES at liver, thymus, intestine, spleen, pancreas

☒ Pin worm eggs, Schistosoma jap (Parasites) YES

Do 3 day extremely high dose of parasite program, including Rascal.

Summary: Anne had a bout of HIV apparently due to sheep liver fluke invasion of the thymus. There was benzene in the thymus. She cleared this up quickly but remained in poor health. Bacteria seemed endless. But killing the tapeworm head may put an end to her various pains. The presence of tapeworm eggs all over her body implies that the tapeworm heads had "hatched" and let out their unfertilized eggs. I believe benzene causes such hatching of stages that have been in capsules.

Two weeks later

She still has the tapeworm.

One week later

She still has pieces of the tapeworm.

One week later

Tapeworms are all NO. She complains of hoarseness and shoulder pain.

☐ Protein 24 (HIV) NO

☐ Ortho-phospho-tyrosine, hCG (Cancer) NO

She will repeat liver cleanses. She already has over 1,000 stones washed out.

Summary: Anne's health is typical of tapeworm sufferers. She will have some very good days and think her bad health is in the past. Then she will be sick again. She has accomplished a lot for herself already. It is heartening to see her determination to get well. She will use our Cold Prevention Program: CFH capsules (thyme plus fenugreek) one a day by summer, two a day by winter, zinc tablets from

Bronson, one a day by winter, Oscillococcinum in case of influenza. Her chest tightness disappeared. She plans to continue cleaning her liver to completion; a taste of good health, even intermittent, keeps her focused on completion.

11 Phylis Zink — HIV and Cancer

Phylis is a 46 year old woman who drove by herself 150 miles for reasons of her history of breast cancer. It was discovered by mammogram. She had a mastectomy and they took out 3 lymph nodes two years ago and has been followed since then by annual mammograms. She has a heart murmur, occasional pain in knees and wrists, and a long history of period-related problems. They have a water softener and use reverse osmosis (R.O.) water for drinking.

☒ Ortho-phospho-tyrosine (Cancer) YES

☒ Protein 24 (HIV) YES

Since these results seemed impossible to her and I was afraid she might leave, do nothing about her status, and never return, I suggested she get a clinical test (P24 antigen test) for HIV.

Six weeks later

She waited two weeks before doing the test and it came back NO (negative) for the HIV virus. This was most unfortunate since she waited another month before returning.

☒ Ortho-phospho-tyrosine (Cancer) YES at liver and breast

The cancer has spread to the liver.

☒ hCG (Pre-Cancer) YES at liver, breast and blood

☒ Protein 24 (HIV) YES at thymus only

Perhaps the clinical test didn't find the virus because the lab examines blood serum, not the white blood cells or their contents. A case must be further advanced for the virus to be so prevalent that the virus is in the blood serum.

☒ Fasciolopsis (Parasite) YES at intestine, liver, thymus

Adults in the liver are giving her cancer; adults in the thymus are giving her HIV. However, she has no sensations over the breastbone nor chest tightness.

☒ Fasciolopsis redia (Parasite) YES at liver and thymus

☐ Sheep liver fluke and all stages (Parasite) NO

☐ Pancreatic fluke and all stages (Parasite) NO

☒ Human liver fluke (Parasite) YES high at liver, thymus, bladder, kidney, breast

☒ Human liver fluke metacercaria (Parasite) YES high at liver, thymus, kidney, bladder, saliva

Notice: she could transmit these very tiny infective stages by kissing! She will start on parasite killing program.

☒ Benzene (Solvent) YES at liver, thymus, breast, etc.

Brushes teeth twice a day with Colgate™, Crest™, and Tom's™ toothpastes–eats cold cereal daily–go off the entire benzene polluted list.

☒ Propyl Alcohol (Solvent) YES at liver, thymus, breast, etc.

Remainder not tested. She will check her cosmetics for propanol and make her own hair spray. She will switch shampoo to borax.

Seven days later

She is having some loose bowels, probably due to parasite killing herbs.

☐ Protein 24 (HIV) NO

☐ hCG (Pre-Cancer) NO

☐ Ortho-phospho-tyrosine (Cancer) NO

☒ Regular leaded gasoline, Petroleum ether (Solvent) YES

Put gas in her car yesterday. She will be much more careful.

☒ Methyl Ethyl Ketone (Solvent) YES

Instead of stopping cold cereal, switched to a health brand, will stop.

☒ Titanium, Thallium, Germanium (Toxic Elements) YES

Tooth fillings.

☐ Toxic Elements (Remainder) NO

See dentist immediately to remove all metals; save grindings for me to add to my thallium collection.

Summary: Phylis cleared up her HIV and cancer in 7 days. But will she complete her program of getting well again? Thallium is to

the body what termites are to a wood frame house—just a question of time before health collapses.

12 Ray Broyles — Cancer and HIV

We first saw Ray two years ago. He was age 40 at that time and had just had an unusual experience. He had always been healthy and energetic. Then for no reason he passed out. He began vomiting, felt extremely weak and had other strange symptoms. His regular doctor prescribed a tranquilizer, Oxazepam™, after ruling out numerous possibilities. However, these attacks recurred, and he lost about 10 pounds in a few months. I did not suspect nor test for cancer. I found the parasite, Trichuris, and heavy metals from tooth fillings as well as tungsten from his electric hot water heater. He was put on a parasite program. He became well but did not clear up the metal problems. He did not stay on a maintenance program for killing parasites. We did not see him till recently. He had no further episodes of passing out but was unable to recover from a recent flu.

This time the parasite test revealed *Fasciolopsis* in the liver. He was put back on the parasite killing recipe. The cancer test, ortho-phospho-tyrosine, was positive, and tungsten was showing its presence in all his body tissues. He soon got rid of his cancer and by changing his water sources and doing dental work he got rid of the tungsten problem. (He stopped all use of electrical frying pans and toasters.) He felt fine, his former self, and was released with food and body product restrictions.

We saw him again a half year later for frequent burping and difficulty swallowing. There was some similarity to his original attacks. There was pain over his chest and heart area, but I did not suspect HIV at that time. The parasite test showed heartworm and dog tapeworm eggs. The cancer test was negative.

He was put on a high dose parasite killing program and dental repair was recommended. This cleared up his health problems, again, temporarily. He was not given food or product restrictions. A half year later he became ill again with prolonged flu and pressure on his chest.

☐ Ortho-phospho-tyrosine (Cancer) NO

☒ Protein 24 (HIV) YES

☐ Fasciolopsis and all stages (Parasite) NO

I did not search his tissues, only the white blood cells. Could I have missed a few?

☒ Sheep liver fluke redia (Parasite) YES at thymus, penis

☒ Sheep liver fluke metacercaria (Parasite) YES at pancreas only

☒ Pancreatic fluke (Parasite) YES at thymus, pancreas

☐ Human liver fluke (Parasite) NO

☒ Benzene (Solvent) YES at thymus

Uses Nivea™ brand cream after shaving - will go off entire list of benzene containing products.

☒ Wood Alcohol (Solvent) YES high at thymus and pancreas

Others not tested at this time. He was to switch off commercial beverages and will take Milk Thistle capsules temporarily, to assist the liver. And he will return to a high dose parasite killing program followed by a maintenance program. He must avoid eating meats in restaurants.

Three days later

☐ Protein 24 (HIV) NO

Virus is gone but he is still very ill.

☒ Benzene (Solvent) YES

Has not stopped eating cold cereals.

Ten days later

His pains are gone. His digestion continues to be a problem. I suspect tapeworm heads have been released in his liver by the solvents; they are shedding eggs. He feels well enough to return to work. He will add Rascal to his daily routine for 2 weeks to kill tapeworms.

☒ Decane, Methyl Butyl Ketone (Solvent) YES

Hasn't stopped eating processed foods.

☒ Toluene (Solvent) YES

Summary: Ray's patience has paid off, in spite of imperfect compliance. If he had accepted the tranquilizer a few years ago, without pursuing the true cause of his illness, namely parasites and solvents, he would be a permanent invalid today.

13	Sybil McAsh	HIV

This 22 year old woman says her main problem is upper and lower back pain. Due to this pain, she finds it difficult to milk or do her upholstery. Four years ago she had mononucleosis, and she has never really gotten well from it. She also complained of the following: 1) her ears feel shut at times and wet; 2) her hands are sometimes numb; 3) she is gassy; 4) her legs hurt frequently; 5) her knees burn after walking; 6) the arches on her feet hurt; 7) she experiences cramping and clotting as well as headaches and a short temper when she menstruates. Except for a few "weird" symptoms, this seemed like a simple case of kidney stones and liver stones. It was quite surprising, then, to see that:

☐ Ortho-phospho-tyrosine (Cancer) NO

☐ hCG (Pre-Cancer) NO

☒ Protein 24 (HIV) YES at thymus; NO at vagina

She has no pain over her sternum, but she has chest tightness when she breathes. She has the HIV virus, although there are NO risk factors for her. I deliberated for some time before breaking the news to her. I explained the logic of it but perhaps she was too upset to comprehend it.

☒ Fasciolopsis (Parasite) YES at intestine and part of thymus

☒ Fasciolopsis redia (Parasite) YES at the same part of thymus as above

Others not tested.

☒ Xylene, Styrene (Solvents) YES

☒ Benzene (Solvent) YES at both parts of thymus

☐ Solvents (Remainder) NO

She will start on parasite program. She will go off the list of items polluted with benzene. She will go off commercial beverages and drink milk, water, single herb teas, fresh squeezed fruit juices and homemade tomato juice without salt added. She will stop using styrofoam cups. We will deal with kidney stones later.

Two weeks later

She states that she suffers from bloating each time she eats or drinks. We will plan to clean her liver. She also gets severe headaches.

☐ Ortho-phospho-tyrosine (Cancer) NO

☐ hCG (Pre-Cancer) NO

☐ Protein 24 (HIV) NO

She is very pleased, as I am, to have vanquished this virus. However, regaining the health of her thymus is still a challenge.

☐ Benzene (Solvent) NO

☒ Decane, TCE (Solvent) YES

She will be more careful in food selection, avoiding cookies and cakes from the store. She will start on the kidney herb recipe to improve her back and leg pains.

Summary: Sybil got rid of her benzene toxicity and also the HIV virus. She is on day 12 of the parasite program. Her metal tooth fillings, as well as her husband's, appear corroded and tarnished on the top surface. She is to remove all metal from her mouth to improve thymus function so she can regain her normal immunity.

Jonathon Kohl	**HIV and Liver Cancer**

This very young man is here with his family mainly for low energy, but nothing more specific than that. He does not feel well, especially after eating. He is attentive and interested in his health. He has no addictions and no risky behaviors. He has chronic Herpes simplex 1 (cold sores). He sleeps eight hours at night but still can't get up in the morning.

☒ Protein 24 (HIV) YES at thymus and penis

This is certainly a shock for all of us; I explained the basis for it as "parasites plus benzene pollution". He took the news in a calm manner.

☒ Ortho-phospho-tyrosine (Cancer) YES at liver

He has cancer, too, of the liver! His parents are distraught.

☐ hCG (Pre-Cancer) NO

☒ Fasciolopsis (Parasite) YES at liver and thymus

☒ Sheep liver fluke redia (Parasite) YES at liver and thymus; NO in saliva

☒ Sheep liver fluke miracidia (Parasite) YES at liver, thymus, saliva and semen

☐ Pancreatic fluke and all stages (Parasite) NO

☒ Human liver fluke (Parasite) YES at liver and thymus

He will start on parasite killing program.

☒ Benzene (Solvent) YES at thymus

☒ Propyl Alcohol (Solvent) YES everywhere

☒ Kerosene (Solvent) YES

He uses kerosene to heat his work area. I suggested electric heat.

☒ Carbon Tetrachloride, Methyl Ethyl Ketone, TCE, Acetone, TCEthylene (Solvents) YES

☐ Solvents (Remainder) NO

He will be off commercial beverages and the benzene list as well as body products with propanol in them.

Summary: Unfortunately, Jonathon did not return. Perhaps his parents were angry with him. His mother tested NO for HIV, ortho-phospho-tyrosine and hCG; his father complained of chest pains but declined to be tested. No doubt, Jonathon still has several years of moderately good health left. Hopefully, he has made some changes in his product usage.

14	Tina VanWinkle	HIV

This is a young couple belonging to a religious group where the common risky behaviors are unthinkable. Tina has been well until recently. This winter she has already had 2 courses of antibiotics and can't get rid of her cough. She feels pain in the chest when she lifts an object. She also had "walking pneumonia" this winter. She is chronically congested in her head as well, all of which is unusual for her. When she placed her hand over her sternum to illustrate this pain, I suspected HIV/thymus disease. They have several young children.

☐ Ortho-phospho-tyrosine (Cancer) NO

☒ Protein 24 (HIV) YES at thymus, vagina and uterus

☒ Fasciolopsis (Parasite) YES at thymus; NO at liver

No other parasites or stages were tested in order to save office time for her husband.

☒ Benzene (Solvent) YES high everywhere

She has high levels of benzene throughout her body. She is eating various brands of cold cereal daily. She will stop immediately. She will avoid other items on the benzene list, although she had not been using most of them.

Husband, Alfred

He has no obvious health problems and complains about nothing. He smokes (a little).

☒ Benzene (Solvent) YES at the liver; NO at thymus

This is quite unusual. Benzene nearly always accumulates at the thymus.

☒ Propyl Alcohol (Solvent) YES at liver

He uses no body products, other than shampoo. His main source of propanol must be cold cereal.

☐ Protein 24 (HIV) NO

☒ Ortho-phospho-tyrosine (Cancer) YES at liver and lung

Note: He has cancer developing at the liver! They both (as well as their children) will stop eating cold cereal. They will start parasite killing program. They will avoid the benzene list.

Thirteen days later

Tina no longer has chest tightness, but her cough has gotten croupy and worse.

☐ Ortho-phospho-tyrosine (Cancer) NO

☐ hCG (Pre-Cancer) NO

☐ Protein 24 (HIV) NO

We are all very pleased.

☒ Hexane dione (Solvent) YES
Stay off commercial beverages.

☒ Methyl Ethyl Ketone, TCE (Solvents) YES

☐ Solvents (Remainder) NO
Note that her benzene problem is gone.

Alfred

Her husband, Alfred, seemed put out and put upon with all the restrictions I placed on him. However, he did accomplish his purpose.

☐ Ortho-phospho-tyrosine (Cancer) NO

☐ hCG (Pre-Cancer) NO

☐ Protein 24 (HIV) NO

☒ Carbon Tetrachloride (Solvent) YES
Stay off cold cereal and commercial beverages. Others not tested.

Summary: This young couple averted disaster, narrowly, as each filled up on solvents by eating cold cereals and drinking commercial beverages. Hopefully, they will be able to teach their children how to avoid both cancer and HIV by avoiding polluted food and products.

15* Lenzy Perez	HIV

Lenzy is a young man, age 28, who has come to correct his HIV positive status. We assured him that in 6 weeks he would get an HIV-NEGATIVE test result if he followed instructions meticulously. He seems incredulous but willing to try. He brought the test results under a code number. The test was done and confirmed at Anonymous AIDS Antibody testing lab. He has a chronic sore throat and some anxiety but otherwise is not ill.

☐ Ortho-phospho-tyrosine, hCG (Cancer) NO

☒ Protein 24 (HIV) YES

☒ Benzene (Solvent) YES at thymus and penis

☒ Kerosene, Methylene chloride (Solvents) YES
He will go off cold cereals and all commercial beverages. He will be vegetarian for 3 months. He will be off the benzene-pollution list I gave him.

☒ Fasciolopsis (Parasite) YES at thymus only; NO at liver and intestine

☒ Fasciolopsis unincubated eggs (Parasite) YES at thymus, penis, spleen, semen

☒ Sheep liver fluke cercaria (Parasite) YES at thymus, penis, spleen

☒ Pancreatic Fluke (Parasite) YES at thymus

☐ Human liver fluke and all stages (Parasite) NO

He will start the parasite killing program. He was concerned that his friend was using marijuana and it might be polluted. I tested it for benzene. It was YES (positive). He will alert his friend immediately.

Seven days later

His sore throat is gone. He feels better. He still has a complexion problem on forehead.

☐ Ortho-phospho-tyrosine, hCG (Cancer) NO

☐ Protein 24 (HIV) NO

He is now HIV-free.

☐ Fasciolopsis and all stages (Parasite) NO

☐ Sheep liver fluke and all stages (Parasite) NO

☐ Pancreatic fluke and all stages (Parasite) NO

☐ Human liver fluke and all stages (Parasite) NO

He is very happy but incredulous also.

☒ Bismuth (Toxic Element) YES at thymus

Off colognes and all fragrant products.

☒ Palladium (Toxic Element) YES

Tooth metal.

☒ Mercury (Toxic Element) YES high at thymus and numerous other tissues

☒ Gallium (Toxic Element) YES at thymus

Tooth metal.

☒ Lead (Toxic Element) YES at thymus

We will test water.

☒ Lutetium, Zirconium (Toxic Element) YES at thymus

He will go off commercial deodorant and other body products. He will continue on parasite program. He needs to have all metal removed from his mouth.

Seven days later

His clinical doctor repeated the HIV antibody test. It was POSITIVE again, as you would expect an antibody test to be.

☐ Ortho-phospho-tyrosine, hCG (Cancer) NO

☐ Protein 24 (HIV) NO

He is on day 14 of the parasite program.

☒ Benzene (Solvent) YES at the edge of thymus

☐ Solvents (Remainder) NO

He will be more diligent about avoiding the benzene list and will bring personal products for testing.

☒ Bismuth (Toxic Element) YES

He has brought several fragrance varieties for testing, but I prefer he not use any commercial variety.

☒ Warts, Candida, CMV, Treponema, Capsules of bacteria (Pathogens) YES

☐ Pathogens (Remainder) NO

End of box 1 and 2. Note: He picked up a small amount of benzene but has not developed numerous infections...only 5 pathogens, total, out of 67 tested! This is as good or better than average for a non-HIV infected person.

Seven days later

He is feeling much better than he did at first. His dental appointment is scheduled.

☐ Ortho-phospho-tyrosine, hCG (Cancer) NO

☐ Protein 24 (HIV) NO

☒ Denatured alcohol, Petroleum ether (Solvents) YES

He will be more careful when putting gas in his car. He is now on a parasite maintenance program. His complexion is clear. He looks well.

☒ Lead (Toxic Element) YES

☐ Lead (Toxic Element) NO in his drinking water

☐ Bismuth (Toxic Element) NO

Uses the cologne tested to be bismuth-free.

☐ Zirconium (Toxic Element) NO

☒ Proteus mir:, B strep, Histoplasma, Salmonella ent, Lepto ent, Haem inf, Bacillus anth (Pathogens) YES at thymus

☐ Pathogens (Remainder) NO

End box 1 and 2. This is a very good record for an average person but not as good as his previous record. Four of these are tooth bacteria. He will do dental work soon.

☒ Uric Acid, Cysteine and Cystine, all 3 phosphates (Kidney Stones) YES

He has an unusually large number of kidney stones. He has not been drinking milk for over a year; he has read it causes mucous and could make his sore throat worse. I reassured him his throat would clear up after dental work. He also needs to reduce phosphate in diet (meat, bread, cereal, sodas) and eat more fruits and vegetables. He plans to buy a vegetable juicer. He will start to drink milk if he digests it OK. He may wait until his stomach parasites are killed so he can digest it better. He will start on kidney herb recipe to dissolve these deposits and also take magnesium oxide, 300 mg, per day. He is ready for HIV antigen test. We will send requisitions.

One week later

☐ Ortho-phospho-tyrosine, hCG (Cancer) NO

☐ Protein 24 (HIV) NO

He will do an HIV antigen test. We did not send requisitions earlier.

One week later

He looks good and feels very well.

☐ Ortho-phospho-tyrosine, hCG (Cancer) NO

☐ Protein 24 (HIV) NO

☒ Mycoplasma, Histopl cap, A strep, Proteus (Pathogens) YES

This is the average number of infections for a well person. He has not completed his dental work yet.

One week later

His clinical HIV antigen test results are back. It states he is NEGATIVE. He is very pleased. He recently had a regular blood test by his clinical doctor; it showed a T cell count of 787.

⊠ Chlamydia tr, Coxsackie B4, Bacillus anth, Pneumocystis carn, Spirillum rub, Trepon pall (Pathogens) YES

He has 6 YES tests out of about 70; this is better than the average healthy person. He has completed his dental work.

Summary: Lenzy says he is enjoying his new lifestyle. He would like someone to talk to about all of this, though, and I hope he finds a few other cured cases with whom to share his joy and anxiety over recurrence. He is planning an expansion of his massage clinic and plans to bring in products to be tested for benzene so that he isn't selling this "death-trap" to anybody. He is a uniquely moral person.

16	Dan Holt	HIV and Anemia

This is a 40 year old man with anemia. For the last 1-2 years he has had a chronic cold-flu syndrome. He is over stressed. He is in engineering. He has pain in the pancreas area and over the heart. He experiences "hot flushes." He has dry skin and lower back pain. He drinks a lot of decaffeinated beverages. He has additional bizarre symptoms.

⊠ Asbestos (Toxic Element) YES

Will test clothes and hair dryers.

⊠ Silver (Toxic Element) YES

Tooth fillings.

⊠ Gold (Toxic Element) YES

In his glasses and tooth fillings.

⊠ Thulium (Toxic Element) YES

In his vitamins.

⊠ Palladium (Toxic Element) YES

Tooth fillings and glasses.

⊠ Zirconium (Toxic Element) YES

Deodorant and toothpaste.

☐ Toxic Elements (Remainder) NO

Remainder were NO. He will start on kidney herb recipe and get plastic rimmed glasses and arrange to get metal tooth fillings replaced by plastic.

BLOOD TEST	Result	Comment
1. RBC	low	anemia, parasites
2. Creatinine	slightly high	kidney
3. Uric acid	slightly high	kidney
4. Calcium	low	He will drink 2% milk, 3 glasses/day and take Magnesium oxide, 1 a day (300 mg, from Bronson Pharm).
5. SGOT, SGPT	low	Take B6 (500 mg) one/day.
6. Cholesterol	very low	cancer risk

Three weeks later

☒ Cysteine, Cystine (Kidney Stones) YES

He has been on kidney herbs for 4 weeks. Continue up to 6-8 weeks.

☒ Echinococcus granulosus cysts adult (Parasite) YES

☐ Echinococcus granulosus eggs (Parasite) NO

☒ Chilomastix (Parasite) YES

☐ Parasites (Remainder) NO

Will start on parasite program

One month later

☐ Cysteine, Cystine (Kidney Stones) NO

☐ Chilomastix, Echinococcus all stages (Parasites) NO

☐ Asbestos, Zirconium, Silver, Gold, Thulium (Toxic Elements) NO

Start on thioctic acid (100 mg), 1 per day.

☐ Solvents (ALL) NO

He says he feels very well. All his symptoms are resolved. Client released. He will stay on vitamin E (400 mg), B6 (250 mg), vitamin C (1000 mg) magnesium (300 mg), thioctic (100 mg) daily.

One month and 2 weeks later

He now has thrush, which his wife has also. He has had it for 6-8 weeks and is on a prescription drug for it.

☒ Protein 24 (HIV) YES at thymus

☐ Ortho-phospho-tyrosine (Cancer) NO

☐ Fasciolopsis adults and redia (Parasite) NO

☒ Fasciolopsis eggs (Parasite) YES at thymus, liver, and penis

☒ Benzene (Solvent) YES high
He uses Tom's™ toothpaste and rubber cement; he will stop. He will repeat parasite killing program at higher dose. He will avoid rare beef.

Two months later

Thrush has returned. He was feeling very well until recently. He has not eaten beef for 22 years or any meat except chicken, turkey and tuna fish. He will go off all but fish and seafood.

☒ Protein 24 (HIV) YES at thymus

☐ Ortho-phospho-tyrosine (Cancer) NO

☒ Fasciolopsis miracidia (Parasite) YES at thymus only

☐ Fasciolopsis adult and remaining stages (Parasite) NO

☐ Sheep liver fluke and all stages (Parasite) NO

☒ Methylene chloride (Solvent) YES at thymus
Drinks Celestial Seasonings™ tea.

☐ Solvents (Remainder) NO
We will test his beverages. He will start on a 5 day high dose parasite program again.

Two weeks later

He still has thrush and general fatigue. He has done the 5 day high dose parasite program and is still on a maintenance program.

☐ Ortho-phospho-tyrosine (Cancer) NO

☒ Protein 24 (HIV) YES

☒ Fasciolopsis miracidia (Parasite) YES at thymus, penis; NO elsewhere

☐ Fasciolopsis adult and remaining stages (Parasite) NO

☐ Sheep liver fluke (Parasite) NO

☐ Pancreatic fluke (Parasite) NO

☒ Candida (Pathogen) YES

☒ Hexane (Solvent) YES
Still drinking Celestial Seasonings™ tea.

☒ Toluene (Solvent) YES

☐ Solvents (Remainder) NO
Go off commercial beverages.

One day later
He still has Candida (yeast infection).

☐ Ortho-phospho-tyrosine (Cancer) NO

☒ Protein 24 (HIV) YES

☒ Fasciolopsis (Parasite) YES at thymus

☒ Fasciolopsis redia and miracidia (Parasite) YES

☒ Sheep liver fluke cercaria, redia, and miracidia (Parasite) YES
He was eating turkey, frozen and cooked. He will stop.

☒ Pancreatic Fluke (Parasite) YES

☒ Candida (Pathogen) YES

Five days later

☒ Benzene, Xylene, Grain Alcohol (Solvents) YES

☐ Solvents (Remainder) NO
He will go off benzene list more carefully.

Five days later
He is still fatigued.

☒ Protein 24 (HIV) YES

☐ Ortho-phospho-tyrosine (Cancer) NO

☒ Fasciolopsis (Parasite) YES
Others not tested.

Five days later

☐ Protein 24 (HIV) NO

☐ Ortho-phospho-tyrosine (Cancer) NO

☐ Fasciolopsis and all stages (Parasite) NO

- ☐ Sheep liver fluke (Parasite) NO
- ☐ Pancreatic fluke (Parasite) NO
- ☐ Solvents (ALL) NO
- ☐ Candida (Pathogen) NO
  Perhaps he has finally conquered this problem by staying off all meats and commercial beverages.

One month later

- ☐ Protein 24 (HIV) NO
- ☐ Ortho-phospho-tyrosine (Cancer) NO
- ☒ Petroleum ether (Solvent) YES
  Car problem.
- ☒ Methyl butyl ketone (Solvent) YES
- ☐ Solvents (Remainder) NO
  He is still using Celestial Seasonings™ teas.

Summary: Mr. Holt was one of my early clients with HIV illness; I did not suspect it nor test for it until he got thrush (Candida in his throat). It was quite difficult for him to eradicate it because his benzene sources were obscure. But he was diligent and finally was successful.

17 Linda Holt HIV

This 37 year old woman is the wife of Dan Holt and had a lot of symptoms. Her eyes are itchy and runny. She suffers from sinus infections and ringing in the ear. Her throat is sore due to asthma and asthma drugs and she has a yeast infection in her throat. Her neck is stiff and the muscles are sore Her shoulders are tense. She suffers from chest congestion, asthma, and had pneumonia two years ago. Her heart area feels constricted. Her stomach is bloated and aching. She has constant lower back pain. Her feet are achy at the end of the day. Her sleep is affected by her breathing and worries. Her energy level is up and down and affected by her asthma. She has frequent headaches. She often has urinary tract infections. She has had depression off and on for the past 20 years. She has a weight problem. She is on Vanceril™, Ventolin™, Seldane™, Humibid LA™, Intal™, Medrol™ (4 mg), Beconase™, Anacin™, and Acetominophen™. She is allergic to cats, dogs, fish, some foods, horses, dust, mold, and grass. (I suspect Sheep liver fluke and Ascaris.)

☐ Protein 24 (HIV) NO

☐ Ortho-phospho-tyrosine (Cancer) NO

☐ Fasciolopsis and all stages (Parasite) NO

☒ Benzene (Solvent) YES high
She will start parasite program and go off items on the benzene-pollution list.

Two months later

She has swelling across her abdomen.

☐ Protein 24 (HIV) NO

☒ Ortho-phospho-tyrosine (Cancer) YES cervix; NO elsewhere

☒ Fasciolopsis (Parasite) YES at liver; NO elsewhere

☒ Fasciolopsis eggs (Parasite) YES at blood and cervix

☐ Fasciolopsis remaining stages (Parasite) NO

☐ Sheep liver fluke (Parasite) NO
Original guess was wrong.

☒ Wood Alcohol (Solvent) YES at cervix
Drinks root beer.

☒ Propyl Alcohol (Solvent) YES at cervix; NO at liver

☐ Solvents (Remainder) NO
Go back on parasite program. Avoid propanol-containing products.

Two months later

☐ Ortho-phospho-tyrosine (Cancer) NO

☒ Protein 24 (HIV) YES

☒ Fasciolopsis (Parasite) YES at thymus

☒ Fasciolopsis eggs and redia (Parasite) YES

☒ Sheep liver fluke adult, cercaria, miracidia (Parasite) YES

☐ Pancreatic fluke adult (Parasite) NO

☒ Pancreatic fluke stages (Parasite) YES

☒ Wood alcohol, Regular gasoline, Benzene, Grain alcohol, Toluene (Solvents) YES

☐ Solvents (Remainder) NO

She will go on high dose parasite program, then on maintenance program. She will be off benzene list and commercial beverages.

Five days later

☐ Protein 24 (HIV) NO

☐ Ortho-phospho-tyrosine (Cancer) NO

☐ Parasites (ALL) NO

☒ TCEthylene (Solvent) YES

Off Celestial Seasonings™ tea.

☐ Solvents (Remainder) NO

One month and 3 weeks later

☐ Protein 24 (HIV) NO

☐ Ortho-phospho-tyrosine, hCG (Cancer) NO

☒ Ascaris (Parasite) YES

Cause of asthma.

☒ Ascaris mega (Parasite) YES

☐ Fasciolopsis and all stages (Parasite) NO

☒ Sheep liver fluke miracidia (Parasite) YES at liver

☐ Pancreatic fluke (Parasite) NO

☐ Human liver fluke (Parasite) NO

☒ Methylene chloride, Pentane, Methyl ethyl ketone (Solvents) YES

She will definitely go off commercial beverages, definitely.

BLOOD TEST	Result	Comment
1. FBS	slightly high	cleanse liver
2. Phosphate	high	dissolving bone. She will drink 3 glasses of 2% milk daily and take 1 Magnesium (300 mg) daily.
3. LDH	high	liver? heart? cancer?
4. RBC	slightly high	check cobalt toxicity
5. Eos	very high (8%)	parasites

One month later

She is congested. She has been on parasite maintenance program, 2 times a week.

☐ Protein 24 (HIV) NO

☒ Styrene (Solvent) YES
Stop using styrofoam products.

☒ Petroleum ether (Solvent) YES
Stop pumping gas.

☒ Decane (Solvent) YES
Off cold cereal.

☐ Solvents (Remainder) NO

☒ Beryllium (Toxic Element) YES high

☒ Benzalkonium (Solvent) YES
Wash plastic cups before using. She does not use toothpaste.

☒ Chromate (Toxic Element) YES
No source found.

☒ Mercury high, Cerium, Tellurium high (Toxic Element) YES
Tooth fillings.

☒ Barium (Toxic Element) YES high
Lipstick.

☒ Vanadium (Toxic Element) YES high
Search for gas leak in house.

☒ Lutetium (Toxic Element) YES
Ventilate painted room.

☒ Formaldehyde (Toxic Element) YES
Foam mattresses. Throw them out.

☐ Toxic Elements (Remainder) NO
Needs to remove metal from mouth, fix a gas leak in the home, get away from gasoline and paint fumes and throw away foam mattresses. Notice how many of these would worsen her asthma.

Summary: Ms. Holt and her husband were undoubtedly infecting each other with the flukes and had to both be free of them before either could stay well. Hopefully, Ms. Holt will work at her health until she can be off some of her drugs and actually begin to feel better. In a family setting one is faced with other person's parasites and pollution in addition to your own. She has done an excellent job.

18	Claudia Holt	HIV

This is the 13 year old daughter of Linda and Dan Holt. The parents are concerned about the HIV virus for their children. Claudia has no health problems.

☐ Protein 24 (HIV) NO

☒ Fasciolopsis cercaria (Parasite) YES at one part of thymus and vagina only

☐ Fasciolopsis remaining stages (Parasite) NO

☒ Benzene (Solvent) YES

She will start parasite program and go off the items on the benzene-pollution list.

One week later

☒ Benzene (Solvent) YES higher than before

☒ Benzene (Solvent) YES high in Future™ floor polish, NuFinish™ (once a year car polish)

They were keeping these items in a closet; will put them in the garage and never again use polish with bare hands.

☐ Fasciolopsis and all stages (Parasite) NO

Two months later

☐ Protein 24 (HIV) NO

☐ Ortho-phospho-tyrosine (Cancer) NO

☒ Hexane dione (Solvent) YES

Drinks ginger ale, switch beverages. Note: benzene is gone.

One month later

☐ Ortho-phospho-tyrosine (Cancer) NO

☒ Protein 24 (HIV) YES

☒ Fasciolopsis eggs and cercaria (Parasite) YES

☒ Sheep liver fluke adult and miracidia (Parasite) YES

- ☒ Pancreatic Fluke (Parasite) YES
  She will go off meat and start parasite program again.
- ☒ Propyl Alcohol (Solvent) YES
  Cosmetics.
- ☒ Benzene, Ether, Toluene (Solvents) YES
- ☐ Solvents (Remainder) NO
  She will stay off commercial beverages.

Five days later

- ☐ Protein 24 (HIV) NO
- ☐ Ortho-phospho-tyrosine (Cancer) NO
- ☐ Fasciolopsis and all stages (Parasite) NO
- ☒ Pancreatic Fluke and stages (Parasite) YES
- ☐ Sheep liver fluke and stages (Parasite) NO
- ☒ PCB (Toxic Element) YES high
  Go off all detergents.

One month and one week later

- ☐ Protein 24 (HIV) NO
- ☐ Ortho-phospho-tyrosine (Cancer) NO
- ☒ Wood Alcohol (Solvent) YES at pancreas
- ☒ PCB (Toxic Element) YES
- ☐ Toxic Elements (Remainder) NO

Summary: Notice how Claudia can easily kill her parasites but promptly picks them up again. I suspect fast food meats to be her main source of infection. She may be typical of the general population, picking up benzene on a daily basis but eliminating it shortly. Only after a time of several years will the thymus be so damaged and liver detoxification mechanisms be so weakened that benzene begins to pile up and set the stage for AIDS.

Lois Holt	**No HIV**

This is the eldest daughter of Linda and Dan Holt. She is irritable and does not wish to be present in an alternative health setting.

☐ Protein 24 (HIV) NO

☐ Ortho-phospho-tyrosine (Cancer) NO

☒ Fasciolopsis cercaria (Parasite) YES at thymus, blood, vagina and brain

☐ Fasciolopsis remaining stages (Parasite) NO
Note brain location for cercaria.

☒ Benzene (Solvent) YES
She will start parasite program.

Two months later

☐ Protein 24 (HIV) NO

☐ Ortho-phospho-tyrosine (Cancer) NO

☒ Methylene chloride (Solvent) YES
She is drinking Minute Maid™ orange juice (pulp free) frozen but will stop. Note: benzene is gone.

One month later

☐ Protein 24 (HIV) NO

☐ Ortho-phospho-tyrosine (Cancer) NO

☒ Sheep liver fluke eggs (Parasite) YES

☐ Fasciolopsis and all stages (Parasite) NO

☐ Pancreatic fluke (Parasite) NO

☒ Benzene (Solvent) YES
Source unknown.

Five days later

☐ Parasites (ALL) NO

One month later

☐ Benzene (Solvent) NO

☐ Propyl Alcohol (Solvent) NO

☐ PCB (Toxic Element) NO

☒ Wood Alcohol (Solvent) YES

☒ Carbon Tetrachloride (Solvent) YES

Summary: This gives us a picture of how a family with HIV may, initially, be coping with it and not get too sick to function. As their solvent exposure and diet changes, so does their parasitism and HIV infection. The young children are still healthy and strong and show no signs of illness. The parents, however, begin to have serious problems. Fortunately, they were all very diligent in their life style changes and have learned to prevent this impending illness.

19	**Sidney Holt**	**HIV**

Sidney was away at college and was not seen until after the rest of the family. He has severe allergies for which he takes several medications. He is trying to hold a job besides going to school. He has stiffness of joints, shoulder pain, lower and upper back pain, knee pain, and a few others. He wears a splint to keep from grinding his teeth.

☒ Cysteine (Kidney Stone) YES

☐ Kidney Stones (Remainder) NO
He will begin with our kidney herb recipe to remove his sulfur crystals and get relief from stiffness and lower back pain.

Two weeks later

He has not gotten any pain relief. In fact, his fatigue has worsened.

☒ Protein 24 (HIV) YES at thymus, penis and brain
We did not discover this at first visit because of focusing on regular problems and not suspecting HIV!

☒ Benzene (Solvent) YES
Uses Vaseline Lip Therapy™—will go off.

☒ Fasciolopsis (Parasite) YES at thymus and intestine

☒ Fasciolopsis redia (Parasite) YES at thymus and blood

☒ Fasciolopsis cercaria (Parasite) YES at thymus and brain
Others not tested. He will start on parasite killing program. He will avoid benzene-polluted products.

Two months later

☐ Protein 24 (HIV) NO

☐ Fasciolopsis and all stages (Parasite) NO

☐ Benzene (Solvent) NO

☐ Propyl Alcohol (Solvent) NO

He has done well. He has his old energy back and can concentrate on studies.

Three months later

He has felt better than in a long time. He is not even getting colds or flu, like others around him. He will stay on parasite maintenance program.

☐ Protein 24 (HIV) NO

☐ Ortho-phospho-tyrosine (Cancer) NO

☐ Fasciolopsis and all stages (Parasite) NO

☐ Sheep liver fluke (Parasite) NO

☐ Pancreatic fluke (Parasite) NO

☒ Methyl butyl ketone (Solvent) YES

☐ Solvents (Remainder) NO

He will switch to milk and water and fresh squeezed juices, no commercial beverages.

Summary: Sidney has done an exemplary job of changing his lifestyle. He appreciated knowing the cause of his problems which were much too numerous for his age. He was also very thankful to have an understanding of this disease in order to escape it in the future.

Jason Willy	**HIV and Lung Cancer**

Jason is a 43 year old man whose medical record, which he brought with him, gave his diagnosis as "undifferentiated large cell carcinoma of the lung with metastases to the left neck and brain area." More recently, the cancer has spread to the liver. His sister-in-law drove him to our office. Jason smokes, and I reminded him that smoking is incompatible with lung health. He is on Dilantin™ and Decatron™ to prevent brain swelling.

☐ Protein 24 (HIV) NO

☒ Ortho-phospho-tyrosine (Cancer) YES at liver, thymus, lung, brain

Note that cancer in the thymus is quite rare.

☒ Fasciolopsis (Parasite) YES at liver, intestine, lung

☒ Fasciolopsis cercaria (Parasite) YES at lung, etc.

☒ Sheep liver fluke (Parasite) YES at thymus; NO at liver

Note: the normal habitat for the Sheep liver fluke is the liver. Is the intestinal fluke keeping it out somehow?

☐ Pancreatic fluke and all stages (Parasite) NO

☒ Propyl Alcohol, Benzene (Solvent) YES at liver, thymus, kidney, etc.

With this critically ill person here from so far away, I made a second office visit possible for him 7 hours later in the same day. He went off all benzene products and propanol products and took a shower in the meanwhile. He also took a massive amount of parasite killing herbs instead of starting at "day one."

Seven hours later

☐ Ortho-phospho-tyrosine (Cancer) NO

His cancer is already stopped. He doesn't believe what I am telling him, but his sister-in-law is ecstatic. He will stay off rare meats.

☒ Cryptocotyl, Hypodereum con (Parasites) YES

End box 1.

☒ Asbestos (Toxic Element) YES high

☐ Toxic Elements (Remainder) NO

He had only one toxic element out of the entire set. They agree to change his clothes dryer belt to a USA model as soon as they get home.

☒ Candida, CMV, Herpes simplex, Flu (Pathogens) YES

☐ Mycoplasma (Pathogen) NO

Only 5 tests done. Since Jason had 4 out of 5 pathogens as I began to test him, I realized he had extremely low immunity due to having benzene and propanol in his thymus. We will wait until his next visit to test the rest of the pathogens. I did not use the word AIDS when talking to him but this is what he has. And the HIV virus is not far away.

Seventeen days later

He did not keep the appointment which was scheduled for 10 days earlier. Perhaps he is not committed to surviving. He appears very ill today.

☒ Protein 24 (HIV) YES

☒ Ortho-phospho-tyrosine (Cancer) YES

He now has his cancer back and HIV in addition. What went wrong? He has been eating meats as usual. He has not checked out his body products for propanol, simply used all of them, nor stayed off benzene polluted products.

☒ Fasciolopsis (Parasite) YES at thymus

☒ Propyl Alcohol (Solvent) YES

Rubbing alcohol used on his arm at hospital to draw blood yesterday - he is advised to bring own alcohol, Vodka.

☒ Benzene (Solvent) YES

Hasn't stopped using toothpaste or Vaseline.

☐ Asbestos (Toxic Element) NO

Changed the dryer belt.

☒ Trich vag, Bacteroides fr, Chlamyd trach, Campyl pyl, Bacillus cereus, Strep pneu, Proteus mir, Herpes simplex 1, Gardnerella vag, B strep, Adenovirus (Pathogens) YES

Because he had Bacteroides fr, he must have Ascaris, since they are always found together. He is still smoking. I emphasized the importance of stopping. At his first visit, Jason had AIDS but without the HIV virus; the picture of AIDS is seen in the 4 out of 5 YES (positive) tests. At his second visit, the parasites had reached adulthood in his thymus and the virus is present; his AIDS is worsened.

Summary: Maybe I was too harsh with Jason about his smoking, so that he won't come back. But if he doesn't stop he can't survive. It is weeks past his appointment time. I am afraid it is only his sister-in-law who wants Jason to survive, not Jason himself.

20	Ralph Smith	Multiple Cancer and HIV

Ralph, age 43, came to our office because of his sarcoidosis which was diagnosed six years ago, although he had it earlier than that. At that time, he had pain on the center front chest so that he couldn't breathe deeply. He was put on cortisone for it and the pain was reduced, but it is still minimally present. This location suggests the thymus. He is still on Prednisone.™

☒ Protein 24 (HIV) YES at thymus and penis; NO in semen and saliva

☒ Ortho-phospho-tyrosine (Cancer) YES at thymus, intestine, lung, bronchii

He has both cancer and HIV! He stated that he had been tested for HIV antibody twice already, both times with negative results.

☒ hCG (Pre-Cancer) YES in all tissues

He is pre-cancerous throughout his body! This was a shock.

☒ Fasciolopsis (Parasite) YES at thymus and liver

☒ Fasciolopsis cercaria (Parasite) YES at thymus, liver, semen, penis

Other flukes not tested. Start on parasite program.

☒ Propyl Alcohol (Solvent) YES high at liver

Since he does not eat cold cereal nor use body products, his only source is shampoo. Considering his high levels, there must be an unknown source of propanol. He will be watchful. He will switch off commercial shampoo.

☒ Benzene (Solvent) YES high throughout his body

Go off the benzene list. This youngish man had tried many things to improve his health. His medical file is ½ inch thick. It seems incredible that so massive a cancerous state could be missed by clinical routines.

Five weeks later

☐ Protein 24 (HIV) NO

Very good news.

☒ Ortho-phospho-tyrosine (Cancer) YES at intestine only

☒ hCG (Pre-Cancer) YES at intestine, lung, bronchii

☒ Fasciolopsis (Parasite) YES at intestine and liver; NO at thymus

☒ Fasciolopsis cercaria (Parasite) YES at intestine and liver; NO at thymus

☐ Benzene (Solvent) NO

☒ Propyl Alcohol (Solvent) YES

He is still using his favorite shampoo but will switch.

Summary: Ralph has solved part of his problem, the HIV virus and benzene pollution. But the propanol level was still high and the flukes were still thriving (due to eating hamburgers) so the cancer continued. He is determined, though, to cure it all.

21	**Bruce Whitlow**	**HIV**

This is a 34 year old male who has a long history of chronic sinus infections and allergies. He reported that his main problems were: chronic sinus and ear problems. He was getting "bubble shots" from Dr. Schaffer a few years ago. Another doctor did a RAST test. He is now on weekly allergy shots. He feels tired and foggy headed. He had elbow soreness in his right arm and he broke his right arm 4 times. He has a weight problem. He quit smoking a month ago. He suffers from lower back pain. He gets headaches, 1-2 times a week. He has had tinnitus on the left side for 10 years. He has to urinate frequently and has a history of prostate infection. He has no pets.

BLOOD TEST	Result	Comment
1. CO2	high (28)	search for air pollutant
2. Uric acid	high	kidney problem
3. Calcium	slightly low (9.1)	He will increase his milk consumption and take Magnesium (300 mg) 1/day and B6 (250 mg) 1/day.
4. LDH	slightly low	fatigue
5. Iron	very low	parasites
6. Cholesterol	slightly high	liver gallstone cleanse
7. Triglycerides	slightly high	kidneys
8. WBC	low	bone marrow toxin
9. RBC	low	anemia—parasites
10.Platelet count	slightly high	parasites
11. Urinalysis	OK	no urinary tract infection

☒ Uric Acid, Mono and di Calcium phosphate (Kidney Stones) YES

Start on kidney herb recipe.

Twenty days later

He reported that his lower back is better.

☐ Kidney Stones (ALL) NO

☒ Mercury (Toxic Element) YES high at bone marrow and lungs
Tooth fillings.

☒ Rhodium (Toxic Element) YES at bone marrow and lungs
Tooth fillings.

☒ Strontium (Toxic Element) YES at bone marrow and lungs
Toothpaste.

☒ Zirconium (Toxic Element) YES at bone marrow and lungs
Off deodorant.

☒ Vanadium (Toxic Element) YES at bone marrow and lungs
Cause of red skin on face—search for gas leak in home. We will test his home air for vanadium after he fixes his gas pipes. He needs all metal removed from his dental ware.

☒ Fasciolopsis adult, miracidia (Parasite) YES

☒ Fasciolopsis redia, cercaria (Parasite) YES at bile duct

☒ Trichinella, Ancylostoma (Parasite) YES
Remainder untested. Start on parasite program.

Seventeen days later

Gas leak has been fixed.

☒ Mercury, Rhodium (Toxic Elements) YES
Has not done dental work yet.

☒ Strontium (Toxic Element) YES high
Off toothpaste.

☐ Vanadium (Toxic Element) NO

☐ Fasciolopsis and all stages (Parasite) NO

☒ Ancylostoma, Echinococcus, Sheep liver fluke, Dipetalonema (high), Dipylidium caninum, Plasmodium vivax, Schistosoma, Leishmania tropica, Necator, Plasmodium falciparum (Parasites) YES
Increase parasite treatment with a 5 day high dose program. This is an unusually high number of parasites, especially after several weeks of parasite treatment. We must test for HIV/AIDS.

☒ Protein 24 (HIV) YES

☒ Benzene (Solvent) YES
Off benzene-pollution list.

Two weeks later

He reported that his sinus problem has not improved.

☐ Rhodium (Toxic Element) NO

☒ Vanadium (Toxic Element) YES high
Has another gas leak.

☒ Zirconium (Toxic Element) YES
Still on toothpaste.

☒ Strontium (Toxic Element) YES high
Uses toothpaste and has not done dental work.

☒ Eimeria, Diphyllobothrium (Parasites) YES

☐ Parasites (Remainder) NO
Continue on parasite maintenance. He plans to clean his liver to get rid of allergies. He is starting on 07 and peroxy for this purpose.

One month later

He has done 3 liver cleanses. He has been feeling a lot better. Energy is up. He got out a total of 750 stones. He took 14 wormwood for 3 days, plus black walnut —30 drops 4 times a day.

☐ Protein 24 (HIV) NO

☐ Eimeria, Diphyllobothrium (Parasites) NO

☐ Vanadium (Toxic Element) NO
He fixed second leak.

☐ Zirconium (Toxic Element) NO

☒ Strontium (Toxic Element) YES
Still using toothpaste.

☒ Mercury, Rhodium (Toxic Element) YES
Has not done dental work. He is leaving on vacation to Europe for a month. He is very pleased with his new energy.

Summary: We did not see Bruce after this, but he stopped in for some vitamins and told the receptionist he was very well. He was back at his old job. He had a wonderful vacation. He was living carefully as we had taught him, and he planned to come back for follow-up when he had managed to do his dental repair.

Brandi Rosette **HIV and Cancer**

This 3 month old baby is ill. She is filled with mucous. She has already had pneumonia once. She frequently does not want to feed - she is on Enfamil™ with iron. She saw her clinical doctor yesterday, he is giving her antibiotic shots twice a week and told her parents he is at a loss to understand her illness. She has very little leg motion. She does not sleep much.

☒ Protein 24 (HIV) YES

☒ Ortho-phospho-tyrosine (Cancer) YES
The baby has cancer and HIV, how tragic.

☒ Propyl Alcohol (Solvent) YES at liver and thymus

☒ Benzene (Solvent) YES
The baby has been on a lotion, Forever Living Aloe Heat Lotion™ since shortly after birth. This lotion tested YES (positive) to both benzene and propanol when rubbed into my arm!

☒ Fasciolopsis (Parasite) YES at liver and thymus

☒ Fasciolopsis eggs (Parasite) YES at saliva

☒ Strep pneu, EBV, Influenza, B strep, Proteus, Gardnerella vag, Chlamydia tr, Candida, CMV, Resp Sync v (Pathogens) YES
One half of box 1 tested. Note: She is YES (positive) to 10 out of 15 pathogens tested, this qualifies as AIDS. She will start on parasite killing program for babies.

Mother, Argella

☐ Protein 24 (HIV) NO

☒ Ortho-phospho-tyrosine (Cancer) YES at liver
Cancer of the liver is in the mother.

☒ hCG (Pre-Cancer) YES at one part of liver only; NO in WBCs

☒ Propyl Alcohol (Solvent) YES
Will go off body products. Other solvents not tested

☐ Fasciolopsis adults (Parasite) NO

☒ Sheep liver fluke adults (Parasite) YES
Others not tested. Note: this is unusual, not to have the adults in the liver. <u>But it is nearly always liver cancer where this unusual situation is seen.</u>

Father, Fred

☐ Ortho-phospho-tyrosine (Cancer) NO

☐ hCG (Pre-Cancer) NO

☒ Protein 24 (HIV) YES

☒ Benzene (Solvent) YES throughout his body

☐ Propyl Alcohol (Solvent) NO
Other solvents not tested. They will keep the baby off all body products except olive oil. She will get only fruits and vegetables and milk, no crackers and other processed foods. The whole family will go off propanol and benzene polluted foods.

Summary: This case nearly brought tears to the eyes of all of us. They have not returned. Parasites and pollution are claiming the life of this beautiful child.

Later: This story has a happy ending. The baby recovered her health; the family was perfectly observant of the rules to keep her healthy. She is now a happy, growing infant.

22*	David Adair	HIV and Lung Cancer

This is a very ill-appearing tall man, with labored breathing and hot hands to the touch. He was concentrating poorly as we greeted each other. His parents drove him here from a neighboring state for his HIV positive diagnosis on the recommendation of a friend. He is extremely lethargic, but not able to sleep. Very little history was taken because he was barely able to sit in a chair.

☒ Protein 24 (HIV) YES at thymus and penis

☒ Ortho-phospho-tyrosine (Cancer) YES at bronchii
Also has lung cancer. He was diagnosed HIV positive 5 weeks ago, after several bumps appeared on his right leg. But he had not been well for two years and has moved back to his parents' home.

☒ Benzene (Solvent) YES at thymus

☒ Methylene chloride (Solvent) YES at thymus

☒ Acetone (Solvent) YES high at thymus

☒ Kerosene (Solvent) YES high

He will go off commercial beverages and drink only milk, water and homemade fruit and vegetable juices. Note: no propanol was found; yet he is producing ortho-phospho-tyrosine in his lung. Could this be an error? Or did I fail to test for propanol? Perhaps it was only present in the liver, not the white blood cells, so I failed to catch it. He was cleaning paint brushes in kerosene recently; he will never do this again. His parents will cook for him and buy the new products he needs.

☒ Fasciolopsis eggs (Parasite) YES at thymus and penis

☐ Sheep liver fluke (Parasite) NO

☐ Pancreatic fluke (Parasite) NO

He will start parasite program. He will switch from soap and detergent to borax concentrate. He will use only our body products. Note: there is no adult fluke in either liver or thymus; his clinical drug for HIV may have killed it. He will be vegetarian for 3 months.

The next day

He is feeling very ill, barely able to sit for the appointment. His mother is anxious, sitting upright. His father is standing, pacing the floor with his hands together.

☐ Protein 24 (HIV) NO

☐ Ortho-phospho-tyrosine (Cancer) NO

Both the virus and cancer are gone. This quick result may be due to his having only fluke eggs in the body when he arrived yesterday.

☒ Herpes simplex 1, Trich vag, Nocardia, Borellia burg, B strep, A strep, Haemophillus inf, Coxsackie B4, Coxsackie B1, Histoplasma, Campyl pyl, Bacillus cereus, Bacteroides fr, Staph aureus, Plantar wart, Gardnerella, Propiono, Adenovirus, Strep pneu (Pathogens) YES

☐ EBV, CMV, Flu, Resp Sync Virus, Chlamydia, Shigella, Proteus, Salmonella (Pathogens) NO

End box 1. Note: he has 19 out of 27 pathogens in an active stage, obviously AIDS. He will use our L-G, 1 tbs. four times a day.

Also vitamin C, 3 grams a day. L-G is an immune booster we use for serious viral conditions.

They left for home, feeling that a test that shows NO (negative) for HIV without showing any improvement in symptoms must surely be worthless and they must prepare for their son's death.

Eight days later

He is less lethargic today.

☐ Protein 24 (HIV) NO

☐ Ortho-phospho-tyrosine (Cancer) NO

☒ PCB (Toxic Element) YES high

Off all detergents; may eat on paper plates and cups using plastic cutlery to avoid soap residue on dishes.

☐ Solvents (ALL) NO

Is complying very well with instructions.

☒ CMV, Gardnerella, B strep, Bacteroides fr, Salmonella ent, Histoplasma cap (Pathogens) YES

☐ EBV, Flu, Resp Sync Virus, Chlamydia, Shigella, Proteus, (Pathogens) NO

Note: he has only 6 positives out of 27 in box 1! He is improving.

☒ Anaplasma, Strep pyog, Mycobact TB, Shigella dys, Campyl fetus, Strep G, Clostridium sept (Pathogens) YES

☐ Mycoplasma, Candida (Pathogens) NO

End box 2. Note: he has only 7 positives out of 40 in box 2. He is making good progress. I suspect teeth are source of most of the bacteria.

Twelve days later

He looks better. He walks without apparent neuropathy. He is taking his own notes on this visit. He has moved back to his own apartment.

☒ TCE (Solvent) YES

Drinks flavored coffee - will stop.

☐ PCB (Toxic Element) NO

Uses borax for everything. He is on parasite maintenance program.

☐ Protein 24 (HIV) NO

☐ Ortho-phospho-tyrosine, hCG (Cancer) NO

☒ A strep (Pathogen) YES at tooth #17
Left lower wisdom tooth.

☒ Klebsiella (Pathogen) YES at tooth #17 and 1
Upper right wisdom tooth.

☒ Corynebacterium, Campyl fetus (Pathogens) YES tooth #1

☒ Pneumocystis carnii (Pathogen) YES at lungs
Note: he has only 5 pathogens that are growing, out of 67 tested, and these are mainly at 2 tooth locations. He needs to see dentist for cavitations at teeth #1 and 17.

☒ Asbestos (Toxic Element) YES
No clothes dryer or hair blower in apartment - test house air.

☒ Bismuth (Toxic Element) YES
Using cologne - he will go off.

☒ Copper, Mercury (Toxic Elements) YES high
Tooth fillings.

☒ Palladium (Toxic Element) YES
Tooth fillings.

☒ Arsenic (Toxic Element) YES high
Remove all pesticide. Remaining toxins not tested. He is advised to remove all metal from his mouth in addition to having cavitations done.

Ten days later

He is smiling now, walking briskly, and taking charge of his own case. He says he has more energy. But his right leg is a problem. He has difficulty walking on it. It is considered to have neuropathy by his clinical doctor. A new dark spot has appeared beside the old spot on his shin. It is thought to be Kaposi's sarcoma by his clinical doctor. His doctor says he has permanent HIV neuropathy. His breathing is still labored and audible.

☐ Protein 24 (HIV) NO

☐ Ortho-phospho-tyrosine, hCG (Cancer) NO

☒ Fasciolopsis (Parasite) YES at skin; NO in thymus, liver, intestine
Cause of Kaposi's.

☒ Fasciolopsis redia (Parasite) YES at skin, blood, bladder

☒ Sheep liver fluke cercaria (Parasite) YES at skin, bronchii

☒ Pancreatic Fluke adults (Parasite) YES at skin, penis and bronchii

☒ Human liver fluke (Parasite) YES at skin and bronchii

He has been eating at Arby's™ but will stop. He will go on our 5 day high dose parasite program. Note: the parasites are growing in the skin, causing the purplish lumps to appear. He did not get his cancer or HIV back because he did not have propanol or benzene in him. He must have another solvent, though. Will check.

☐ Moniezia tapeworm head (Parasite) NO

☒ Herpes 1 (Pathogens) YES at skin

☒ Resp Sync Virus, B strep, Staph aureus, Adenovirus, Nocardia, Candida (Pathogens) YES at skin and bronchii

He needs to get his dental work done.

☒ Wood Alcohol, Methylene chloride (Solvents) YES at skin

He has been drinking an herb tea blend. He will stick to single herbs.

☐ Arsenic (Toxic Element) NO

Carpets were steam cleaned.

☒ Asbestos (Toxic Element) YES

He brought air samples.

☒ Asbestos (Toxic Element) YES bedroom air, kitchen air

☐ Asbestos (Toxic Element) NO living room air, bathroom air

The kitchen has a radiator, the bedroom is next to the kitchen. We will test the paint on the kitchen radiator for asbestos with a wet towel rubbing.

Nine days later

His breathing is still audible. He has made a dental appointment; is on his way there. He has done a 5 day high-dose parasite program and is on maintenance again.

☒ Pinworm eggs, Strongyloides larvae (Parasites) YES

☐ Parasites (Remainder) NO

☒ Petroleum ether, Regular gasoline (Solvents) YES

Gassed up car this morning. He will be more careful at gas stations.

Seven days later

He appears normal in walking and in energy but his breathing is still audible. His leg is worse, with increased purple blotches.

☐ Protein 24 (HIV) NO

☐ Ortho-phospho-tyrosine, hCG (Cancer) NO

☒ Hexane (Solvent) YES

He has been using artificial creamer for coffee but will stop.

☒ Asbestos (Toxic Element) YES

Brought paint chips from radiator in the kitchen - are YES (positive) for asbestos - remove radiator.

☒ Campylobacter pyl and Campylobacter fet (Pathogens) YES

Causes varicose veins. May contribute to purple blotches.

☒ Salmonella para (Pathogen) YES

☒ Strep G, Diplococcus pn, and Staph mitis (Pathogens) YES

Tooth bacteria.

☒ Mycobacter TB (Pathogen) YES

Lung bacteria.

☒ Klebsiella, Corynebact diph, Blepharisma, Anaplasma (Pathogens) YES

He is in process with dental work and appears well enough to repeat the clinical HIV test soon.

One month later

He has not been ill; he looks well. He had part of his dental work done this morning, but there is still quite a bit more to do.

☐ Protein 24 (HIV) NO

☐ Ortho-phospho-tyrosine, hCG (Cancer) NO

We will give him a requisition to do his clinical HIV antigen test today.

☐ Benzene (Solvent) NO

☐ Propyl Alcohol (Solvent) NO

- ☒ TCE (Solvent) YES

  Eats flavored croutons - will stop. He is on the parasite maintenance program, 2 times a week.

- ☐ Herpes zoster, Candida, Measles (Pathogens) NO

- ☒ Herpes simplex 1, Mycoplasma (Pathogen) YES at thymus

- ☒ CMV (Pathogen) YES

  I picked some possible infections but only got 50% YES (positive), definitely not the picture of AIDS. His legs have healed; his doctors decided not to biopsy after all.

Ten days later

His clinical HIV test results arrived. They are NEGATIVE.

Five weeks later

He had remaining cavitations done yesterday and is scheduled for metal removal from dental ware in several weeks. His symptoms of "HIV neuropathy" are probably due to mercury toxicity. He is also very stiff after sitting. He also lost his peripheral vision. He has not had any illness in the past month. He has started drug testing studies at a hospital. His T count is still under 300. He has been on AZT for 6 months.

- ☐ Protein 24 (HIV) NO

- ☐ Ortho-phospho-tyrosine, hCG (Cancer) NO

- ☐ Benzene (Solvent) NO

- ☒ Propyl Alcohol (Solvent) YES

  Is still using prescription shampoo; will use borax. He will stay on parasite maintenance program. Next time we will check for tapeworm stages and toxins.

Summary: David got rid of his cancer and HIV virus in 24 hours but getting rid of his AIDS was much more difficult. With his parents' assistance and his own stick-to-it-iveness he succeeded.

Verna Albright	**HIV**

Verna, age 30, came for rather mild sounding symptoms such as fatigue and insomnia. She felt lightheaded and often depressed. It all started with an acute sore throat and influenza about 6 months ago, and she can't seem to recover. She is on the birth control pill but it does not prevent her severe menstrual pain. She had acute mononucleosis a few months ago.

☐ Ortho-phospho-tyrosine (Cancer) NO

☒ Protein 24 (HIV) YES at thymus and vagina

This positive HIV test is quite a shock to both of us. I reassured her that it can be quickly cleared up and will not come back provided she understands the illness well enough to avoid it. She seems angry with my finding. It would be best to schedule a regular clinical test for her.

☐ Fasciolopsis adults (Parasite) NO

☒ Fasciolopsis cercaria (Parasite) YES at liver, thymus, blood

☒ Sheep liver fluke eggs (Parasite) YES at liver, thymus, blood

☒ Sheep liver fluke (Parasite) YES at liver, thymus, uterus

This is the probable cause of menstrual pains (other parasites not tested.

☒ Benzene (Solvent) YES at thymus and vagina

☒ Hexane (Solvent) YES

Remainder not tested.

Summary: Verna seemed quite eager to leave the office in spite of our reassurances. She has not returned in 4 months. We scheduled clinical tests for her but received no test results back. We hope she returns eventually. Her anger is understandable.

23	Milton Essey	HIV

Milton, age 21, came with his mother, perhaps against his will, since he wrote very little on his symptom sheet. His mother said they had been doctoring for 7 years already and could not find his problem. He has chronic stomach problems and nausea and fatigue. He can't eat until after one o'clock in the afternoon to reduce distress. I suspect roundworm and Salmonella.

☐ Ortho-phospho-tyrosine (Cancer) NO

☒ Protein 24 (HIV) YES at thymus, blood and genital tract

☒ Benzene (Solvent) YES

Uses no benzene polluted roducts but chews tobacco which may have benzene—I have asked for a sample. Other solvents not tested.

☒ Fasciolopsis (Parasite) YES at thymus; NO at liver, colon, etc.

I should have checked stomach. My error.

☒ Fasciolopsis redia (Parasite) YES at thymus and liver

Other parasites not tested. He will start on parasite killing program. He will remove all solvents, cleaners, Vaseline, and automotive things from his house.

Five days later

☐ Ortho-phospho-tyrosine (Cancer) NO

☐ Protein 24 (HIV) NO

☐ Mycoplasma (Pathogen) NO

☐ Benzene (Solvent) NO

☒ Propyl Alcohol (Solvent) YES

☐ Solvents (Remainder) NO

Summary: We were all thrilled with Milton's (or perhaps his mother's) accomplishment. I thought they were both so upset and angry with my findings that they would not return. But he carried out his instructions perfectly. They removed a lot of "automotive stuff" in cans from their basement. He didn't say much at either visit, but his smile said it all at the end. I hope he also eliminates propyl alcohol and that his quest for normal health is ended.

Sami Jacobs	**HIV**

We had been seeing Sami, age 33, for a year before suspecting anything as serious as HIV illness. Since she was from two states away, she had barely completed her scheduled dental work even after a year. Two months ago she arrived very ill.

☐ Protein 24 (HIV) NO

☐ Ortho-phospho-tyrosine (Cancer) NO

☒ Mycoplasma (Pathogen) YES at vagina only

☐ Fasciolopsis adults (Parasite) NO

☒ Fasciolopsis eggs (Parasite) YES at vagina only

☒ Benzene (Solvent) YES

☒ Wood Alcohol (Solvent) YES

☐ Solvents (Remainder) NO

The presence of these solvents was equally shocking to both of us. She has been living carefully and "naturally" as the environmentally ill person that she is. Note that the intestinal fluke was not multiplying in her thymus yet. In fact, it appeared likely she had picked up the egg stage from her husband (as well as *Mycoplasma*!) She will get our new benzene-pollution list and repeat parasite program.

Two months later

Sami is again very ill in spite of having been on a parasite maintenance program all this time.

☐ Ortho-phospho-tyrosine (Cancer) NO

☒ Protein 24 (HIV) YES

Now has the HIV virus.

☒ Benzene (Solvent) YES high

Has been using Vaseline Lip Therapy™.

☐ Solvents (Remainder) NO

☒ Fasciolopsis (Parasite) YES at thymus and intestine

☒ Fasciolopsis miracidia (Parasite) YES

☒ Sheep liver fluke (Parasite) YES at thymus

☒ Sheep liver fluke cercaria (Parasite) YES

☒ Pancreatic Fluke (Parasite) YES at thymus and pancreas

She will go on a 5 day high dose parasite killing program, again. She will try to avoid all benzene polluted products this time. She has been using Tea Tree Oil™ and related products for years and loved them so much she did not want to talk about them, for fear I would "take them away". She must go off them.

Summary: Sami has had "environmental illness" for a number of years. The human liver was not meant to detoxify solvents and other harsh chemicals advertised as "progress" by their manufacturers. Our environmentally ill persons are like the canaries that go down into the coal mines to test the air; they pay with their lives so those behind them can enjoy spotless dishes and do cold water laundry. This is progress?

24	**Alma Olivas**	**HIV**

Alma is 26 years old and has had a fever of unknown origin for several years. She brought considerable paper work documenting her past illnesses. She has night sweats, is nauseated, and her neck feels swollen. She is extremely fatigued.

☐ Ortho-phospho-tyrosine (Cancer) NO

☒ Protein 24 (HIV) YES at thymus and vagina

☒ Fasciolopsis (Parasite) YES at thymus and intestine

☒ Fasciolopsis cercaria (Parasite) YES at thymus and blood
Other parasites not tested.

☒ Benzene (Solvent) YES
Uses Vaseline™ and will stop.

☐ Solvents (Remainder) NO

Her husband, Cruz

☐ Ortho-phospho-tyrosine (Cancer) NO

☐ Protein 24 (HIV) NO

☒ Fasciolopsis (Parasite) YES at intestine only

☐ Fasciolopsis other stages (Parasite) NO

☐ Solvents (ALL) NO
Note: There are no reproductive stages of Fasciolopsis in Cruz due to the absence of solvents. They will both start on parasite killing program and avoid benzene-polluted products.

Two weeks later

Alma's fevers continue on and off. She has had a very bad cold.

☐ Ortho-phospho-tyrosine (Cancer) NO

☐ Protein 24 (HIV) NO

☐ Fasciolopsis and all stages (Parasite) NO

☐ Benzene (Solvent) NO

☒ Palladium, Tellurium (Toxic Elements) YES

☐ Toxic Elements (Remainder) NO

She will replace her metal tooth fillings to improve her immunity.

☒ mono-Calcium Phosphate (Kidney Stone) YES

☐ Kidney Stones (Remainder) NO

She will change her diet to include 3 glasses of milk, at least 2% and increase fruit and vegetables. She will reduce meat consumption and eat nothing rare. She will start on kidney herb recipe.

Summary: This may have been a very useful experience for Alma and Cruz. In two weeks they learned how to rid themselves of parasites and avoid HIV and cancer for the future. Since they are from several states away, they may not return. Hopefully, they are sticking to their new lifestyle.

25	Bill Lippencott	HIV

Bill is a graduate student in physics and needs superior health to accomplish his goals. When his mood or concentration are not at their peak his performance is poorer and quite noticeable to himself. He is health conscious and has no risky behaviors. We saw him last fall, 4 months ago for a mood and energy problem and now it is back.

☐ Ortho-phospho-tyrosine, hCG (Cancer) NO

☒ Protein 24 (HIV) YES at thymus and penis

This was very shocking news. However, he was able to understand the explanations that followed and felt reassured that he would not be victimized by this disease.

☒ Benzene (Solvent) YES at thymus, penis

☐ Solvents (Remainder) NO

He will go off the benzene-polluted list of products.

☐ Fasciolopsis adults (Parasite) NO

☒ Fasciolopsis miracidia (Parasite) YES at thymus, blood

He will take our parasite killing program.

Eleven days later

☐ Protein 24 (HIV) NO

☒ Methylene chloride (Solvent) YES and in cornflakes

Benzene is gone but he picked up a new food solvent.

One month later

He can tell he is not feeling right again.

☐ Solvents (ALL) NO

☒ Fasciolopsis cercaria (Parasite) YES at liver, thymus and brain

☒ Pancreatic Fluke (Parasite) YES at pancreas

☒ Sheep liver fluke (Parasite) YES at pancreas

☒ Sheep liver fluke miracidia (Parasite) YES at thymus

Note: Bill has picked up rather a lot of fluke parasites. The source is uncertain. He will do a 5 day high dose parasite program.

One month later

☐ Protein 24 (HIV) NO

☒ TCEthylene (Solvent) YES

☒ Pentane (Solvent) YES

Will stop drinking apple juice, the probable source.

Two months later

His bowel movement is strangely disturbed, very much slowed down but not hard or difficult (I suspect tapeworm.)

☒ Hexane (Solvent) YES

☒ Taenia solium scolex (Parasite) YES at intestine and muscles; NO in white blood cells!

☒ Hymenolepis nana, Hymenolepis dim cystic (Parasites) YES

These intermediate stages of tapeworms are buried in the muscle but have been activated, possibly by the erosive action of the powerful solvents, pentane, hexane and benzene he has had exposure to. He will take a heroic dose of parasite herbs.

Two weeks later

He still has tapeworm activity.

☒ Propyl Alcohol, Acetone, K-1 kerosene (Solvents) YES

They are drinking Springdale Spring Water™ (it tested positive for benzene, propyl alcohol and acetone). He will switch to tap water and kill tapeworm stages again with a new formulation called Rascal (see *Sources*).

Summary: This young man was beginning to be ill with HIV disease but conquered it before serious damage was done to the thymus. Notice that in spite of his best efforts to avoid toxic food and products, he continues to suffer from them. There is very little safe food available that does not require cooking. And, in Bill's case, even the water was polluted. Only a massive clean-up policy mandated by the government can stop the tide of pollution flooding our food and water.

Three weeks later

He is feeling better but has some shoulder pain. He took a super high dose of the parasite herbs for 3 days.

☒ Taenia solium scolex (Parasite) YES at intestine

☒ Decane (Solvent) YES

☐ Solvents (Remainder) NO

He needs to clean his liver and stay on Rascal as part of his parasite maintenance program.

Two weeks later

☒ Decane (Solvent) YES

Has been eating cholesterol-free food; will stop.

☒ Gasoline (Solvent) YES

Mark Ikeda	**HIV**

Mark, age 40, came with his wife, Susette, for seemingly minor problems. His main complaint was pain on the chest, right over the thymus. I felt dismayed as he described in detail what are classical HIV symptoms. He had it about 10 years, he stated. He also has severe colon problems and a chronic sinus problem.

☐ Ortho-phospho-tyrosine, hCG (Cancer) NO

☒ Protein 24 (HIV) YES at thymus; NO at penis

He was incredulous to find he was HIV positive; I hastened to reassure him that HIV could quickly be vanquished by fairly simple means.

☒ Fasciolopsis (Parasite) YES at thymus; NO at colon

☒ Fasciolopsis eggs (Parasite) YES at thymus, saliva, semen

☒ Fasciolopsis cercaria (Parasite) YES at thymus, saliva, semen

Other flukes not tested. Mark has been a fairly heavy rare meat eater; he must now stop and order only fish or seafood at a restaurant. At home they must cook all meat as well as if it were pork.

☒ Benzene (Solvent) YES at thymus and intestine

☒ Propyl Alcohol (Solvent) YES everywhere in his body

Remainder not tested. Mark has an early case of HIV disease; it has not infected his penis yet, in spite of possibly 10 years of exposure to benzene. Has he been an occasional consumer of benzene-polluted products? He will stop using his shampoo and shaving products and go off the list of benzene-polluted products. He will start on the parasite killing program.

Susette Ikeda	**HIV and Breast Cancer**

Susette came with her husband, Mark (above), for simple arthritis, shoulder pain, and shortness of breath. But she had frequent nausea with fatigue attacks, and her arm pain extended into the armpit. Also, her shortness of breath was accompanied by chest tightness. She placed her hand over the breastbone where the thymus gland is located. These were ominous symptoms. She had already heard her husband's bad news of being HIV positive. I explained to her that HIV is not a sexual disease, although it can be transmitted that way.

☒ Ortho-phospho-tyrosine (Cancer) YES at side of breast

(The side under the armpit.) She stated the breast was often painful with striking pain running from under the armpit.

☒ hCG (Pre-Cancer) YES high everywhere

☒ Protein 24 (HIV) YES at thymus and vagina

Susette had a much worse condition than Mark, with both cancer and the HIV virus.

☒ Fasciolopsis (Parasite) YES at liver and thymus

☒ Fasciolopsis cercaria (Parasite) YES at liver, thymus, blood, saliva

☐ Sheep liver fluke (Parasite) NO

Other flukes not tested.

☒ Benzene, Propyl Alcohol (Solvents) YES high throughout her body

Other solvents not tested. She will switch off her shampoo and hair spray and use our brands. She will go off the list of benzene polluted products. She will start on parasite killing program. She will avoid eating rare meats. Both Susette and Mark need to be parasite free since they could give it to each other.

Summary: Susette and Mark's appointments were some of the last to be included in this book so their follow-ups were missed.

26,27 Amy & Charles Furtner — HIV

Amy Furtner is a young mother of three children. She was referred to us by her doctor for mysterious illness. She had already seen numerous clinical doctors who wanted to put her on antibiotics, anti inflammatories, antidepressants and the like. Since she had been a very active healthy person, neither she, nor her husband Charles wanted to settle for this. Her husband was with her. Her main problem was pain in her joints (every joint I could name) but she also had belching and muscle wasting which seemed more ominous. The children appeared healthy but Charles had chronic fatigue. Amy had already taken out amalgams and root canals and tried various detoxifying routines and had gotten significantly better after that. She is now 100% better than she was, Charles said, but still has a lot of pain.

☐ Ortho-phospho-tyrosine (Cancer) NO

☒ Protein 24 (HIV) YES at thymus and vagina, NO elsewhere

They were very shocked. They said the referring doctor would not like this. He wouldn't give her an HIV test although they had asked for one.

☒ Fasciolopsis adults (Parasite) YES at thymus, NO at intestine and elsewhere

☒ Fasciolopsis cercaria (Parasite) YES at thymus, blood, vagina, NO at intestine and elsewhere

☐ Fasciolopsis remaining stages (Parasite) NO
Other parasites not tested.

☒ Benzene (Solvent) YES at thymus, NO at blood, vagina, intestine

☒ TCEthylene (Solvent) YES at kidney, NO elsewhere

☐ Solvents (Remainder) NO
She will start on parasite program, together with the whole family. She wants to bring her children for testing next time. She will be off the benzene pollution list.

Twelve days later

Soon after starting the parasite program she felt pressure on her upper chest and the front of her neck. She used to have these symptoms a year ago.

☐ Protein 24 (HIV) NO
She and her husband are happy with the news.

☐ Fasciolopsis and all stages (Parasite) NO
Continue on parasite program as per instruction sheet.

☒ Uranium (Toxic Element) YES at lungs and trachea
Her husband was quickly checked for uranium also. He too was YES (positive) at lungs and trachea. They will try to improve ventilation through crawl space.

☐ Solvents (ALL) NO
She has one child, about three years old, with her. The child was NO (negative) for benzene.

Seven days later

☐ Protein 24 (HIV) NO

☐ Ortho-phospho-tyrosine (Cancer) NO

☐ Fasciolopsis and all stages (Parasite) NO

☐ Sheep liver fluke and all stages (Parasite) NO

☐ Pancreatic fluke and all stages (Parasite) NO

☒ Oxalate, mono-Calcium Phosphate, Cysteine (Kidney Stones) YES

☐ Kidney Stones (Remainder) NO

She will stop drinking tea and go on kidney herb recipe. She will start to drink 3 glasses of 2% milk unless her symptoms worsen. She thinks her other doctor will not like this; he thinks milk causes a lot of problems. I suggested she sterilize her dairy foods herself.

☐ Uranium (Toxic Element) NO

They opened the crawl space windows.

Sixteen days later

☐ Ortho-phospho-tyrosine (Cancer) NO

☒ Protein 24 (HIV) YES

She has the virus back again. She did not continue the parasite program after the last visit. Will do so.

Two weeks later

She has all three children with her. Her eyes are giving her problems.

☐ Protein 24 (HIV) NO

☐ Ortho-phospho-tyrosine (Cancer) NO

☒ TCEthylene, MEK (Solvents) YES very high

She has been drinking store bought fruit juices. Will stop.

☐ Solvents (Remainder) NO

☐ Fasciolopsis and all stages (Parasite) NO

☐ Sheep liver fluke adults (Parasite) NO

☒ Sheep liver fluke cercaria (Parasite) YES at thymus, vagina only

☐ Pancreatic fluke (Parasite) NO

Others not tested.

Charles Furtner

We will test her husband to check for possible sexual transmission.

☐ Fasciolopsis and all stages (Parasite) NO

☒ Sheep liver fluke adults (Parasite) YES

☒ Sheep liver fluke cercaria (Parasite) YES at thymus, blood, penis

☐ Pancreatic fluke (Parasite) NO

Note: sexual transmission seems very likely.

Child Debbie, about 3

☐ Solvents (ALL) NO

☐ PCB (Toxic Element) NO

☒ Fasciolopsis adults (Parasite) YES

☒ Fasciolopsis redia (Parasite) YES

☒ Fasciolopsis miracidia (Parasite) YES

She will be put on parasite program, going up to 4 wormwood capsules and 6 drops of Black Walnut Hull Tincture.

Child Brian, about 6

☐ Protein 24 (HIV) NO

☐ Ortho-phospho-tyrosine (Cancer) NO

☒ Fasciolopsis adult (Parasite) YES

☒ Fasciolopsis eggs (Parasite) YES

☐ Fasciolopsis other stages (Parasite) NO

☒ PCB (Toxic Element) YES high

☒ Acetone (Solvent) YES high

☒ Petroleum ether (Solvent) YES high

Car fumes? They will go off detergent and store bought fruit juice for the whole family. Brian will start parasite program, going up to 6 wormwood capsules and 10 drops Black Walnut Hull Tincture.

Child Beverly, about 10

☐ Protein 24 (HIV) NO

☐ Ortho-phospho-tyrosine (Cancer) NO

☒ Benzene (Solvent) YES at thymus

☒ TCEthane (Solvent) YES

☒ Petroleum ether, Toluene (Solvent) YES high

☒ Hexane, TCEthylene (Solvent) YES

☐ Solvents (Remainder) NO

She will stop drinking fruit juice, and avoid gasoline smells which she is fond of. Mother will go off detergent use.

☒ Fasciolopsis adult (Parasite) YES at thymus, NO at intestine

☒ Fasciolopsis redia (Parasite) YES

☐ Fasciolopsis other stages (Parasite) NO

She will be on parasite program going up to 6 wormwood capsules and 10 drops of Black Walnut Hull Tincture.

Note how close to having the HIV virus she is. Perhaps she already has been getting it intermittently.

Amy Furtner, thirteen days later

☐ Protein 24 (HIV) NO

☐ Ortho-phospho-tyrosine (Cancer) NO

☐ Fasciolopsis and all stages (Parasite) NO

☐ Sheep liver fluke (Parasite) NO

☐ Pancreatic fluke (Parasite) NO

☒ Xylene (Solvent) YES

Off "organic" apple juice, homemade OK.

☐ Solvents (Remainder) NO

☒ A. strep (Pathogen) YES at tooth #17

Probable cause of joint pain.

☒ Proteus (Pathogen) YES

Always present with oxalate kidney stones. Stay on kidney herbs six weeks.

☒ Clostridium tet (Pathogen) YES at tooth #17

Cause of stiffness in muscles.

☒ Pneumocystis carnii (Parasite) YES

☐ Pathogens (Remainder) NO

She will get upper left wisdom tooth X-rayed and cleaned up.

Summary: Amy could be proud of her parenting. She got her three children back to perfect health. She said she could hardly remember when they had been happy or playful. Now, only thirteen days after starting treatment, they were playing with each other. She

and her husband love to watch them from the side: they don't hit each other; they seem content with themselves and their own things. Her joint pain is no better. Hopefully, the dental clean up and parasite maintenance program will be the last of her problems.

Charles Furtner

Back to the first visit. He has no health problems, except occasional fatigue.

☐ Protein 24 (HIV) NO

☐ Ortho-phospho-tyrosine (Cancer) NO

☒ Benzene (Solvent) YES at thymus

☒ Methylene chloride (Solvent) YES at kidney

☒ MBK (Solvent) YES
Other solvents not tested.

☒ Fasciolopsis miracidia (Parasite) YES at blood, intestine

☐ Fasciolopsis adults and other stages (Parasite) NO

☐ Sheep liver fluke and stages (Parasite) NO
He will go on parasite killing program and benzene removal along with Amy to protect her and the family as well as himself.

Twenty five days later

Amy had stopped the parasite program, and so had he.

☒ Protein 24 (HIV) YES
He was shocked by this result.

☐ Ortho-phospho-tyrosine (Cancer) NO

☒ Benzene (Solvent) YES
He uses rubber cement. Will bring it in for testing and switch brands. He will return to parasite program and benzene restrictions.

Two weeks later

Amy's tests were NO.

☒ Protein 24 (HIV) YES
But Charles still has the virus.

☐ Ortho-phospho-tyrosine (Cancer) NO

☐ Benzene (Solvent) NO

☒ Xylene, Toluene (Solvent) YES
Other solvents not tested.

☐ Fasciolopsis and all stages (Parasite) NO

☒ Sheep liver fluke adults (Parasite) YES

☒ Sheep liver fluke cercaria (Parasite) YES at thymus, blood, penis

☐ Pancreatic fluke (Parasite) NO
Note: Both Fasciolopsis adults and benzene are missing from this HIV incident, so it seems quite likely that the virus can survive for short periods without its parasite host.

Thirteen days later

☐ Protein 24 (HIV) NO

☐ Ortho-phospho-tyrosine (Cancer) NO

☒ TCE (Solvent) YES

☐ Solvents (Remainder) NO

☐ Fasciolopsis and all stages (Parasite) NO

☒ Fasciolopsis redia (Parasite) YES

☒ Sheep liver fluke adult (Parasite) YES

☐ Pancreatic fluke (Parasite) NO

Summary: Here we see how a whole family becomes host to fluke parasites. The parents probably transmit it to the children by kissing and transmit it to each other as well. But they all have "fluke disease" due to solvent build up. We cannot expect our bodies to detoxify solvents; it is an unreasonable expectation since these solvents are unnatural to the biosphere; therefore we must avoid them. This family showed exemplary compliance and intelligence.

28* Allan Gies	HIV

Allan is a young man of 38, diagnosed with HIV virus three years ago. He came from two thousand miles away specifically for his HIV status. A former girlfriend also has HIV positive status, and he believes he "picked it up" from her. He has been in a doctor's care since then. He appears well. On his symptom list he mentions chest tightness, rashes, occasional night sweats, fatigue, a weight loss of 20 pounds since infection. His only medication is preventive antibiotics. He found a dentist to remove his mercury amalgams before arriving. He has brought a recent blood test with him:

BLOOD TEST	Result	Comment
WBC	very low (3.4)	bone marrow toxin
RBC	very low (3.2)	anemia–parasites and bone marrow toxin
MCV	high (101)	Ascaris?
Platelet count	low (131)	bone marrow toxin
Lymphs	low (17%)	bone marrow toxin
Eos	very high (7%)	parasites
Phosphate	low (2.3)	needs vitamin D

He has also had an immune cell analysis. His helper/suppresser ratio is near zero.

☒ Protein 24 (HIV) YES at thymus

☐ Ortho-phospho-tyrosine (Cancer) NO

☐ hCG (Pre-Cancer) NO

☒ Aflatoxin (Toxic Element) YES high at thymus, elsewhere

We will test his foods for aflatoxin.

☒ Benzene (Solvent) YES

He will go off benzene list.

☒ Fasciolopsis (Parasite) YES

☐ Sheep liver fluke (Parasite) NO

☐ Pancreatic fluke (Parasite) NO

☐ Human liver fluke (Parasite) NO

This low level of fluke infestation probably accounts for his small number of symptoms.

☒ Ascaris (Parasite) YES

☒ CMV, Mycoplasma, Candida (Pathogens) YES

☐ Herpes 1, Bacteroides fragilis, Haemophilus infl (Pathogens) NO

It is unusual for *Bacteroides fragilis* to be absent when *Ascaris* is present. I also tested a dozen other pathogens, of which he had six, suggesting AIDS. He has had thrush for some time. He will start on the parasite program.

He has brought water samples from home, as well as air samples.

☒ Hot water sample (Environment) YES in white blood cells
His hot water has something toxic in it.

☐ Cold water sample (Environment) NO
He plans to live with a relative when he returns home in order to avoid both the water and a pet he has.

Two days later

☐ Protein 24 (HIV) NO
His virus is gone.

☐ Aflatoxin (Toxic Element) NO
Stopped commercial fruit juices. They probably contained aflatoxin from the inevitability of some moldy fruit getting into the batch intended for juice making.

☒ Mercury, Nickel (Toxic Elements) YES at thymus
His dentist apparently did not get all the amalgam out. He will need to repeat dental work. He is dismayed. Start on thioctic acid, two three times per day.

☒ Arsenic (Toxic Element) YES
We tested his dust sample from home to find the source of arsenic in his immune system, it was NO (negative). He will ask motel service to stop using pesticide in his room.

☒ Wood Alcohol (Solvent) YES
Stop coffee.

☐ Benzene (Solvent) NO
He is complying with benzene list.

☒ Nocardia, Beta strep, Alpha strep, Mumps, Staph aureus (Pathogens) YES
Out of 18 tested this is an improvement already!

Two days later

☐ Protein 24 (HIV) NO

☐ Fasciolopsis and all stages (Parasite) NO
These parasites are gone.

☒ Aflatoxin (Toxic Element) YES high
Suspect grapes.

☒ Benzene (Solvent) YES

Suspect bacon.

☒ Oxalate (Kidney Stones) YES

☐ Kidney Stones (Remainder) NO

Start kidney herbs.

☒ Samarium, Tellurium, Gallium, Barium, Iridium, Tantalum, Rhodium, Thallium (Toxic Elements) YES

Only dental fillings could give these metals.

☒ Anaplasma, Bordetella, Besnoitia, Central spores, Clostridium sep, Coryne xer (Pathogens) YES

Out of 12. He is not improving further, due to dental problem.

Five days later

His hot water that he tested positive to was analyzed.

☒ Tungsten, PCB (Toxic Elements) YES in hot water

☐ Cadmium, PVC, Lead (Toxic Elements) NO in hot water

He was sent to be retested for HIV using the Protein 24 test.

Four days later

☒ Benzene (Solvent) YES

He is still eating benzene polluted foods like ice cream. Will stop. His clinical Protein 24 test for HIV was still positive.

Summary: Allan had to leave for home at this point. We were both disappointed at the clinical results. This was my first attempt to retest so early (nine days); perhaps it takes longer than that for the clinical test to confirm mine. He will also start on vitamin D (50,000, two per week forever) to raise his serum phosphate level. Allan did a perfect job of killing parasites and getting rid of HIV. But correcting his immune problem will depend on redoing dental work to get thallium and mercury out of his body, and staying off benzene polluted items.

Eight weeks later (based on saliva sample)

He is still free of HIV but is getting frequent infections. He has not redone dental work yet nor distanced himself from pet. Must get on with this.

Six weeks later

Allan has tested NEGATIVE in a clinical Protein 24 antigen test. We are pleased with his vigilance. He is staying off toast and taking B_2 daily.

29,30 Jane, Donald Elliot	**HIV**

We saw Jane six months ago for cancer, which she cleared up at that time. Now she returned with her husband, Donald. She was concerned about his fatigue and irritability which she felt was not normal. She had stayed irregularly on the parasite killing program but had been using commercial body products and no diet restrictions. She is concerned about her own choking spells during mealtime.

☐ Ortho-phospho-tyrosine (Cancer) NO

Cancer has not returned.

☒ Protein 24 (HIV) YES

This was both shocking and distressing. Her immediate thought was could she have gotten HIV from Donald. I assured her that sex was not a primary source. Most likely she picked up HIV through a parasite stage still alive in the rare steaks they are both fond of.

☒ Propyl Alcohol (Solvent) YES

Off the propyl alcohol list.

☒ Benzene (Solvent) YES

Off the benzene list.

☒ Fasciolopsis (Parasite) YES at thymus

Go on high dose parasite program.

Husband, Donald

☐ Ortho-phospho-tyrosine (Cancer) NO

☒ Protein 24 (HIV) YES at thymus, penis, liver, prostate; NO at intestine

Donald was also shocked and mystified over his possible source of the virus. He wondered whether he could be getting it from their pet dog.

☒ Benzene (Solvent) YES at thymus

He will go off the benzene list.

☐ Propyl Alcohol (Solvent) NO

☒ Fasciolopsis (Parasite) YES at thymus and intestine
He will start on parasite program. He wanted their dog tested. They will bring him on Sunday, when there are no people around.

Dog, Buster

☐ Ortho-phospho-tyrosine (Cancer) NO

☒ Protein 24 (HIV) YES
This is my first observation of HIV in a pet. Dogs and cats are not natural hosts for *Fasciolopsis.*

☒ Benzene, Propyl Alcohol, others (Solvents) YES
They will bring in his food for testing; there is some in the car because they are from two states away.

☒ Benzene, others (Solvents) YES in dog food
Donald is furious over pollution in pet food. They will purchase several varieties and find a clean one.

☒ Fasciolopsis (Parasite) YES
I suspect solvents make this possible. They purchased several other dog food brands, but all had solvents. They will feed Buster table scraps.

Seven days later

Jane

☐ Ortho-phospho-tyrosine (Cancer) NO

☐ Protein 24 (HIV) NO
She is very relieved.

☐ Benzene (Solvent) NO
Although the source was not identified.

☒ Propyl Alcohol (Solvent) YES
She has not switched shampoo but will try.

☐ Fasciolopsis and all stages (Parasite) NO
She will stay on parasite maintenance.

Donald

☐ Ortho-phospho-tyrosine (Cancer) NO

☐ Protein 24 (HIV) NO

☒ Benzene (Solvent) YES

There may be a chemical in his office that has benzene. He will bring several for testing.

☐ Propyl Alcohol (Solvent) NO

☐ Fasciolopsis and all stages (Parasite) NO

Buster

☐ Ortho-phospho-tyrosine (Cancer) NO

☒ Protein 24 (HIV) YES

☒ Benzene (Solvent) YES

He is still getting some commercial feed. He is a big dog; there aren't enough table scraps.

Summary: Both Jane and Donald got rid of their virus and parasites before their dog did, probably because of the benzene problem for Buster. But they plan to find pure food for him so he is no longer infectious. They would like to know if he was really their source of infection. They have not stopped eating red meats but cook it thoroughly now. This was my first encounter with a pet carrying HIV. It seems a likely source for them since the dog licks them and he is a house dog.

Erik Gerger **HIV and Cancer**

Erik is 26 years old and has only minor problems. He is here for his underweight condition; he is 25 lbs. underweight. There is a cat in his house. He needs ten hours of sleep at night but still has low energy.

☒ Ortho-phospho-tyrosine (Cancer) YES

He has cancer, but he is incredulous and anxious to leave. There isn't time to search for its location.

☒ Protein 24 (HIV) YES high

He has a very high level of HIV virus. This seems even less likely to him. But I prevailed upon him to stay long enough to get his instructions.

☒ Fasciolopsis adults and redia (Parasite) YES at thymus

☐ Sheep liver fluke (Parasite) NO

☐ Pancreatic fluke (Parasite) NO
Others not tested. He will start on parasite killing program.

☒ Benzene (Solvent) YES at thymus
Uses Tom's™ toothpaste.

☒ Hexane (Solvent) YES

☐ Solvents (Remainder) NO
He is instructed to go off commercial beverages and avoid the benzene list.

Summary: Erik has not returned. I hope he at least stopped using benzene-polluted products, and is staying on a parasite maintenance program. But it's too much to hope for. Note that propanol was not listed as YES and yet ortho-phospho-tyrosine is present. Nor is Fasciolopsis listed as present in the liver. Were these tests missed? If not, this would be a unique case of cancer without both of its two chief causes. I will search for more such exceptions.

Vince Lombardo	**HIV**

This is an 11 year old boy with asthma. He is also a bed wetter (he probably has roundworm in his bladder as well as his lungs). He is overweight. They have a water softener.

☒ Protein 24 (HIV) YES

☒ Ortho-phospho-tyrosine (Cancer) YES
Vince has both the HIV virus and cancer! It seems impossible to his parents.

☒ Fasciolopsis adults (Parasite) YES at thymus

☒ Fasciolopsis other stages (Parasite) YES high at thymus

☐ Sheep liver fluke (Parasite) NO

☐ Pancreatic fluke (Parasite) NO

☐ Ascaris (Parasite) NO
Since all asthma cases have Ascaris, I would presume this case is not true asthma; or possibly I didn't test for the lung stage of Ascaris. He will start parasite program.

☒ Benzene (Solvent) YES

☒ MBKetone (Solvent) YES

☒ Denatured alcohol (Solvent) YES

☐ Solvents (Remainder) NO

They will go off the benzene list and commercial beverages. The rest of the family tested NO to both HIV and ortho-phospho-tyrosine.

Summary: This family did not return. Was propanol missing in the test? Did I not check for Fasciolopsis in the liver? Here is another case of ortho-phospho-tyrosine being produced, namely cancer, but the two causes both being absent; perhaps they are intermittent, as could be expected in the very early stages of these diseases.

31 Alita Sokolis HIV

Alita Sokolis is 25 years old and came in with a variety of pains in unusual places. She had seen 3 clinical doctors and 2 specialist doctors for the pain over her ovaries. A laparoscopy revealed nothing. She has a history of asthma and pain and tightness in her chest (this is suggestive of HIV). She also has constant headaches.

☐ Ortho-phospho-tyrosine, hCG (Pre-Cancer) NO

☒ Protein 24 (HIV) YES at thymus and vagina

☒ Fasciolopsis (Parasite) YES at intestine, thymus, ovary and uterus

Finding the adult human intestinal fluke in the ovaries is extremely rare. Probable cause of pain at ovaries.

☒ Fasciolopsis eggs (Parasite) YES at thymus, ovary, uterus and saliva

☒ Sheep liver fluke (Parasite) YES at liver, thymus and ovary

Others not tested. Alita has a dreadful infestation of large flukes. She will start on the parasite killing program.

☒ Benzene (Solvent) YES throughout her body

Others not tested. She will go off the benzene list. She has been using Blistex™.

Two weeks later

She feels much better but has begun to have headaches on one side of her face (right side). Chest pain is gone but slight pain over ovaries is still present.

- ☐ Ortho-phospho-tyrosine, hCG (Cancer) NO
- ☐ Protein 24 (HIV) NO
- ☐ Fasciolopsis and all stages (Parasite) NO
- ☐ Sheep liver fluke (Parasite) NO
- ☒ Pancreatic Fluke (Parasite) YES
  Ate a hamburger recently but will stop eating them.
- ☒ Wood Alcohol (Solvent) YES
  Won't drink Koolade™ and artificial sweeteners.
- ☒ t-Butyl Nitrite (Solvent) YES
- ☐ Solvents (Remainder) NO
- ☒ Antimony (Toxic Element) YES
  Off colognes.
- ☒ Vanadium (Toxic Element) YES high
  Search for gas leak in home.
- ☒ Thallium (Toxic Element) YES
- ☐ Germanium (Toxic Element) NO
  Thallium may be coming from pesticides, not tooth fillings, since germanium is NO. Will repeat at next visit.
- ☒ Fiberglass (Toxic Element) YES high
  Search for a hole in wall or ceiling of home. Others not tested.

Summary: Alita has improved her health greatly and cured her HIV infection. Now that she sees better health is possible, she is determined to make the necessary changes to recover from all her problems.

32	**Renee Williams**	**HIV**

We have seen Renee several times a year for the last 10 years. In this time she has made changes when a crisis occurred but nothing fundamental. They still have a water softener. They still are cooking with aluminum and copper pots. She still has a mouth full of mercury. She wears a lot of make-up and metal on her skin. She also has a stressful life with a full-time job. Each health crisis seems a bit more severe than the last one. Today she has arrived with numbness in her hands. This implicates heavy metals in the brain, particularly mercury from her numerous corroded tooth fillings. However, I will check for solvent toxicity today since she has a very short appointment and I have stressed the tooth fillings in the past.

☒ Propyl Alcohol (Solvent) YES

May have cancer.

☐ Ortho-phospho-tyrosine (Cancer) NO

A relief.

☐ Protein 24 (HIV) NO

☒ Mycoplasma, E coli, A strep, Myco TB, Plantar wart, Diplococcus pn, Papilloma, Anaplasma (Pathogens) YES

☐ Pathogens (Remainder) NO

This is more than the average number of active bacteria for a well person. I recommend getting her metal tooth fillings replaced and a course of parasite treatment as well as replacing her cosmetics with propanol-free varieties. I believe this is falling on deaf ears, however.

Six weeks later

Renee is much worse. Her hands are hot and swollen. Her legs are sore. She has seen her clinical doctor who recommends vigorous treatments for rheumatoid arthritis.

☐ Ortho-phospho-tyrosine (Cancer) NO

☒ Protein 24 (HIV) YES

Does not surprise me but startled her—disbelief soon calms her.

☒ Fasciolopsis (Parasite) YES at thymus

☒ Fasciolopsis cercaria (Parasite) YES at thymus and heart

☒ Fasciolopsis miracidia, redia, eggs (Parasite) YES

☒ Sheep liver fluke and miracidia (Parasite) YES

☐ Pancreatic fluke (Parasite) NO

Others not tested. She agrees to start the parasite killing program.

☒ Pathogens (8 Tested) YES

She is positive to 8 out of 8 pathogens tested. This is AIDS. She doesn't hear what I am saying.

☒ Benzene, Propyl alcohol (Solvents) YES

I encouraged her to stay off the benzene list and propanol-containing products. She is asked to follow-up in 5 days.

Eleven days later

Renee's hands are no better but my first concern is her thymus health.

☐ Ortho-phospho-tyrosine (Cancer) NO

☐ Protein 24 (HIV) NO

This convinces her that all my tests are invalid since her hands are no better. But she is also afraid to leave this unconventional approach because it has served her so well for 10 years.

☒ Fasciolopsis adults and cercaria (Parasite) YES at thymus

☒ Pancreatic fluke (Parasite) YES at thymus

Continues to eat fast food hamburgers.

☐ Propyl Alcohol (Solvent) NO

Good progress—found propanol-free cosmetics.

☒ Benzene (Solvent) YES

Possibly nail polish.

One week later

Swelling in her hands persists.

☐ Ortho-phospho-tyrosine (Cancer) NO

☐ Protein 24 (HIV) NO

☒ Uric Acid (Kidney Stone) YES

Start on kidney herb recipe. Stay on parasite maintenance program.

Two weeks later

Joints of hands are hot and swollen. She can make no progress without removing the mercury and heavy metals from her dental ware and getting rid of benzene so her natural immunity can conquer the bacteria in her joints.

☐ Protein 24 (HIV) NO

☐ Ortho-phospho-tyrosine (Cancer) NO

☒ Fasciolopsis cercaria (Parasite) YES

Still eating hamburgers.

☐ Sheep liver fluke (Parasite) NO

☐ Pancreatic fluke (Parasite) NO
She will continue on the parasite program.

☒ Benzene (Solvent) YES
Eats ice cream. She is advised again to get metal removed from her dental ware.

Summary: Renee is very close to permanent invalidism, taken from her high activity level and put in a wheelchair. She has delayed too long with all the necessary changes. Will she conquer her ice cream and hamburger habit? We hope it won't be too late. Notice that she became free of the HIV virus while she still had adults and cercaria in the thymus. Is it the other stages that bring the virus?

33	Neil York	HIV

We have seen Neil, age 67, for four years, along with his wife. They stay in moderately good health, especially Neil. But today he complains of fatigue, nothing specific. He describes his chest as feeling "drawn."

☒ Gold (Toxic Element) YES

☐ Toxic Elements (Remainder) NO
He has never replaced his gold dental ware. I suggest going off peroxide and tooth-paste to reduce gold erosion until he gets them replaced. Also start on thioctic acid (100 mg), 4 a day, to draw gold from his tissues.

Two months later

He has not improved. His respiratory problem is worse. He is worried about asthma.

☒ Gold (Toxic Element) YES
Must get on with dental work.

☒ EBV (Pathogen) YES

☒ Protein 24 (HIV) YES
Note: I missed this test at his earlier visit, although there was a clear chest symptom! My error.

☒ Fasciolopsis (Parasite) YES at thymus

☒ Fasciolopsis miracidia (Parasite) YES at thymus, penis
Others not tested.

☒ Benzene (Solvent) YES
Using car polish with bare hands.

☒ Propyl Alcohol (Solvent) YES
Will switch to our shampoo. He will repeat a 5 day parasite program. He will go off benzene products.

Two weeks later

☒ Ortho-phospho-tyrosine (Cancer) YES

☐ Protein 24 (HIV) NO
He now has cancer instead of the HIV virus.

☒ Fasciolopsis (Parasite) YES at liver; NO at thymus, etc.

☐ Benzene (Solvent) NO

☒ Propyl Alcohol (Solvent) YES
He will go off all products on the propanol-polluted list. He will repeat a 5 day parasite program.

Two weeks later

☐ Solvents (ALL) NO
He is feeling much better

Summary: We are quite endeared to Neil because he appreciates us so much. He had a close encounter with HIV virus which would have given him AIDS in half the usual time because of his metal problem. Hopefully, he will part with that corroded gold soon.

34 Delia Heron	HIV

This 30 year old woman had a baby 7 months ago. After delivery she got more and more tired. Her first child is 5. She had one problem after another after this second baby. She has only been home 2 weeks at a time since then, always needing to be hospitalized. Finally, she had open heart surgery and got a valve put in. A clot in her leg occurred and infections in the valve. She was rehospitalized. Her latest hospitalization was for general illness but culturing showed nothing. She is feeling very bad all the time.

Today, she has just arrived from the hospital where she was released at 9 am. This is a very young looking, frail woman with a very blonde complexion. Even as a child medicine was not tolerated. She is very allergic to penicillin; she got desensitized to it but got more reactive to it later when she was given some.

She now has an aortic valve due to bacterial endocarditis (I suspect a chronic tooth infection). She has a tooth that is broken off, but it didn't get fixed. She had braces in her teens. She has been having diarrhea recently since she was started on Cleocin™ antibiotics.

☐ Ortho-phospho-tyrosine (Cancer) NO

☒ Protein 24 (HIV) YES at thymus, liver, brain, etc.
She and her parents are incredulous that she could be HIV positive. They are very devout. They may not take me seriously after this disclosure.

☐ Fasciolopsis adults (Parasite) NO

☒ Fasciolopsis miracidia (Parasite) YES at thymus; NO elsewhere

☒ Fasciolopsis redia (Parasite) YES at thymus; NO elsewhere

☐ Sheep liver fluke (Parasite) NO

☒ Mycoplasma, Papilloma #4, Resp Sync Virus, CMV, Staph aureus, Proteus, Haemoph, Adenovirus, Nocardia, Salmonella, B strep, Gardnerella, Chlamydia, Bacillus cereus, Strep pneu, Histoplasma (Pathogens) YES

☐ Influenza A and B, Herpes simplex, Papilloma plantar, Trich, Coxsackie 4, Borellia, Campyl, Bacteroides fr (Pathogens) NO
This is certainly the picture of AIDS (16 positives out of 25 tests).

☒ Benzene (Solvent) YES at thymus
Will stop using toothpaste and other products on benzene list.

☒ Propyl Alcohol (Solvent) YES at thymus; NO at liver

☒ PCB (Toxic Element) YES high
Off detergent—switch to borax.

☐ Solvents (Remainder) NO

☒ Mercury (Toxic Element) YES high
Needs tooth fillings out. She will begin parasite program.

One day later

Her father called to say Delia was having burning over her chest. This is a typical result of killing parasites in the thymus. I encouraged him to interpret this as a good result.

One week later

She is very weak but able to sit.

☐ Protein 24 (HIV) NO

She now has a chance to survive.

☐ Fasciolopsis and all stages (Parasite) NO

☒ Pentane (Solvent) YES

Drinks Classic Coke™ and Pepsi Free™—will go off.

☐ PCB (Toxic Element) NO

Switched off detergents.

☐ Mycoplasma, Flu A and B, CMV, Chlamydia, B strep, A strep, Resp Syn, Gardnerella, Propion, Papilloma #4, Campyl Haemoph, Histoplasma, Trich, Proteus, Herpes simplex, Adenovirus, Staph aur, Strep pneu, Bacteroides fr, EBV, Papilloma, Borellia, Nocardia, Coxsackie B4, Bacillus cereus (Pathogens) NO

☒ Shigella flex (Pathogen) YES

Cause of stomach problem—take citric acid 1/8 tsp., 4 times a day in water, juice or boiled milk; also Lugol's iodine, 6 drops 4 times a day in ½ glass water (after meals and bedtime).

☒ Salmonella, Coxsackie B4 (Pathogens) YES

Her picture has improved greatly. She has only 3 infections out of 29 tested. We will encourage her to get dental work done so she can recover. She will begin taking Milk Thistle, 3 a day and thioctic, 4 a day.

Summary: We saw Delia only twice. At her first visit we could see she had both benzene and propanol accumulated in her tissues. In addition, she had PCBs at high levels and mercury at high levels. She was a very ill person with no time to lose. However, she did not return and we have heard no more about her. We had not sufficiently warned her about meat eating and all the benzene polluted products. I fear she got her illness back and decided that our treatment was worthless. Notice that propyl alcohol has <u>*not*</u> *accumulated in the liver; it is present in the thymus! What are the factors determining which organ lets it accumulate? Does the parasite precede the solvent to the chosen organ?*

Craig Newbold **HIV**

Craig is a young man, age 24, whose parents and wife came with him. He has extreme fatigue and a heart problem: irregularity. He had been healthy until age 18. He is exposed to a lot of cigarette smoke.

☐ Ortho-phospho-tyrosine (Cancer) NO

☒ Protein 24 (HIV) YES

This came as a surprise to us all. Perhaps his family felt critical of Craig for aspects of his lifestyle they were assuming. I could sense a hostile attitude. I thought they might not return, and this would surely seal Craig's fate. For this reason, we scheduled a clinical HIV test for Craig. Perhaps, I reasoned, if he sees it on a printed form it will have more impact, and he will return to improve his situation.

Summary: Craig never returned. They did not pick up the requisition for the blood test. There was insufficient time to warn him about benzene and meat eating. Hopefully, he will someday return and it will not be too late.

Gerald Lacy **HIV**

We have seen Gerald several times over the past 10 years. 7 years ago he had a low WBC (white blood cell count) 3.9%. 3 years ago he still had a low WBC (3.9%). At this time thallium was found in his white blood cells. He is here for a routine check-up. He is not suffering from fatigue or illness.

☐ Ortho-phospho-tyrosine, hCG (Cancer) NO

☒ Protein 24 (HIV) YES at thymus and penis

Surprisingly, Gerald noticed no illness.

☒ Benzene (Solvent) YES throughout his body

☒ Propyl Alcohol (Solvent) YES

☒ Carbon tetrachloride (Solvent) YES

Others not tested. He will go off the benzene list, also the propanol list. He will switch to borax. They have been eating a lot of cold cereal but will stop.

☒ Fasciolopsis (Parasite) YES at liver, thymus, intestine, penis

Rare to see adult flukes here.

☒ Fasciolopsis eggs (Parasite) YES at thymus, saliva, etc.

Others not tested. He will start on parasite program.

Note: Gerald had the condition necessary for cancer: propanol accumulation and an adult fluke in the liver. Why is he not making either hCG or ortho-phospho-tyrosine? Maybe the cancer must begin in the intestine, i.e. only the intestine can make hCG. This was a rare opportunity to study this question, but time did not permit.

Jennifer Arthur	**HIV**

This 44 year old woman came in with a long list of pains and weaknesses. Her neck, upper arms, shoulders, upper and lower back, thighs and ankles, knees, feet, and urinary tract were all involved. Her clinical doctor had given her a diagnosis of fibromyalgia. It all began 4 years ago. She also listed pain in the web of her hand between the thumb and forefinger, under the collar bone, and upper chest. This suggests HIV disease. There is a water softener.

☐ Ortho-phospho-tyrosine (Cancer) NO

☒ Protein 24 (HIV) YES

☒ PCB (Toxic Element) YES high

☒ Mycoplasma, Candida (Pathogens) YES

Others not tested. Jennifer was immediately unhappy with these findings and did not want to hear any more. I was not able to reassure her that she could eliminate this herself and be in control of her health. The *Mycoplasma* infection was the probable cause of all her aches and pains. Hopefully, she will seek help as she sickens.

35 Sandra Carson HIV

Sandra is 29 and was diagnosed as HIV positive at a hospital in a neighboring town. She will bring in her medical summary. She also has a long list of pains, including chest pain. During her menstrual period her whole body hurts from top to toe. She has a chronic headache.

☐ Ortho-phospho-tyrosine (Cancer) NO

☒ Protein 24 (HIV) YES high at thymus and vagina

She feels pressure over breast bone.

☒ Fasciolopsis (Parasite) YES at thymus; NO at liver, intestine

☒ Sheep liver fluke cercaria (Parasite) YES at thymus, vagina, blood

☒ Pancreatic fluke (Parasite) YES at pancreas

She will start on parasite killing program.

☒ Herpes simplex 1, Gardnerella, Adenovirus, Propiono, CMV, Bacteroides fr, Proteus, Campyl pyl, Shigella, Haem inf, B strep, Bacillus cereus, Salmonella, Borellia, Trich, Nocardia, A strep, Coxsackie B 1, Staph aur, Histoplasma, Strep pneu, Papilloma 4, Chlamydia, Coxsackie B 4, EBV (Pathogens) YES

☐ Influenza A and B, Resp Syn V, Plantar wart (Pathogens) NO

This is certainly the picture of AIDS. She is positive to 25 out of 28 pathogens tested.

☒ Benzene (Solvent) YES at thymus and vagina

Switch from Colgate Tartar Control™ toothpaste to baking soda for tooth cleaning. Observe the rest of the benzene pollution list.

Three days later

She felt an unusual sensation over her upper breast bone for a while after starting on parasite herbs, but now it is gone. Probably due to parasite killing; this is common.

☐ Ortho-phospho-tyrosine (Cancer) NO

☐ Protein 24 (HIV) NO

She no longer has the HIV virus; it took her only 3 days to accomplish this. We will give her requisitions for retesting soon.

☐ Fasciolopsis and all stages (Parasite) NO

☒ Sheep liver fluke cercaria (Parasite) YES at thymus
Ate hamburger against instructions, but will stop.

☐ Pancreatic fluke (Parasite) NO

☐ Solvents (ALL) NO
She will start on kidney herb recipe for her lower back pain.

Summary: Sandra did not return after her second visit, probably for financial reasons. Her friend was paying the bills. She had already financially ruined herself. Possibly she did not wish to have her HIV status changed since she did not wish to go off Social Security support. She was not well enough to hold a job. If her HIV status had changed she may have lost all means of survival. We hope she is abiding by the rules for living that we gave her and that she can enjoy life again. We, in turn, lost an opportunity to prove to the clinical profession that she had reverted to HIV-NEGATIVE status.

Jerome Palash	**HIV**

Jerome, age 47, came in for a rash on his leg, a sore throat, chronic fatigue and some depression, all of which seemed to be rather mild symptoms. However, he had never been ill before in his life, so this unusual combination had him concerned. He then began to have a low grade fever daily and felt a tightness in his neck and jaw. His clinical doctor sent him for further testing but nothing was found to explain the problems. He had a blood test done by his doctor, which he brought. Blood Test results: The urinalysis shows a severe chronic urinary tract infection, with blood and bacteria in the urine. There is also a trace of protein which may explain the sudden hair loss he occasionally got. There were oxalate crystals present (kidney stones or deposits) and some urobilinogen, implicating the liver. His clinical doctor had done two urine cultures looking for bacteria. Both were negative. They had never done a "morning, fasted state" urinalysis, when such problems are more evident.

☒ Salmonella (Pathogen) YES in the stomach
This is the usual cause of fevers of unknown origin or intermittent fevers. A pharmacist or his clinical doctor could provide him with Lugol's iodine solution. He was to take 6 drops in half a glass of water after meals and at bedtime for three days. He will get Salmonella back if he consumes dairy products without sterilizing them first.

☒ Strep pneu (Pathogen) YES at his wisdom teeth

Remainder of box 1 NO. He will start on kidney herbs as well.

Twelve days later

The fever subsided initially, but now is back, higher than before. His headaches and stiffness were gone for a week but now all are back. Clearly, there is an ongoing cause that I have missed.

☐ Salmonella (Pathogen) NO

☒ Strep pneu (Pathogen) YES high

Respiratory infection.

☒ Coryn dipth, Troglo (Pathogens) YES

Remainder of box 2 NO.

☒ Oxalate (Kidney Stones) YES

He has not cleared up stones yet.

☐ Kidney Stones (Remainder) NO

His symptoms seem too severe for these small findings. We will test for cancer.

☐ Ortho-phospho-tyrosine (Cancer) NO

We have run out of office time; will search for toxins and parasites next time (in one week).

Two months later

He is still getting occasional fevers. He is less fatigued and thought he was getting well; this is probably due to the supplements and kidney herbs.

☒ Dipetalonema (Parasite) YES

☒ Fasciolopsis (Parasite) YES at intestine and thymus

Will test for HIV.

☒ Fasciolopsis redia (Parasite) YES at thymus; NO elsewhere

☒ Fasciolopsis miracidia (Parasite) YES at thymus; NO elsewhere

He will start on parasite killing program.

☒ Benzene (Solvent) YES high

Uses Melaluca™ products (Tea Tree)—does not want to give them up.

☐ Solvents (Remainder) NO

He has been a health conscious person, never eating "junk food."

☒ Protein 24 (HIV) YES

He is disturbed and angry with this information and will not return.

Summary: After this experience, I decided to test all persons for HIV as well as cancer at the beginning of their very first visit. I did not suspect his HIV POSITIVE status. He had no risk factors. Hopefully, he has gone off the Tea Tree oil products and has recovered. But he was not given the whole benzene list and will surely get sick again.

36	Shirley Stafford	HIV and Liver Cancer

Shirley has a healthful lifestyle, without alcohol or nicotine. But she developed a pain over the upper mid-chest (she put her hand right over the thymus gland) and visited her regular doctor. The doctor wanted her to have a mammogram. Her left arm feels heavy. She also has low back pain that runs down her left leg.

☒ Protein 24 (HIV) YES at thymus and vagina

This was almost self-evident, considering the chest pain. My explanations seemed odd to her. She has no known risk factors.

☒ Ortho-phospho-tyrosine (Cancer) YES at liver only

She has cancer of the liver as well.

☒ Fasciolopsis (Parasite) YES at liver and thymus; NO at intestine

☒ Fasciolopsis redia (Parasite) YES

Others not tested. She will start on parasite program.

☒ Benzene (Solvent) YES

Go off all items on the benzene list.

☒ Propyl Alcohol (Solvent) YES at one part of the liver only; NO at WBCs!

Note: I could have easily missed the propanol if I had not searched the liver for it. She will go off shampoo and use ours.

Two weeks later

Shirley has not been ill since the last visit. Her arm feels normal now: it had felt heavy before. The pain over her breastbone is gone now.

☐ Protein 24 (HIV) NO

☐ Ortho-phospho-tyrosine (Cancer) NO

☒ Kerosene (Solvent) YES
Be more careful when pouring it.

☐ Solvents (Remainder) NO

☒ Asbestos (Toxic Element) YES
Will test home air. Suspect washing machine belt.

☒ Formaldehyde (Toxic Element) YES
New recliner chair and foam pillows.

☒ Mercury (Toxic Element) YES at thymus

☐ Toxic Elements (Remainder) NO
She is advised to replace her metal tooth fillings with metal-free plastic ones. She will do away with new furniture.

Two weeks later

Her low back pain is unimproved. She has brought 2 belts for testing. One of the belts was YES for asbestos. She will start on kidney herbs for low back pain.

Two weeks later

She has scheduled her dental work.

☐ Protein 24 (HIV) NO

☐ Ortho-phospho-tyrosine (Cancer) NO

☒ hCG (Pre-Cancer) YES

☒ Propyl Alcohol (Solvent) YES
She began using Listerine™; will stop.

☒ Arsenic (Toxic Element) YES

☐ Asbestos (Toxic Element) NO
The new belt is asbestos free. She will remove pesticide from home.

Summary: It is always a delight to work with a client who can dispose of new furniture or carpets without regrets when health is at stake. Our culture teaches us to value our material things, not our health. Shirley was inspiring to our office with her ease of choosing health before gold crowns and expensive new furniture.

37	**Helen Douthet**	**HIV and Cancer**

We have seen Helen in the past five years for painful joints, high blood pressure, and thyroid problems, but she has been in reasonably good health. After a long absence, she arrived at the office looking very pale and thin. She has just returned from the Mayo Clinic. She said they were unable to diagnose her with anything significant in spite of her critical condition. She had not made an appointment but was only purchasing vitamins. I coaxed her to take my first test panel.

☒ Ortho-phospho-tyrosine (Cancer) YES at thymus, bone marrow, liver, intestine and brain!

☒ Protein 24 (HIV) YES at thymus, brain, pancreas, blood
She has widely disseminated disease. How could this be missed by clinical medicine?

☐ Fasciolopsis adults (Parasite) NO

☒ Fasciolopsis miracidia (Parasite) YES at thymus, bone marrow and liver

☒ Fasciolopsis redia (Parasite) YES at thymus, bone marrow, and blood

☒ Benzene (Solvent) YES
She will begin parasite program immediately and go off benzene and propyl alcohol containing products and return in 2 days for a follow-up. She seemed too ill to do more testing now.

Two days later
She looks exceedingly ill, can barely walk.

☒ Ortho-phospho-tyrosine (Cancer) YES at thymus, intestine

☒ Protein 24 (HIV) YES at thymus and bone marrow
Notice how both illnesses have shrunk their territory in her body.

☒ Fasciolopsis miracidia (Parasite) YES
Continue parasite program.

☒ Benzene (Solvent) YES high

The level is much higher than two days ago, she has obviously had a recent high exposure. She has brought some cans, her water and an air sample (of house dust) to test.

☒ Benzene (Solvent) YES in Scotchguard™ for fabrics (a spray can), laundry room air (laundry room has an odor), and in her filtered water at sink (purified drinking water)

☐ Benzene (Solvent) NO in Carbona™ spot remover, Energine™ cleaning fluid and plain cold tap water

In view of the possibility that the purified drinking water is contaminated with benzene, she will use purchased drinking water. She does not trust her tap water. She is still an emergency case and needs to follow-up in 3 days.

Three days later

She seems a bit better.

☐ Protein 24 (HIV) NO

☐ Ortho-phospho-tyrosine (Cancer) NO

☒ Fasciolopsis redia (Parasite) YES at thymus, bone marrow

She has had discomfort over her middle abdomen to the point of pain during this week.

☒ Benzene (Solvent) YES and in WD40™

Uses it on exercise bike—will stop.

Four days later

She is still very ill but feels some improvement. She has partly cleaned the house of chemicals. She has had a "full" feeling on front of neck, still noticeable.

☐ Protein 24 (HIV) NO

☐ Ortho-phospho-tyrosine (Cancer) NO

She will not eat pork or beef and will not handle meat in the house. She does not eat turkey or chicken because of her sensitivity to Salmonella (gets sick right away).

☐ Fasciolopsis and all stages (Parasite) NO

☒ Benzene (Solvent) YES high

She is using facial cleanser, a heating pad, shower water, shampoo, Polysorbate 80™ She will stop until we test each one for benzene.

☒ Strep pyog, Pseudomon aer, Diplococc pn, Gaffkya (high), Clostridium (high) (Pathogens) YES

Remainder not tested. Note: all five of these are typically found in teeth. She has a mouth full of metal - mostly gold. She had too many infections (5 out of 6 tests), so I did not continue testing. The implication of AIDS was obvious. She resisted suggestion of dental work. But she will call the dentist regarding cavitations at teeth #1 and #32. I tried to impress on her the need for speedy removal of tooth infections and benzene.

Four days later

Although Helen is not interested in removing the metal from her mouth, she has just returned from seeing the dentist. The dentist found no X-ray evidence of any tooth abscess or cavities, but Helen did have several cavitations cleaned. She is feeling considerably better for the first time.

☒ Benzene, xylene, acetone, wood alcohol, propyl alcohol (Solvents) YES

She will switch to grain alcohol as general cleanser and continue parasite program.

Three days later

She is still getting some low days. She still weighs under 100 pounds but feels she may have gained 1 pound.

☐ Benzene, ether, propyl alcohol (Solvents) NO

☒ Dipetalonema, Echinococcus, E. hist, Echinoporyph, Fishoedrius (Parasites) YES

☒ Pancreatic Fluke (Parasite) YES

Remainder: NO (Box 1). She tested YES for cholesterol crystals and needs to cleanse her liver of gallstones.

Five days later

She is feeling better than 1 week ago, but she still has her ups and downs.

☒ Fishoedrius, Myxosoma (Parasites) YES

☒ Necator (human hookworm) (Parasite) YES high

☒ Moniezia (Parasite) YES high

Tapeworm head, probably escaping from its cyst after solvent action.

☒ Leishmania mex, Taenia sag (Parasites) YES

☐ Parasites (Remainder) NO

☒ Mycoplasma (Pathogen) YES high (systemic)
Probable cause of general aching.

☐ Protein 24 (HIV) NO

☐ Ortho-phospho-tyrosine (Cancer) NO

☒ Fasciolopsis miracidia (Parasite) YES at thymus

☒ Propyl Alcohol (Solvent) YES high
Went back to using commercial shampoo.

☐ Benzene (Solvent) NO

☐ Solvents (Remainder) NO
Stay on parasite maintenance program.

Five days later

☒ Benzene (Solvent) YES

☒ Propyl Alcohol (Solvent) YES
Using untested body chemicals. Will stop.

Six weeks later

☐ Protein 24 (HIV) NO

☐ Ortho-phospho-tyrosine (Cancer) NO

☒ TCE (Solvent) YES
Off commercial beverages.

☐ Solvents (Remainder) NO
Stay on parasite program.

Six weeks later

She is very much better. She has been on chelation treatment for 1 week. She is on a parasite maintenance program.

☐ Solvents (ALL) NO

☐ Protein 24 (HIV) NO

☐ Ortho-phospho-tyrosine (Cancer) NO

☐ Fasciolopsis and all stages (Parasite) NO

☒ Sheep liver fluke (Parasite) YES

☐ Pancreatic fluke (Parasite) NO

She will stay off rare meat.

Summary: Helen had a very close brush with death. Her great dependence on body chemicals of all kinds (lotions, etc.) contributed to this near tragedy. At one point her weight was 93 pounds, and I feared we had seen her for the last time. If she had followed her friends' advice to hospitalize herself or had returned to the Mayo Clinic, she would not have survived. Although she appeared well at the last visit, her failure to remove dental metal could shipwreck her health in the future.

38	Sing Tong	HIV

This 27 year old man came in complaining of fatigue, minor depression, and occasional swimmer's ear. He was concerned about his HIV status and wanted to be tested in my unconventional way in spite of getting an HIV negative result recently.

☒ Protein 24 (HIV) YES high at thymus and blood

☐ Ortho-phospho-tyrosine (Cancer) NO

☒ Benzene (Solvent) YES

Off the benzene-pollution list.

☐ Fasciolopsis adults, eggs, miracidia (Parasite) NO

☒ Fasciolopsis cercaria (Parasite) YES at thymus and blood

☒ Fasciolopsis redia (Parasite) YES at one part of thymus and blood

☒ Echinococcus granulosus (Parasite) YES

☐ Parasites (Remainder box 1) NO

☒ E coli (Pathogen) YES at blood

Constipation or a fissure or even hemorrhoids can let these colon bacteria into the bloodstream.

☒ Klebsiella (Pathogen) YES at one part of thymus (the same), blood and penis

☐ Pathogens (Remainder) NO

He worked in a restaurant for 7 years and handled a lot of meat. He will start on parasite killing program.

One week later

He has more energy. He felt a sensation over the thymus the first few days on the parasite program. This is common.

☐ Protein 24 (HIV) NO

☐ Benzene (Solvent) NO

☐ Fasciolopsis and all stages (Parasite) NO

☒ Echinococcus granulosus eggs (Parasite) YES

☐ Echinococcus granulosus adult (Parasite) NO

☒ Gyrodactylus, Leucocytozoon, Leishmania mex, Plasmodium falc, Schistosoma, Trypanosoma lew, Trichinella (Parasites) YES

☒ Taenia pisiformis cysticercus (Parasite) YES

Has tapeworm disease.

☐ Parasites (Remainder box 2) NO

He will increase parasite program to 4 capsules of cloves three times a day for 4 days.

☐ E coli, Klebsiella (Pathogens) NO

☒ Thorium (Toxic Element) YES

☐ Toxic Elements (Remainder) NO

He will seal cracks in basement floor. Note: benzene is gone. He is eating more healthful food, also. He has cleaned the house and basement of all solvents, paint, varnish and cleaners.

One week later

Sing feels fine.

☐ Echinococcus all stages, Gyrodactylus, Leucocytozoon, Leishmania mex, Plasmod falc, Schistosoma, Trypanosoma, Trichinella, Taenia pis (Parasites) NO

He will stay on parasite maintenance program.

☐ Thorium (Toxic Element) NO

Has put in a crawl space fan.

☐ Benzene (Solvent) NO

☒ Shigella flex (Pathogen) YES

☒ Strep G (Pathogen) YES

Needs cavitation cleaned at tooth #1.

One month later

☐ Solvents (ALL) NO

☐ Ortho-phospho-tyrosine (Cancer) NO

☐ Protein 24 (HIV) NO

Summary: Sing was a model HIV client. He had previously been given an HIV antibody test which was NEGATIVE, but he was not surprised to find he was POSITIVE when he came to us. He was anxious to understand all the features of HIV-illness and to learn how to take care of himself. Although he had vanquished the virus in 6 days, he returned to improve his immunity and he did accomplish everything in about 6 weeks.

39	Jimmy Smith	HIV

This 45 year old man has had strep throat for about 2 weeks and can't clear it up. His ears have painful stabs with pain running down his neck on both sides (obviously tooth infections). He has a tingling on the front top chest wall. He experiences pain in his left heel when getting up in the morning, but it's not acute during the day. He has soreness in the base of his breast bone. He experiences headaches (needs a liver cleanse). He has stiffness and reduced motion at his elbows and general body stiffness. He will take the kidney herb recipe for his foot pain.

☒ Proteus (Pathogen) YES
Off nickel–probably tooth metal–take histidine, 1/day, 500 mg. Histidine is a nickel chelator but this is not a good solution for a dental problem, of course.

☒ Papilloma, Plasmodium, Hemophil inf (Pathogens) YES
He is testing positive to the first four pathogens in a row, suggesting HIV illness—will check.

☒ Protein 24 (HIV) YES
We will postpone kidney cleanse and do parasite program.

☐ Ortho-phospho-tyrosine (Cancer) NO

☒ Fasciolopsis (Parasite) YES at thymus, intestine; NO at liver

☒ Fasciolopsis miracidia (Parasite) YES at thymus, kidney

☒ Benzene (Solvent) YES

☒ Propyl Alcohol (Solvent) YES

Others not tested. They might have paint thinner in the house. We will test air. He uses nothing on the benzene list. He will switch off his shampoo and use ours. He will start on parasite killing program.

One week later

☐ Solvents (ALL) NO

☐ Ortho-phospho-tyrosine (Cancer) NO

☐ Protein 24 (HIV) NO

☐ Fasciolopsis and all stages (Parasite) NO

☐ Sheep liver fluke (Parasite) NO

☒ Cystine, phosphates (Kidney Stones) YES

He eats a lot of meat, namely phosphate; he will switch to fish that at least have built in bones (calcium). Start on kidney herb recipe.

Three weeks later

His throat feels better but he has minor sternal pain occasionally (probably heart parasites). There is no change in his ankle and heel pain. Soreness at the base of breast bone persists. He has fewer headaches and less stiffness.

☐ Toxic Elements (ALL) NO

Surprisingly good.

☒ Acanthocephala (Parasite) YES

Do a 5 day high dose parasite program and start on readiness program for liver cleanse.

☒ Dirofilaria (Parasite) YES

Dog heartworm, cause of chest pain.

☒ Loa Loa (Parasite) YES

Also causes chest pain. Others not tested.

One month later

Jimmy has tingling and soreness over his chest wall and neck again. He had 1-2 weeks that were OK.

☐ Protein 24 (HIV) NO

☐ Ortho-phospho-tyrosine (Cancer) NO

☐ Fasciolopsis and all stages (Parasite) NO

☐ Pancreatic fluke (Parasite) NO

☒ Sheep liver fluke (Parasite) YES at thymus
Probable cause of tingling.

☒ Sheep liver fluke metacercaria and cercaria (Parasite) YES
He will avoid eating meat in restaurants and stick to fish and seafood. He will repeat a 3 day high dose parasite program.

☒ Benzene (Solvent) YES
Off ice cream.

☒ Xylene (Solvent) YES
Off Sprite™.

☒ TCEthylene, Acetone, Toluene (Solvents) YES
Probably 7UP™. He will avoid all commercial beverages.

One month later

He still has tingling over his abdomen occasionally and a lot of bloating. He also had the flu for a week again.

☒ TCE (Solvent) YES
Drank a small amount of pop again—will stop.

☐ Protein 24 (HIV) NO

☐ Ortho-phospho-tyrosine (Cancer) NO

☐ Mycoplasma, Candida (Pathogens) NO

☒ CMV, Gardnerella, Adenovirus, B strep, Shigella, Nocardia, Trich vag, Borellia, Plantar wart, Coxsackie B1, Strep pneu, A strep, Herpes zoster, Salmonella ent, Staph aureus, Bacillus cereus, Histoplasma, Proteus mirab, (Pathogens) YES
End of box 1. This is the picture of AIDS, but without HIV.

☒ Fasciolopsis redia (Parasite) YES at thymus

☒ Fasciolopsis cercaria (Parasite) YES

☐ Sheep liver fluke (Parasite) NO

☐ Pancreatic fluke (Parasite) NO

☒ Clonorchis (Parasite) YES

He has been eating McDonald's hamburgers and will definitely stop this time. He will repeat the 5 day high dose parasite program and start on maintenance after that.

Two weeks later

He had continuous influenza. He is on Kephalexin™ antibiotic and cough medicine.

☐ Solvents (ALL) NO

☐ Protein 24 (HIV) NO

☐ Ortho-phospho-tyrosine (Cancer) NO

☒ Iridium (Toxic Element) YES at thymus

Tooth fillings—remove metal from mouth.

☒ Hafnium (Toxic Element) YES at thymus

Source unknown.

☒ Palladium high, Nickel high at thymus, Gadolinium at thymus, Scandium (Toxic Elements) YES

Tooth fillings.

☒ PVC (Toxic Element) YES at thymus

Works with building materials.

☐ Toxic Elements (Remainder) NO

He needs all dental metal replaced with metal-free plastic.

☒ Herpes zoster, Mycop, EBV, Bacillus cere, Human papilloma 4, Lepto int, Eikanella, Lacto acid, Klebsiella, Gaffkya, Bacill anthrac, Anaplasma, Mycob. TB, Pseudo aer, Strep mit, Tobacco mosaic virus, Haemoph inf (Pathogens) YES

This is the picture of AIDS.

Summary: Jimmy has done an excellent job of removing solvents from his foods and products. He has gotten rid of the HIV virus but not his AIDS. He has been advised to get the metals out of his mouth in order to stop them from fluxing into the thymus. We are waiting anxiously for him to complete this job so his immunity can recover.

Vivian Van Hise	**HIV**

This 19 year old woman came in complaining of chest pain over her sternum. She has had this for 2-3 years and feels it mostly when

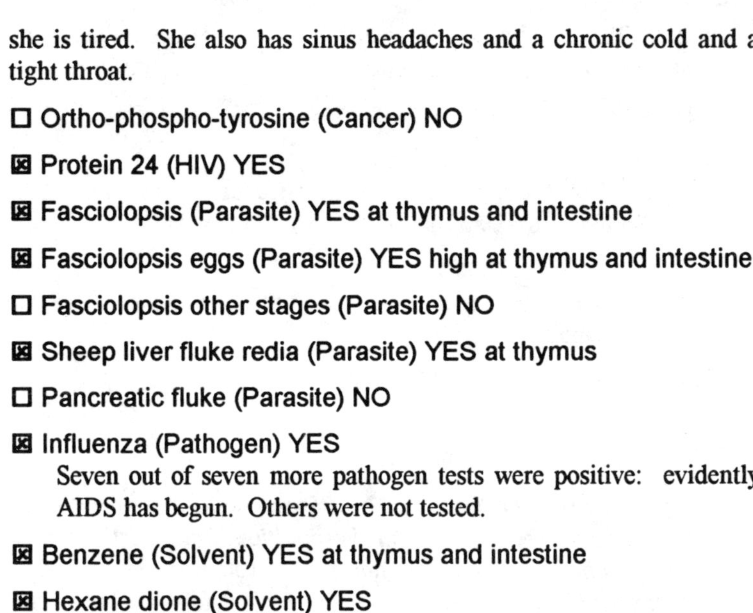

she is tired. She also has sinus headaches and a chronic cold and a tight throat.

☐ Ortho-phospho-tyrosine (Cancer) NO

☒ Protein 24 (HIV) YES

☒ Fasciolopsis (Parasite) YES at thymus and intestine

☒ Fasciolopsis eggs (Parasite) YES high at thymus and intestine

☐ Fasciolopsis other stages (Parasite) NO

☒ Sheep liver fluke redia (Parasite) YES at thymus

☐ Pancreatic fluke (Parasite) NO

☒ Influenza (Pathogen) YES

Seven out of seven more pathogen tests were positive: evidently AIDS has begun. Others were not tested.

☒ Benzene (Solvent) YES at thymus and intestine

☒ Hexane dione (Solvent) YES

Drinks Mountain Dew™ — will stop.

☒ Styrene (Solvent) YES

Avoid eating out of styrofoam.

☐ Solvents (Remainder) NO

She will stay off all items on the benzene list and avoid commercial beverages. She will make her own orange juice and vegetable juice and freeze them. She will start parasite killing program.

Summary: Vivian has not returned after 3 months. These are big expenses for so young a person. She has been dealt with unfairly by society. Pollution problems are not of her making. At age 19 she is desperately in need of good health. We hope she is working at wellness for herself.

Stella Rowley	**HIV and Cancer**

This 23 year old woman came in because of her chronic yeast infection, menstrual cramps she has suffered from "all her life," migraines, bunions, and heart arrhythmia. She also noted that she has sinus problems during the fall and spring. Her right wrist is sore. She has occasional constipation and diarrhea; her right knee is sometimes sore. She is on several medications for her various ailments, way too many for her age.

☒ Ortho-phospho-tyrosine (Cancer) YES

☒ Protein 24 (HIV) YES
She has both cancer and HIV illness unbeknownst to her, but she is not too surprised. I am surprised at her calmness.

☒ Propyl Alcohol (Solvent) YES high
Eliminate propanol polluted products like cold cereal and shampoo.

☒ Benzene (Solvent) YES high
Off benzene list.

☐ PCB (Toxic Element) NO

Summary: She arrived with HIV test results that were NEGATIVE. Apparently, however, she had the intuition that something was quite wrong with her but could not get it established clinically. We recommended a vegetarian diet for her, which appealed to her anyway. She has not returned, and three months have passed. Hopefully, she has followed some of the advice we gave her. Her finances may not have been adequate for her to return for follow-up.

40	Dawn Generes	HIV

This 51 year old woman had the following problems: 1) her feet kill her. She works at a hospital and is on her feet all day. At night there is a cramp in them. They burn and ache all the time. She has tried different shoes. The pain is not in her toes but higher up, to about 6 inches above the ankle, mostly on her right foot. This started about 5-10 years ago and has worsened in the past 2 years; 2) her sinuses are clogged and she feels like there is something in her throat; 3) she has a low energy level; 4) she is holding water in her hands and feet; 5) she has lower back pain, for which she sees a chiropractor; 6) her knees hurt; 7) she has elbow pain—it hurts her to pick up a quart jar; 8) her left hip and leg are painful; 9) she has gum disease; her front teeth are badly eroded and she has loose teeth.

She will go on a tooth program which consists of:

- Flossing 1 time/day (use monofilament nylon fish line, 2 to 4 pound test)

- Brushing 2 times/day. At one brushing use potassium iodide (white iodine, see *Recipes*) from a pharmacist. Use 4 drops on a tooth brush. At second brushing use 17½% hydrogen peroxide, food grade, again 4 to 5 drops on tooth brush. If spilled on skin, wash it off.
- Also, take 3 glasses of 2% milk/day (sterilized by boiling), 1 magnesium oxide (300 mg)/day; 500 mg B6/day, and vitamin D 1/day for three weeks, then 2 a week forever. Obtain vitamin D from dentist (50,000 units).

She will start on kidney herb recipe.

One month later

Her legs are very restless. She works the night shift and will use ornithine to sleep and arginine as a caffeine substitute to keep awake.

☐ Protein 24 (HIV) NO

☐ Ortho-phospho-tyrosine (Cancer) NO

☒ Ancylostoma duod, Dientamoeba, Echinostoma rev, Eimeria ten (Parasites) YES

Has pigeons and chickens.

☐ Parasites (Remainder) NO

Stay on parasite killing program.

Six weeks later

She is experiencing pain over her sternum.

☐ Ortho-phospho-tyrosine (Cancer) NO

☒ Protein 24 (HIV) YES

☐ Fasciolopsis adult (Parasite) NO

☒ Fasciolopsis cercaria (Parasite) YES at thymus, vagina, blood

☐ Pancreatic fluke (Parasite) NO

☐ Sheep liver fluke (Parasite) NO

☒ Propyl Alcohol (Solvent) YES at thymus; NO at liver!

☒ Benzene (Solvent) YES high at thymus and vagina

☐ Solvents (Remainder) NO

Note: The propanol is in her thymus, not her liver. She does not eat junk food or drink commercial beverages so has no other solvents in her! She will go off the benzene list, off shampoo and hair spray. She will use our varieties.

Six weeks later

She is "fantastically better," she says.

☐ Ortho-phospho-tyrosine, hCG (Cancer) NO

☐ Protein 24 (HIV) NO

☐ Fasciolopsis and all stages (Parasite) NO

☒ Sheep liver fluke cercaria (Parasite) YES at blood; NO at liver and thymus

She had a roast beef sandwich at Hardee's™ a few days ago. Go on 3 day high dose parasite program followed by maintenance, and stay off restaurant meats.

☐ Propyl Alcohol (Solvent) NO

☐ Benzene (Solvent) NO

☒ Beryllium (Toxic Element) YES

Gasoline, car exhaust.

☒ Gold (Toxic Element) YES

Change wrist watch to plastic.

☒ PCB, Holmium (Toxic Elements) YES

Switch to borax and washing soda instead of detergent.

☒ Formaldehyde (Toxic Element) YES high

There is no foam furniture or mattresses in the house—they are remodeling the hospital where she works.

☐ Toxic Elements (Remainder) NO

Summary: Dawn has succeeded in every way to improve her health, a tribute to her intelligence and good attitude.

41	Diane Barron	HIV

This 22 year old woman had numerous serious problems. She had a chest X-ray that showed spots that are thought to be tuberculosis. She suffers from cataracts in one eye and sinus problems. She has a hearing loss in her left ear and her throat is frequently dry and sore. Her shoulders have dull aching pain and her wrists crack with sharp pains as well as her hands. Her chest feels heavy, congested and she has occasional sharp pains there. She has an irregular heartbeat, possibly mitral valve prolapse. She suffers from stomach ulcers and easily feels nauseated. She has chiropractic adjustments weekly for sharp pain between the shoulders. Her leg muscles ache and twitch, especially when she is tired. Her knees pop easily and ache. She may have bunions and her feet ache. She sleeps a lot but also has occasional insomnia. Her energy level is consistently low and her concentration is much less than it used to be. She has frequent bad headaches that make her sick to her stomach. She has frequent urinary tract infections. She suffers from depression and bulimia. She works in a dental office. This is an odd assortment of symptoms, especially for so young a person, typical of HIV illness.

☐ Ortho-phospho-tyrosine (Cancer) NO

☒ Protein 24 (HIV) YES

☒ Fasciolopsis (Parasite) YES at intestine only

☒ Fasciolopsis eggs (Parasite) YES at thymus, vagina, and blood

☐ Fasciolopsis other stages (Parasite) NO
Other parasites not tested. Start on parasite program.

☒ Benzene (Solvent) YES at thymus and vagina
She uses Tea Tree Oil Shampoo.™ Will stop and use our recipe.

☐ Solvents (Remainder) NO
Note: She has no build-up of other solvents yet. Presumably her liver can still detoxify them quickly.

One month later

☐ Ortho-phospho-tyrosine (Cancer) NO

☐ Protein 24 (HIV) NO

☐ Fasciolopsis and all stages (Parasite) NO

☐ Sheep liver fluke (Parasite) NO

☐ Pancreatic fluke (Parasite) NO
Continue parasite program.

☒ Arsenic (Toxic Element) YES
Pesticide Deacon™ everywhere in the house; remove.

☒ Radon (Toxic Element) YES high
House is partly over crawl space and partly over basement—open crawl space vents.

☒ Molybdenum (Toxic Element) YES
Automotive chemicals?

☒ Gold (Toxic Element) YES

☒ Gadolinium (Toxic Element) YES

☐ Toxic Elements (Remainder) NO
She has no gold tooth fillings, but works with gold crowns in dental office that give off vapor and dust.

☐ Benzene (Solvent) NO

☒ Hexane (Solvent) YES
Off commercial beverages.

☒ Acetone (Solvent) YES
Dental glue.

☒ Ether (Solvent) YES
Dental materials.

☒ Methylene chloride (Solvent) YES
Commercial beverages.

☒ TCEthylene (Solvent) YES
Flavored foods.

☒ Her house air, and office air (Unknown pollutant) YES
Note: She has some pollutant in her house air as well as office air. She will try to clean them up by removing all chemicals.

☒ Candida (Pathogen) YES
Yeast. Needs to raise her immunity.

Summary: Diane has gotten rid of her HIV virus but still has a lot of cleaning up to do before she gets as well as a young person of 22 should be. She needs to eliminate radon from her home or move. She needs to change her occupation to a less hazardous one. She needs to remove all metal from her mouth and body. I will discuss these items in the future as she gets more adjusted to her current restrictions. She is doing well and staying free of benzene.

42* Gene Liggan HIV

This 36 year old man has been suffering from fevers and night sweating for several months. He recently ran a temperature of 104°. This went on for a week; the attacks lasted 4-5 hours, then he had one week of remission, then another week of attacks. He saw a clinical doctor who did many tests. He feels very good now in comparison. His HIV virus was found about 4 months ago. He stopped drinking and smoking. He lost about 16 pounds during that ill period, but has gained it back. He had his mercury fillings taken out a year ago when he began seeking out alternative therapies for his mysterious illness. He has a rash on his left cheek and chronic thrush. He brought a thick file with medical records. He has been health conscious for some time and is happy to find us.

☒ Babesia (Parasite) YES

☒ Echinococcus granulosus eggs and cysts (Parasite) YES
He has a dog now but has had cats in the past.

☒ Fasciolopsis (Parasite) YES at thymus, kidney

☒ Fasciolopsis miracidia (Parasite) YES at thymus, kidney

☐ Fasciolopsis other stages (Parasite) NO
He has been trying to get AZT. Note: miracidia are not in the blood, possibly due to taking a sulfa drug recently for about 3 days (he is on it preventively).

☐ Ortho-phospho-tyrosine (Cancer) NO
A few days ago his immunologist gave him a tuberculosis shot, pneumonia, and tetanus shot.

☒ Protein 24 (HIV) YES

☒ Trich (Pathogen) YES
Cook and eat in metal-free pots and cutlery to reduce nickel intake.

☒ Shigella flex, Proteus, EBV, A strep, CMV, Papilloma 4, Coxsackie B1, Troglo, Pseud aerug, Strep G, Plasmod cyno, Staph aureus (Pathogens) YES
He has 13 YES (not counting HIV) out of 27 tested. This is mild AIDS. He has had shooting pains in certain teeth.

☒ Benzene (Solvent) YES throughout his body

He has done a lot of painting and remodeling. He will clear his house of all old paint cans, old brushes, etc. We will test house air for benzene. He will start parasite program.

Three days later

☐ Protein 24 (HIV) NO

☐ Fasciolopsis and all stages (Parasite) NO

He is very pleased but somewhat incredulous.

Three days later

He has been very energized (more so than in the last 2 years); he has to force himself to go to bed, yet he is relaxed and his mood is good. He sleeps well. Cheek skin is better. He has minor fissures at the corner of his mouth. He has no night perspirations anymore. His fevers seem gone. He had been at 102°-104° He also had a very low temperature at times (94°-95°). He is not coughing much at all anymore. He feels his chest is very clear; he quit smoking 4 months ago but it did not clear up his chest.

☐ Protein 24 (HIV) NO

☐ Babesia, Echinococcus all stages (Parasites) NO

☒ Haemoproteus, Multiceps ser, Prosthogonimus, Pneumocystis car, Trypanosoma gam (Parasites) YES

He had a duodenal ulcer, was on Xantac™ and Mylanta™ by the bottle, then a lot of baking soda about a year ago. Remaining parasites (box 2) NO.

☒ Adenovirus (Pathogen) YES

Remainder box 1: NO.

☒ Strep pneu (Pathogen) YES at two teeth

☒ Anaplasma (Pathogen) YES

Remainder box 2: NO. He is still on antibiotics. This is no longer the picture of AIDS.

☐ Benzene (Solvent) NO

☒ Uranium (Toxic Element) YES high

Living quarters are very dusty. He has ringing in his ear and some pain at 2 teeth. Needs to do dental work.

One month later

He has gained 10 pounds. He has felt less stressed and his energy was very good until yesterday. Some days he is still slightly lethargic. His minor rash on his cheeks persists. His tongue is very sore and swollen. He has not done dental work yet.

☐ Ortho-phospho-tyrosine (Cancer) NO

☐ Protein 24 (HIV) NO

☒ Leishmania mex (Parasite) YES
Other Leishmanias: NO.

☒ Haemophilus infl, Shigella (Pathogens) YES

☐ Pathogens (Remainder) NO

One month later

His thrush has cleared up, but he has a slight headache and lower leg pain.

BLOOD TEST	Result	Comment
1. T cells and T-helpers	Low	
2. Monos	high (12%)	
3. Chloride	high	
4. Calcium	very low	He will drink 3 glasses of 2% milk/day and take magnesium oxide (300mg), one a day.
5. BUN, Creatinine	slightly high	kidney problem
6. SGOT, SGPT	very high	possibly due to drugs

He works with other people; they have a lot of respiratory problems. He will go on the respiratory health program:

1. CFH 2/day in winter (this is a combination of thyme and fenugreek herbs).
2. One Bronson Zinc tablet (60 mg) daily.
3. Oscillococcinum when chills are felt.

☒ Kerosene (Solvent) YES

☒ Methylene chloride (Solvent) YES
Has been drinking soda, will stop.

☐ Solvents (Remainder) NO

☐ Fasciolopsis adults (Parasite) NO

☒ Fasciolopsis eggs (Parasite) YES at pancreas

☐ Sheep liver fluke adults (Parasite) NO

☒ Sheep liver fluke miracidia (Parasite) YES at liver; NO elsewhere

Repeat 5 day high dose parasite program. Go off beef (he has been eating some prime rib rare beef).

☒ Candida (Pathogen) YES

☐ Protein 24 (HIV) NO

Is free of benzene. He will do an HIV antigen test at clinical lab.

Five days later

His temperature is 102° today. He also has an injured ankle. He has been having a normal or low temperature in the mornings, but it goes up about a degree in the evenings. He isn't feeling as well as he should, with a lot of aching in his legs, especially from the knees down.

☐ Protein 24 (HIV) NO

☐ Ortho-phospho-tyrosine (Cancer) NO

☒ Fasciolopsis eggs (Parasite) YES at thymus only

☐ Fasciolopsis other stages (Parasite) NO

Continue on parasite program.

☐ Candida, Shigella, Salmonella, (Pathogens) NO

☒ Mycoplasma, Influenza A and B (high) (Pathogens) YES

Note: His influenza is activated and he will be on Oscillococcinum for five days.

One week later

His clinical HIV antigen test result has arrived. It is negative.

His temperature in the morning is 98.8°. He went to the emergency room the other night with wheezing and was diagnosed with bronchitis. He was put on antibiotics.

☐ Fasciolopsis and all stages (Parasite) NO

☐ Sheep liver fluke (Parasite) NO

☐ Pancreatic fluke (Parasite) NO

Continue parasite maintenance program and pet parasite program. He has a cat.

☐ Solvents (ALL) NO

☐ Protein 24 (HIV) NO

☐ Ortho-phospho-tyrosine (Cancer) NO

☒ Staph aureus, Strep G (Pathogens) YES at tooth #1
Needs cavitation cleaned.

Summary: Gene was quite elated with his HIV negative status. He is advised to see dentist to clear bacteria which are a chronic drain on his health. He will continue on his restricted life-style and come in for a checkup every month.

43	Valri Nesbit	HIV

This 27 year old woman came in with a long list of problems including tinnitus, a low grade fever for several months, a general feeling of illness for several months, the source of which no clinical tests can uncover. She has chest pain at mid-sternum (probably HIV) and has been nauseated a lot lately. She has intermittent tachycardia (heart problem), tingling of the hands and feet, a minor sleep problem and a daily headache. She is on oral Mycostatin™ for her vaginal ,yeast infection which she has had for a long time. This all began after moving to a new building at work.

☐ Ortho-phospho-tyrosine (Cancer) NO

☒ Protein 24 (HIV) YES at thymus and vagina

☒ Fasciolopsis (Parasite) YES at thymus

☒ Fasciolopsis cercaria (Parasite) YES at thymus and blood

☐ Fasciolopsis other stages (Parasite) NO

☒ Benzene (Solvent) YES
She uses Vaseline Lip Therapy.™ She will remove all solvents from her basement and kitchen and other sources. She will start a parasite killing program and go off the benzene-pollution list.

Two weeks later

Her fevers subsided but she is still feeling sick with hot flushes. She still feels sternal pain radiating out on each side of the breast bone.

☐ Ortho-phospho-tyrosine (Cancer) NO

☐ Protein 24 (HIV) NO

☐ Fasciolopsis and all stages (Parasite) NO

☐ Sheep liver fluke (Parasite) NO

☐ Dog heartworm (Parasite) NO

☒ Loa Loa (Parasite) YES high

Source of sternal pain and heart problem. Remaining parasites not tested.

☐ Benzene (Solvent) NO

☒ Mercury (Toxic Element) YES

☐ Toxic Elements (Remainder box 1) NO

Valri has made a lot of progress in two weeks. She will get metal tooth fillings replaced with plastic.

Three weeks later

She feels better but still has a low-grade fever (about 99°). Her sternal pain is gone. She has fatigue and muscle aches as well as headaches in the afternoon when she starts to feel hot.

☒ Mineral oil (Toxic Element) YES

Off all lotions and soaps. Use our recipes.

☐ Solvents (Remainder) NO

☒ Lead (Toxic Element) YES high

Test water and air.

☐ Toxic Elements (Remainder box 2) NO

She is on the parasite maintenance program.

☐ Protein 24 (HIV) NO

☐ Ortho-phospho-tyrosine (Cancer) NO

☐ Loa Loa (Parasite) NO

She will start on kidney herb recipe.

Two weeks later

She went back to work. Her water tested YES (positive) to lead by commercial lab test which her husband ordered immediately when she told him about it after her last visit. She has ear pressure.

☐ Protein 24 (HIV) NO

☐ Ortho-phospho-tyrosine (Cancer) NO

☐ Loa Loa (Parasite) NO

☒ Fasciolopsis adults (Parasite) YES at intestine
Ate hamburgers. Others not tested.

☒ Wood Alcohol, Toluene, Methyl ethyl ketone (Solvents) YES
Off commercial beverages.

☒ Methyl butyl ketone (Solvent) YES
Off flavored foods.

☐ Solvents (Remainder) NO
Note the return of Fasciolopsis, but not in the thymus or liver. It is in the intestine, where it "belongs." Note: there is no benzene or propanol in her.

☒ Candida (Pathogen) YES
Yeast; she needs to raise her immunity.

One month later

She is doing a lot better and has no more fever; she has returned to a normal life and is not eating fast food meals or red meats.

☐ Protein 24 (HIV) NO

☐ Ortho-phospho-tyrosine (Cancer) NO

☒ Fasciolopsis redia (Parasite) YES

☒ Sheep liver fluke cercaria, eggs (Parasite) YES
She is on parasite maintenance program but is eating turkey, and chicken; will stop.

☒ Influenza (Pathogen) YES

☒ Candida (Pathogen) YES
Has been on Mycostatin™ for the past 3-4 months.

☒ Pentane (Solvent) YES
Possibly in beer she drank last night.

☐ Solvents (Remainder) NO

Summary: Valri did an admirable job of curing her illnesses. The restrictions may eventually be too constraining for her so that she will repeatedly get HIV and/or cancer. Hopefully, our meat supply will get cleared up of this parasite in the not-too-distant future. At her last visit, her husband, John, came with her, in order to clear the whole family of this parasite.

Husband, John

☒ Lead (Toxic Element) YES

They are working on the lead-in-water problem. (He had been incredulous of our results with Valri until the lab reported presence of lead, he stated.)

☒ Carbon Tetrachloride (Solvent) YES

Uses disinfectants.

☐ Solvents (Remainder) NO

☒ PCB (Toxic Element) YES

Off detergent. He will stop drinking commercial beverages.

☐ Fasciolopsis and all stages (Parasite) NO

☐ Pancreatic fluke (Parasite) NO

☒ Sheep liver fluke cercaria (Parasite) YES

He has always eaten rare steak but will stop.

☐ Protein 24 (HIV) NO

☐ Ortho-phospho-tyrosine (Cancer) NO

Fortunately for Valri, John is supportive at least when he is able to observe the testing and follow the logic himself. Together, they may be able to keep Valri well.

Kim Maddox	**Near HIV and Breast Cancer**

Kim is a middle age mother of several children. She has had a mole on her breast enlarge and get red and sore. The breast felt full and uncomfortable. It is the same breast where she had many breast infections while nursing babies. The mole is now scaling and flaking.

☒ Ortho-phospho-tyrosine (Cancer) YES

☒ Fasciolopsis (Parasite) YES at liver and intestine

☒ Fasciolopsis cercaria, miracidia (Parasite) YES at breast and blood

She will start on parasite program.

Eight days later

☐ Ortho-phospho-tyrosine (Cancer) NO

☐ Fasciolopsis and all stages (Parasite) NO

Continue parasite program.

One month later

She is fatigued and feels pressure on her chest.

☒ Fasciolopsis (Parasite) YES at thymus; NO in liver and elsewhere

☒ Fasciolopsis cercaria (Parasite) YES at thymus and edge of breast

☐ Ortho-phospho-tyrosine (Cancer) NO

☐ Protein 24 (HIV) NO

☒ Mycoplasma, CMV (Pathogens) YES

☒ Benzene (Solvent) YES

Uses Melaluca™ toothpaste, a Tea Tree product.

☒ Propyl Alcohol, Acetone (Solvents) YES

Note: The adult fluke is not in the liver and there is no cancer, in spite of the presence of isopropanol. The adult fluke and cercaria are in the thymus (one part of it) and yet the HIV virus is not present. Does HIV only come with redia in the thymus? She is advised to stop using Tea Tree™ products and go off the entire benzene pollution list as well as shampoo and commercial beverages.

Six days later

☐ Fasciolopsis and all stages (Parasite) NO

☒ Benzene (Solvent) YES

Still uses Melaluca™ products.

☐ Propyl Alcohol, Acetone (Solvent) NO

Note: She is very fond of Tea Tree products and does not wish to go off them. She sees that she got rid of her cancer the first time without going off them and this proves to her keen mind that she does not absolutely have to go off it.

Seven days later

☐ Solvents (ALL) NO

She is off Melaluca™ products.

Summary: Hopefully Kim hasn't ruined her health by having benzene in her thymus for a prolonged time. She just loved her Melaluca™ products and wished them no evil. Perhaps she stopped in time. She is a conscientious, health-minded, intelligent person.

One week later

She has had a Herpes attack and feels critical of my methods since she feels she should be well by now. She is also losing her hair and has pressure on the chest.

☒ Fasciolopsis (Parasite) YES at one part of the thymus

☒ Fasciolopsis cercaria (Parasite) YES at the same part of the thymus and edge of the breast

☐ Fasciolopsis other stages (Parasite) NO

☐ Protein 24 (HIV) NO

☐ Ortho-phospho-tyrosine (Cancer) NO

Note: She has the setting for HIV, with adults in the thymus, but does not show the virus. Perhaps it is at its very beginning. Perhaps the redia stage must also be present.

☒ Benzene (Solvent) YES

Is using Tom's™ toothpaste instead of Melaluca™; will switch to baking soda.

☒ Propyl Alcohol (Solvent) YES

Cannot give up the products she is accustomed to.

☒ Acetone (Solvent) YES

She will go back on parasite program and give up all toothpaste and body products this time.

One week later

☐ Fasciolopsis and all stages (Parasite) NO

☒ Benzene, Acetone (Solvents) YES

Returned to Melaluca™.

☐ Propyl Alcohol (Solvent) NO

She is accustomed to pure borax shampoo now and likes it.

One week later

☐ Solvents (ALL) NO

Including benzene. She has gone off her Melaluca™ products and wants to inform the company of their benzene pollution. She wants a written, signed statement from me verifying the presence of benzene in Melaluca™ products. I sympathized with her but declined because she should get a commercial laboratory to verify benzene; my technique would not be accepted by the company anyway. She is justifiably angry about this.

One month later

☒ PCB (Toxic Element) YES

Does not like using borax for dishes so went back to detergent but will go back to borax.

One week later

She still has breast pain.

☐ Fasciolopsis and all stages (Parasite) NO

☐ Protein 24 (HIV) NO

☐ Ortho-phospho-tyrosine (Cancer) NO

☒ PCB (Toxic Element) YES

Prefers detergent. I reminded her to continue on parasite maintenance program and stay off the entire benzene list.

Final Summary: We need many more persons like Kim who are so shocked that health foods and health products are polluted that it simply is unbelievable. Hopefully, she will turn her anger on the correct culprits after she has accepted the truth.

44	**Gracie Maddox**	**HIV**

Gracie is Kim Maddox's daughter, age 18, whose life is being ruined by chronic fatigue and undiagnosed illness. She is very pleasant and amenable to change in anything that will brighten her life and promise her a future. Because of her mother's history I suspect solvent toxicity.

☒ Benzene, Isopropyl alcohol, Acetone, Wood alcohol (Solvents) YES, high

Note: wood alcohol accumulates in the pancreas and upsets sugar regulation, the so-called "low blood sugar syndrome." The sugar substitute, Equal™ and soft drinks are two large sources of this solvent. She will stop these and go off Melaluca™ products and propanol sources. However, her mother claims she has been ill in a chronic, low level way, since puberty, before she was using these things.

☒ Fasciolopsis adults (Parasite) YES at thymus and vagina

Has a lot of pain with periods and irregularity.

☐ Fasciolopsis other stages (Parasite) NO

With benzene and the fluke present in the thymus, she must have the HIV virus!

☐ Protein 24 (HIV) NO

Possibly, a stage of the fluke brings the virus and no stages are currently present. Possibly, the virus is already present in the thymus but has not yet been triggered? Perhaps it is too early. Whatever the reason, we are very pleased. She will start parasite program.

One week later

☐ Fasciolopsis and all stages (Parasite) NO

☐ Protein 24 (HIV) NO

☐ Ortho-phospho-tyrosine (Cancer) NO

☒ Benzene, Isopropanol, Wood alcohol, Acetone (Solvents) YES

She has not gone off Melaluca™ products since her mother doesn't believe this is the source. I prevailed upon her to be serious in her effort to get well and stop taking risks.

One week later

☐ Solvents (ALL) NO

She stopped using Melaluca™ products but is not convinced it has anything to do with her chronic illness since she had it (the illness) long before she was using the product.

One month later

She is feeling ill and has cramps with her period.

- ☐ Fasciolopsis and all stages (Parasite) NO
- ☐ Pancreatic fluke (Parasite) NO
- ☒ Sheep liver fluke (Parasite) YES at uterus

  Cause of cramps. She will stay on parasite maintenance program and avoid eating meat.
- ☐ Solvents (ALL) NO
- ☒ PCB (Toxic Element) YES

  Off detergent.

Two weeks later

She is more fatigued than before.

- ☒ Gadolinium (Toxic Element) YES
- ☒ Palladium (Toxic Element) YES
- ☐ Toxic Elements (Remainder) NO

  She is advised to remove the one small tooth filling she has and get it replaced with metal-free plastic.
- ☒ Styrene (Solvent) YES

  Handles styrofoam in her job.
- ☒ Fasciolopsis redia (Parasite) YES
- ☒ Cat Liver fluke (Parasite) YES
- ☒ Ascaris, horse variety (Parasite) YES

  Remainder box 1 NO.

  She will start a 5-day high dose parasite program.

Six weeks later

She is suffering headaches.

- ☐ Ascaris, Cat Liver fluke (Parasite) NO
- ☐ Sheep liver fluke (Parasite) NO
- ☒ Sheep liver fluke redia (Parasite) YES
- ☐ Pancreatic fluke (Parasite) NO
- ☒ Pentane (Solvent) YES at thymus

  Stop drinking commercial beverages.

☒ Benzene (Solvent) YES

She is eating Bryer's™ ice cream and using Melaluca™ products again. She will stop but is not convinced because her mother is using them and is not ill.

☐ Ortho-phospho-tyrosine (Cancer) NO

☒ Protein 24 (HIV) YES

Now has the HIV virus. Note: There are no intestinal fluke stages at present. Can HIV be transmitted from them to sheep liver fluke or another fluke? This would be very unfortunate. Or did she have an intestinal fluke stage as recently as yesterday? She is not too upset about this result since she has little confidence in it anyway.

Two weeks later

☐ Protein 24 (HIV) NO

☐ Ortho-phospho-tyrosine (Cancer) NO

☐ Fasciolopsis and all stages (Parasite) NO

☐ Sheep liver fluke (Parasite) NO

☒ Pancreatic Fluke (Parasite) YES

The cause of chronic fatigue.

☒ Toluene, Hexane (Solvents) YES at pancreas

Drinking soda pop again.

☐ Solvents (Remainder) NO

She has only been drinking one bottle of commercial beverage a week. She will stop.

One month later

She is very fatigued and having some vision loss. She does not feel her health has improved by coming to us.

☐ Protein 24 (HIV) NO

☐ Ortho-phospho-tyrosine, hCG (Cancer) NO

☒ Wood Alcohol (Solvent) YES high

Cause of vision loss.

☒ Methylene chloride (Solvent) YES high

Drinking commercial orange juice.

☒ Kerosene (Solvent) YES

☐ Solvents (Remainder) NO

I am somewhat frustrated with this young woman's poor recovery. She should be able to tolerate more than she does. She is more health conscious than most. Perhaps she has tapeworm cysts coming out.

☒ Moniezia scolex (Parasite) YES at intestine

Says bowel does not wish to move, in spite of normal consistency, typical of Moniezia.

☒ Moniezia eggs (Parasite) YES

Start on special herbal combination for tapeworm, Rascal, take for 14 days as directed on label and include with parasite maintenance program once a week.

Summary: Gracie's history of on-again off-again illness and pollution is quite difficult to deal with. It is particularly common amongst young HIV patients. It is probably due to the extra-ordinary restrictiveness of the diet and habits I recommended. Perhaps there are unknown factors, even beyond parasites such as tapeworm, and solvents, that are involved with health. Yet there are plenty of cases where health returns with a "bang" after the tapes are cleared (provided restrictions are kept in place). One must ask: Is there permanent liver or thymus damage? Cases like Gracie's may help me understand this, eventually.

45	Joseph Haidu	HIV

Joseph arrived from the Southwest for his HIV positive condition. I assured him that he would be completely well soon. He has limited time (six days) in this area. He is seeing a clinical doctor frequently, is on antibiotics preventively, and is quite anxious about his condition. He is about 35. He does not appear very ill.

☒ Protein 24 (HIV) YES at thymus and penis

☐ hCG (Pre-Cancer) NO

☐ Ortho-phospho-tyrosine (Cancer) NO

☐ Fasciolopsis adults (Parasite) NO

☒ Fasciolopsis eggs (Parasite) YES throughout body and in saliva

We will get a saliva specimen for microscope study.

☒ Sheep liver fluke (Parasite) YES at thymus; NO at liver

Others not tested.

☒ Benzene (Solvent) YES throughout his body

☒ Propyl Alcohol (Solvent) YES at liver and thymus

He will start on parasite killing program. He will go off the benzene list and propanol containing body products such as shampoo.

☒ Wood Alcohol (Solvent) YES

☒ Decane (Solvent) YES

☐ Solvents (Remainder) NO

He will go off commercial beverages.

☒ Mercury, Nickel (Toxic Elements) YES at thymus

Tooth fillings.

☒ PCB (Toxic Element) YES at thymus

Off detergent. Others not tested. He is advised to remove all metal from his mouth and replace it with metal-free plastic. Joseph appears dismayed over this necessity. He plans to postpone this action.

☒ Influenza, EBV, CMV, Resp Syn V, Plantar Wart, B strep, Histopl cap, Adenovirus, Haem inf, Campyl pyl, Staph aur, Propio, Bacillus cer, Coxsackie B-1, Nocardia, Proteus mir, Strep pn, A strep, Gardner vag (Pathogens) YES

☒ Herpes zoster, Hep B (Pathogens) YES at thymus

End of box 1. This is obviously AIDS, since he has 21 YES out of 27 tests.

Two days later

☐ Ortho-phospho-tyrosine, hCG (Cancer) NO

☐ Protein 24 (HIV) NO

☐ Propyl Alcohol (Solvent) NO

☐ Benzene (Solvent) NO

☒ Hexane dione, Grain alcohol (Solvents) YES

He has used no alcoholic beverage. However, he is taking our Black Walnut Hull Tincture drops in the parasite program, which are 25% alcohol. Must take it in warm beverage.

☒ Salmonella typhi, Eikanella cor, E coli, Clostr tet, Bacill anth, Erwin coro, Blephar, Coryne dip, Neisseria, Coryne xer, Strep pyog, Sphaerot nat, Strep G, Trep pall, Veillon disp (Pathogens) YES

End box 2. He has 15 YES out of 40 tested, obviously still the picture of AIDS.

Two days later

☐ Ortho-phospho-tyrosine, hCG (Cancer) NO

☐ Protein 24 (HIV) NO

☒ Propyl Alcohol (Solvent) YES

Used Listerine™.

☐ Benzene (Solvent) NO

☒ Butyl Nitrite (Solvent) YES

Source unknown. Others not tested.

☒ Sodium Fluoride (Toxic Element) YES

In Listerine™?

☒ Thallium and Germanium (Toxic Elements) YES

This is a surprise! And explains, in part, his extremely low immunity even after the benzene and parasites are gone. He will save the dentist's tooth grindings for me to test for thallium.

☒ Antimony (Toxic Element) YES

Used Kiss My Face™ soap.

☒ Aluminum (Toxic Element) YES

Soap.

☒ Fiberglass (Toxic Element) YES

Is at a friend's house and will leave soon.

☒ Radon (Toxic Element) YES high

Possibly from friend's house.

☒ PVC (Toxic Element) YES

Possibly from friend's house.

☒ Formaldehyde (Toxic Element) YES
Got a foam mattress from the hospital will throw out.

Two days later

This is a follow-up to assess Joseph's improvement in immunity.

☐ Propyl Alcohol (Solvent) NO

☐ Benzene (Solvent) NO

☒ TCEthylene and several more food solvents (Solvent) YES
Others not tested. He has been drinking Celestial Seasonings™ tea and bottled water (probable sources).

☒ Pancreatic fluke adults (Parasite) YES at thymus

☒ Pancreatic fluke stages (Parasite) YES at thymus
Others not tested. He has eaten a hamburger (probable source). He is advised to be a vegetarian for 3 months to eliminate hazard of reinfection.

☒ Pathogens (MANY) YES
He tested positive, again, to 25 of 27 tests, a most devastating picture of AIDS. He was advised to return as soon as possible to this area in order to get his dental work done so his immunity can increase.

Summary: Joseph has accomplished his goal of eliminating the HIV virus but has not accomplished his goal of recovering from AIDS. He will probably be ill soon and will need to be hospitalized. Hopefully, he will get his dental work done before he is incapacitated and terminally ill.

46	**Lil Zwick**	**HIV**

Lil has been coming to our office for 1½ years for assorted problems. She had already cleared up a number of toxic pollution problems resulting from pesticide in their well water and arsenic and gas leaks in the house. She has also gone through a parasite killing program, liver cleansing, and kidney cleansing. She had complete dental work to remove metal and infections. She appeared in robust good health today but complained of a burning sensation at the top of her esophagus which she attributed to heartburn (she put her hand over her thymus, I suspect HIV).

☐ Ortho-phospho-tyrosine, hCG (Cancer) NO

☒ Protein 24 (HIV) YES at thymus and genital tract

☒ Fasciolopsis (Parasite) YES at thymus and vagina

☒ Benzene (Solvent) YES at thymus and vagina
Will avoid meats and all the items on our benzene list. The source is not obvious.

☒ Bismuth (Toxic Element) YES
Off skin lotion.

☒ Aluminum (Toxic Element) YES
Off deodorant.

☒ PVC (Toxic Element) YES
Source of PVC unknown. She will go back on the parasite program. She will also avoid isopropanol.

Six weeks later
Her chronic fungus problem is much better.

☐ Protein 24 (HIV) NO

☐ Ortho-phospho-tyrosine, hCG (Cancer) NO

☐ Parasites (All flukes) NO

☒ Taenia solium scolex (Parasite) YES
Tapeworm, start on Rascal for 3 bottles.

☒ Influenza (Pathogen) YES
All other respiratory pathogens were NO.

Summary: She feels like her old self again, able to work hard, physically; she has no more "heartburn." Notice how easy it is to acquire the HIV virus or a precancerous condition and how easy it is to get rid of it. Many healthy persons have probably gone through the cycle of getting it and losing it numerous times.

Marilyn Werdick	**HIV Illness and Pancreatic Cancer**

Marilyn Werdick came with a diagnosis of pancreatic cancer at age 50. It happened suddenly, with stomach trouble two months ago. She thought it was due to her pain medicine for lower back pain. CAT scan showed area of pancreas that was suspicious. Biopsy showed pancreatic cancer. Surgery was begun but they just sewed her back up. She is on morphine. She is still smoking but promised to stop.

☒ Protein 24 (HIV) YES at thymus, vagina, pancreas

☒ Ortho-phospho-tyrosine (Cancer) YES at pancreas

☒ Fasciolopsis (Parasite) YES at liver and thymus

☒ Fasciolopsis eggs (Parasite) YES at thymus, NO elsewhere

☐ Sheep liver fluke (Parasite) NO

She has no sensations over the breast bone.

☒ Gardnerella, Flu, Plantar Wart, Strep pn, Trichomonas, Adenovirus, Campylobacter, Alpha Strep, Proteus v, Papilloma 4, Bacillus cereus, Nocardia, Staph aureus (Pathogens) YES

☐ Bacteroides fr, Haemoph inf, Herpes 1, CMV, Borellia, EBV, Shigella, Histoplasma, Chlamydia, Coxsackie B4, Salmonella, Resp Sync V (Pathogens) NO

Stopped here (this is less than half the test). This shows AIDS-like lost immunity. Too many pathogens are growing in her. Her body must be full of solvent.

☒ Benzene, Wood Alcohol, Hexane, Pentane, Propyl Alcohol (Solvents) YES

She was started on parasite killing program. She will be off all commercial beverages and cosmetics and benzene sources.

Four days later

She missed her appointment.

Twelve days later

She died (telephone call).

Summary: Marilyn had none of the risk factors associated with HIV. She was just an ordinary middle-age woman who didn't drink alcoholic beverages. If she had acted quickly, she would most likely have survived and gotten reasonably well again. Perhaps she missed her appointment because of embarrassment over not being able to stop smoking. Maybe I was too hard on her about it. We did not hear any details surrounding her death. Notice the adult fluke in the thymus where T cells are made. The thymus is a small gland and the fluke is a large parasite; it is like having an elephant in the kitchen. How could the thymus do its work? People often feel strange sensations at the top of their breast bone when flukes are in it, but she didn't. Cancer and

<u>HIV illness are first cousin diseases.</u> Cancer results when propanol builds up in the body. AIDS develops when benzene builds up.

47 Harlan Wilson	HIV

This 76 year old man has been coming to our office for the past year, for a variety of ailments including heart disease and pain in his hips as well as his hearing loss. He had already done a parasite killing program and had cleaned up his teeth. Suddenly he tested POSITIVE for HIV infection in my office in a routine test.

☒ Protein 24 (HIV) YES

☒ Campylobacter, Coxsackie virus, Nocardia, Chlamydia, Staph aureus, Klebsiella, Gaffkya, Clostridium tet (Pathogens) YES

☒ Wood Alcohol (Solvent) YES
Off commercial beverages and chemical sweeteners.

☒ Benzene (Solvent) YES

☐ Solvents (Remainder) NO

☒ Fasciolopsis eggs (Parasite) YES at thymus

☐ Fasciolopsis adults and other stages (Parasite) NO
He has been eating hamburger and pork sausage. He will go on a parasite killing program. He had neglected the maintenance program for several months. His pulse is irregular; he will stay off caffeine.

One week later

☐ Protein 24 (HIV) NO

☐ Ortho-phospho-tyrosine (Cancer) NO

☐ Benzene (Solvent) NO

☐ Wood alcohol (Toxic Element) NO

☐ Nocardia, Chlamydia, Coxsackie 4, Gaffkya, Klebsiella (Pathogens) NO

☒ Staph aureus, Clostr tet (Pathogens) YES
Tooth bacteria, cause of heart problem. He is much better. We will search for teeth responsible next time.

One month later

His pulse is still irregular. He is on new heart medication from his clinical doctor.

☒ Chlamydia, Bacter fr, Coxsackie B1 (Pathogens) YES

☐ Pathogens (Remainder box 1) NO

☒ Ascaris, Treponema (Parasites) YES

☐ Ascaris megalo (Parasite) NO

☒ Staph aureus (Pathogen) YES high

Probable cause of heart disease. Remainder not tested. Ascaris worms always bring Bacteroides fragilis bacteria and the Coxsackie viruses. He has not seen dentist yet.

Five months later

He had a check up recently with his clinical doctor who pronounced him well and told him that his blood test was good.

☐ Protein 24 (HIV) NO

☐ Ortho-phospho-tyrosine (Cancer) NO

☒ hCG (Pre-Cancer) YES at intestine

He is just beginning a cancer!

☒ Fasciolopsis adults (Parasite) YES at intestine and one part of the liver

He has been eating hamburger and chicken. He will go back on parasite program, 5 day high dose.

☒ Propyl Alcohol (Solvent) YES

Has been using commercial shampoo; will switch to borax.

Summary: Notice how easy it is to pick up the intestinal fluke parasite and how easy it is to start a cancer or get HIV from it. But it also takes propyl alcohol to start a cancer and benzene to start HIV. Hopefully, our meat supply and other foods will be cleared of parasites and solvents soon, so the risks are removed.

48	Joyce Stegeman	HIV, Breast Cancer, Colon Cancer

Joyce has been going to a clinical doctor for 2 months, but no diagnosis has been reached. She reported the following problems: 1) fatigue; 2) hunger and nausea both; 3) warmth in head (mild fever?), occasional chills; 4) sounds like wind tunnel inside the head (roaring); 5) loose bowels, 3 to 4 times daily; 6) weight loss; 7) weakness; 8) tired and restless at same time; 9) some numbness. Slight inflammation of the liver was seen by one doctor.

☒ Fasciolopsis (Parasite) YES at gallbladder, liver, thymus; NO at intestine

☒ Fasciolopsis redia (Parasite) YES

☒ Ortho-phospho-tyrosine (Cancer) YES at colon and breast
She had intense stinging in her colon and in both her breasts and under armpits 2 months ago, but it went away.

☒ Protein 24 (HIV) YES
This came as a surprise. She was tested clinically for HIV a few months ago; it was NO (negative). She seemed relieved to hear these findings; that is, that she was HIV positive; she thought she'd had it for some time.

☒ Dipetalonema, Echinococcus granulosus, Fischoedrius, Haemoproteus, Toxoplasma (Parasite) YES
Start on parasite program.

Four days later

☐ Fasciolopsis (Parasite) NO

☐ Ortho-phospho-tyrosine (Cancer) NO

☒ Benzene (Solvent) YES at muscle, bone, thyroid, thymus
She is using Tom's™ fennel toothpaste. Will go off.

☒ Tin (Toxic Element) YES at muscle, bone, thyroid, thymus
Toothpaste.

Three days later

☐ Tin (Toxic Element) NO

☒ Benzene (Solvent) YES
She has been off toothpaste. She will go off the whole benzene list. She is too fatigued to go to work.

Six days later
She is feeling more like herself. No hot spells, but she is not well.

☐ Benzene (Solvent) NO

☐ Protein 24 (HIV) NO

☒ Dipetalonema, Pancreatic fluke (Parasite) YES; remainder of box 1 NO

Summary: Joyce had both cancer and the HIV virus. Small wonder that her symptoms were too confusing for clinical doctors to reach a diagnosis. By the time I saw her I was routinely testing everybody for Protein 24 in their white blood cells (immune system); P24 is a small chip off the core of the virus. When the intestinal fluke was gone, both cancer and HIV were gone! She had the solvent benzene accumulated in her; propanol was not tested at the first visit so it can't be ruled out of the picture. Joyce got her health back. Her illness had made her financially broke, so she did not come back. She was only in her early 30's. We hope she is staying off benzene and propanol sources.

Debra Ells	**HIV, Colon, Stomach Cancer, Liver Cancer**

This is a 41 year old woman who came in for a long list of problems: 1) Cysts and rashes on skin. She has had them removed from back of neck, ears, chin, breast and even fingers. (My guess is these are PCB caused.) 2) Swelling at joints all over body. 3) Pain everywhere: elbows, shoulders, wrists, hands, chest, lower back, legs, knees, feet, and headaches. This suggests gallstones and rheumatoid arthritis but the chest pain doesn't fit into this picture. I will test for HIV (She is using Advil™ as a pain killer. It doesn't help much.) 4) Stomach problem.

She had a hysterectomy for excessive bleeding in her early 20's and her ovaries were removed 5 years ago. A total mastectomy was done 8 years ago for multiple cysts and she got breast implants but had to have them removed for leakage later.

I discussed with her the need to do all 5 of our routines and that she would probably be much better in 3 months. These would be: 1) Kidney cleanse; 2) Parasite killing; 3) Toxic element removal; 4) Bacteria and virus elimination; and 5) Liver cleanse.

Since her urinalysis showed crystals in the urine, we would start with a kidney cleanse.

☒ Ortho-phospho-tyrosine (Cancer) YES at colon, liver, and stomach

I explained to Debra that this unexpected result would change the order of our program; we would kill parasites first. She said her brother had died of cirrhosis of the liver; she was not too surprised she had liver cancer!

☒ Fasciolopsis (Parasite) YES at thymus, blood, colon, stomach; NOT IN LIVER!

☒ Fasciolopsis cercaria (Parasite) YES at thymus and stomach only

☐ Fasciolopsis remaining stages (Parasite) NO

This picture suggests HIV/AIDS illness together with cancer. There are probably other flukes, like the liver fluke and pancreatic fluke at the extra locations. But I did not test since she had enough shock from hearing about the cancer. I postponed the tests for 2 days. She will start on parasite killing program.

Two days later

☐ Ortho-phospho-tyrosine (Cancer) NO

☐ Fasciolopsis and all stages (Parasite) NO

When I gave her this exceptionally good news, she was not happy since she did not feel any differently; she had no pain relief and she expressed her disappointment.

☒ Arsenic (Toxic Element) YES

☒ Europium, Lutetium, Yttrium, Ytterbium (Toxic Elements) YES

☐ Toxic Elements (Remainder) NO

Since health supplements and drug tablets were implicated, plus her carpets, she could not believe my explanations. I decided to postpone this part of her corrective programs and go directly to HIV testing.

☒ Protein 24 (HIV) YES at genital tract and thymus

She did not believe this result, nor was she willing to go for a conventional HIV test at the Health Department. I could see she was very angry and would not come back to see me. I emphasized the primary importance of staying on a parasite killing maintenance program. I did not manage to warn her of the solvents benzene and propyl alcohol, or of the danger of eating undercooked beef, chicken and turkey.

Summary: It is understandable when a sick person finds our methods and results too strange to believe. Hopefully, as illness worsens, she will get tested and find her way back here. Note: In HIV cases, the adult fluke has developed from a metacercaria in the THYMUS, not in the LIVER.

49* Alex Solis	HIV

Alex is a short, stocky person, brought by his sister from a nearby state. Alex is somnolent, sleeping 23 out of 24 hours. He did not speak for himself but was able to walk alone. He has been HIV POSITIVE for about a year. In the past he was very healthy. He was hospitalized for 6 weeks in Kentucky and is on medication for Toxoplasma, TB, etc.

☒ Protein 24 (HIV) YES at thymus and penis; NO at urine, saliva, etc.

☐ Ortho-phospho-tyrosine, hCG (Cancer) NO

There is no cancer or precancer.

☒ Fasciolopsis (Parasite) YES at intestine, thymus; NO at liver

☒ Benzene (Solvent) YES at thymus, intestine; NO at liver

He will start parasite program and go off all benzene-polluted products on my list. Since his sister is very health-oriented, the source of benzene in such high quantities was not obvious. They will bring in their water supply for testing.

Two days later

☐ Protein 24 (HIV) NO

The virus is gone.

☒ Benzene (Solvent) YES

We're not sure where this is coming from—he is drinking a tonic made by a relative, using cold tap water and fresh herbs; also using spring water (fresh from the spring). Both of these are here for testing:

☒ Benzene (Solvent) YES in Tonic, YES in Water

This came as a shock since they do not live near a toxic dump. The sample bottles may be contaminated. They will immediately get new samples and have them sent overnight mail.

☒ Candida, Influenza, Mycoplasma, Salmonella ent, CMV, Hepatitis B (Pathogens) YES

6 out of 8 pathogens tested YES. This low immunity indicates AIDS. Note: It was especially easy for Alex to kill all parasites, taking only 2 days, instead of 5. Perhaps his herbal concoction is also a parasiticide. But he will stop using it and switch to using faucet water immediately.

One day later

☐ Protein 24 (HIV) NO

☒ Benzene (Solvent) YES

☐ Benzene (Solvent) NO in faucet water

They have also been drinking distilled water from the grocery store. They will go off this and use ONLY faucet water.

☒ Aluminum (Toxic Element) YES

☒ Mercury (Toxic Element) YES

Needs to remove metal from mouth.

☒ Asbestos (Toxic Element) YES high

Sister is using a hair blower; will stop.

☒ Cobalt, PCB (Toxic Elements) YES

Off detergent. They will use pure borax only, for all purposes and use no detergent.

☒ All 6 drugs, Vitamin B6 (Samples) YES

His white blood cells are working on removing one or more things in these. Change brands and bring in for testing.

Two days later

☐ Protein 24 (HIV) NO

☐ Benzene (Solvent) NO

☒ TCEthylene, Hexane dione (Solvents) YES high

Restaurant food.

☐ Solvents (Remainder) NO

Note: Alex is well enough to sit for a longer period of time for testing. The entire solvent test was done this time, not only the benzene test. Note how few other solvents he has, a tribute to his sister's home cooking and food selection.

☒ Oxalate, all Phosphates, Uric Acid (Kidney Stones) YES

Start on kidney herbs. Note how many kidney stone varieties he has!

Two days later

Memory and mental function is very much better. Fatigue is slightly better. He is still sleeping 21 out of 24 hours. He is able to smile. He converses a bit with his sister.

☐ Protein 24 (HIV) NO

☐ Benzene (Solvent) NO

☒ Wood Alcohol (Solvent) YES

☐ Solvents (Remainder) NO

☒ PCB (Toxic Element) YES

Was using some Dr. Bronner's Baby Supermild Soap™; will stop and use borax only.

☒ Radon (Toxic Element) YES

Move into a different hotel room. End of box 1.

☐ Pneumocyst carnii, TB, Paragonimus Westermanii (Parasites) NO

☒ Taenia solium scolex (Parasite) YES in liver

☒ Taenia pisiformis cysticercus (Parasite) YES in liver

Start on Rascal; take 4 capsules 3 times a day for about 3 weeks.

Three days later

He feels he is getting better. Still sleeping about 16 hours out of 24. He speaks to me for himself. He produced an entire sentence.

☐ Protein 24 (HIV) NO

☐ Ortho-phospho-tyrosine, hCG (Cancer) NO

☐ Benzene (Solvent) NO

☐ Propyl Alcohol (Solvent) NO

☒ Urocleidus (Parasite) YES

☒ Trypanosoma gambiense, Trypanosoma equip (Parasites) YES

Sleeping sickness.

☒ Trypanosoma lewisi, Trypanosoma brucei, Trypanosoma rhodesiense, Trichuris (Parasites) YES

☐ Trypanosoma cruzi (Parasite) NO

☒ Naegleria (Parasite) YES high

Note: Naegleria is a brain parasite. He has 2 kinds of "sleeping sickness." He has been in Africa in the past. These infections may account for his extreme somnolence. He is continuing the parasite program.

Two days later

☒ Trypanosoma lewisi, Trypanosoma brucei (Parasites) YES

☐ Trypanosoma cruzi, Trypanosoma rhodesiense, Trypanosoma equip, Trypanosoma gambiense (Parasites) NO

☐ Naegleria (Parasite) NO

☒ Schistosoma mansoni (Parasite) YES high

☐ Protein 24 (HIV) NO

☐ hCG (Pre-Cancer) NO

☐ Benzene (Solvent) NO

☐ Propyl Alcohol (Solvent) NO

☒ Benzene (Solvent) YES in water samples

Water samples of both spring water and cold faucet water were sent from his home. Both tested YES for benzene. This seems extremely enigmatic to his sister. She will remove all possible source of pollution after she gets home and we will then retest the water for her. Since Alex is improving, they have my permission to be away on a 1 week vacation.

One week later

Alex is walking about and converses with his sister and others who speak to him. He is very much better.

☐ Protein 24 (HIV) NO

☐ Ortho-phospho-tyrosine, hCG (Cancer) NO

☒ Histoplasma, Chlamydia trachomatis, Herpes simplex 1, Adenovirus, 2 Coxsackie viruses, Measles (Pathogens) YES

End box 1. Note: He still has 7 out of 27 pathogens tested; he still has low immunity but not AIDS.

Two days later

He is conversant when awake but is still sleeping approximately 18 hours.

☐ Taenia pisiformis cysticercus (Parasite) NO in all tissues

☒ Taenia saginata cyst (Parasite) YES at liver

He will stay on Rascal as originally directed. Then he will take it 2 days a week.

Summary: Alex is ready to go home. He will stay in his sister's home until follow-up time in one month. His sister has done an admirable job in reclaiming Alex from his imminent comatose condition. Hopefully, they will not run into a polluted-water problem while at her home. They will continue their parasite program and diet and product restrictions. They were given blood test requisitions at last visit; will test for HIV antigen P24. They are very pleased with Alex's new found health.

About ten days later

Report received from clinical laboratory for Alex Solis: HIV antigen NEGATIVE.

50	Calvin Parker	HIV

This 34 year old man was diagnosed as HIV POSITIVE about 5 years ago. He started taking AZT 4 years ago. He is alternating between AZT and DDI plus Bactrim™. He was referred by a cancer client. He is not visibly ill.

☒ Protein 24 (HIV) YES at thymus, kidneys, semen and urine

☐ Ortho-phospho-tyrosine, hCG (Cancer) NO

☒ Fasciolopsis (Parasite) YES at thymus, liver and intestine

☒ Fasciolopsis eggs (Parasite) YES high at urine and saliva

Others not tested. Start on parasite program.

☒ Benzene (Solvent) YES at thymus only (low level)
He will go off all benzene-polluted items on my list.

One week later

He is getting a CBC and T cell count every 3 weeks. He is on day 7 of the parasite program.

☐ Fasciolopsis and all stages (Parasite) NO

☒ Hexane dione (Solvent) YES
Flavored food.

☒ Ether (Solvent) YES
He will be more careful when pumping gasoline.

☐ Solvents (Remainder) NO
He does not have benzene in him today; this is good progress.

☒ Silver (Toxic Element) YES

☒ Thallium (Toxic Element) YES high
Remainder not tested. Thallium is probably coming from his metal tooth fillings, probably as a pollutant of mercury. He needs all metal removed from mouth.

☒ Influenza, Shigella flex, Adenovirus, Mumps, Coxsackie B4, Histoplasma (Pathogens) YES

☒ Haemophilus infl (Pathogen) YES at part of thymus only

☒ Staph aureus (Pathogen) YES at part of thymus only

☒ Herpes simplex 1 (Pathogen) YES
Also visible in mouth. End of box 1. He has 9 out of 27 tests positive, moderate AIDS. He will take 1 dose of Oscillococcinum at bedtime for flu.

Two weeks later

He has a dental appointment. He has not had an illness, and this past week his energy returned.

☐ Protein 24 (HIV) NO

☐ Ortho-phospho-tyrosine, hCG (Cancer) NO

☒ Methyl propanol (Solvent) YES
Will test chocolate which is his weakness.

☒ Formaldehyde (Toxic Element) YES
Will test house air.

☐ Toxic Elements (Remainder) NO

☒ Staph aureus, Clostridium sept, Pseudomonas, Clostridium bot, Erwinia caro, Strep G, Haemophilus inf, Troglodytella, Mycobacterium TB, Treponema pneu, Pneumocystis carn, Veillonella, Sphaerotilus natans (Pathogens) YES

End box 2. At least 5 of these are tooth bacteria; they should disappear after dental work.

One week later

He has had no illness. All the metal is out of his mouth. He still has plastic crowns (maybe they will be OK and not need replacement). He is feeling very much better with less fatigue. He found a dentist near his home to do the necessary work.

☐ Protein 24 (HIV) NO

☐ Ortho-phospho-tyrosine, hCG (Cancer) NO

☐ Solvents (ALL) NO

☒ Formaldehyde (Toxic Element) YES and in living room air

He has 2 pieces of new fabric furniture in living room; he will separate furniture placing them into two different rooms and test the air in each room to find out which piece is fuming formaldehyde. He has been on Rascal for a week.

☐ Taenia pisiformis, Taenia solium (Parasites) NO

☒ Staph aureus, Haemophilus influenzae, Herpes zoster (Pathogens) YES

☐ Pathogens (Remainder) NO

He has only 3 infections growing in him out of 67 tested! This is better than average. The dental work has had a profoundly beneficial effect. He is ready for his clinical HIV antigen test.

One week later

He has had no illness.

☐ Protein 24 (HIV) NO

☐ Ortho-phospho-tyrosine, hCG (Cancer) NO

☐ Aflatoxin (Toxin) NO

☐ Formaldehyde (Toxic Element) NO

Removing furniture worked! Stay on Rascal, take for 1 day a week.

☐ Herpes zoster (Pathogen) NO

One month later

His clinical test results came back POSITIVE for HIV.

Summary: Calvin was an exemplary client; he did everything correctly. What went wrong? Why did his clinical test say positive when mine said negative? There are several possible explanations, but the best course of action is to repeat my test, correct any regression that might have occurred, and then repeat the clinical test once more.

51	**Maurice Johnson**	**HIV**

Maurice is a 44 year old man with a prostate problem. He gets up more than once during the night to urinate. He had a severe prostate infection in his early 20's. He has been experiencing swelling for about 6 months. He also has occasional lower back pain. He will start on the kidney herbs for these symptoms. He will take it full strength for 3-4 weeks and then ½ half strength for 3 months. He also experienced some chest pain 3 years ago, so severe he thought it was a heart attack.

☒ Protein 24 (HIV) YES

☐ Ortho-phospho-tyrosine, hCG (Cancer) NO

☒ Benzene (Solvent) YES

☒ Fasciolopsis (Parasite) YES
Start on parasite killing program. He will avoid all items on the benzene-polluted list.

One day later

☐ Protein 24 (HIV) NO

☒ Propyl Alcohol, 1 Methyl Propanol (Solvents) YES
Shaving supplies and mouthwash.

☐ Benzene (Solvent) NO

☐ Solvents (Remainder) NO

☒ Schistosoma haematobium (Parasite) YES
Probable cause of prostate problem.

☒ Taenia pisiformis cysticercus (Parasite) YES

☒ **Dirofilaria immitis (Parasite) YES**
Probable cause of chest pain experience.

☐ **Loa Loa (Parasite) NO**
Others not tested.

☒ **Antimony (Toxic Element) YES**
Off colognes and fragrant body products.

☒ **Fiberglass (Toxic Element) YES**
Check insulation, make sure it is covered, no holes.

☒ **Aluminum, Aluminum Silicate (Toxic Elements) YES**
Off deodorant and soap.

☒ **Mercury (Toxic Element) YES**
Needs all metal out of mouth.

☒ **PCB (Toxic Element) YES**
Off detergent, use borax only.

☒ **Nickel (Toxic Element) YES**
Tooth fillings.

Summary: Since Maurice is from another far away country, he cannot return for several months to follow-up. He plans to be very compliant. He was not surprised at his HIV positive status and, in fact, is somewhat relieved to hear about his real problem. It was easy for him to shed the parasite and the HIV virus and to avoid benzene.

52 Orlo Kremer — HIV and Kaposi's

(Orlo Kremer's file covering his first few visits was lost, so I am writing this introduction from memory.)

Orlo is a terminally ill young man in his mid-thirties who was brought to our office by his friend. During critical periods his friend would bring him to his own home and care for him. Orlo had no interest in alternative therapy but his friend did, and insisted on his taking vitamins and herbs. This had gone on for several years before coming to my office. In his near terminal state, Orlo offered little resistance physically but still resisted emotionally. His diagnosis had never been clear but his friend suspected AIDS. Not until Orlo broke out into purple spots all over his right arm was Kaposi's diagnosed.

Upon arrival, Orlo was barely ambulatory, breathing with difficulty but he had not stopped smoking. His friend appealed to me to come down as hard as possible on Orlo for this. Normally, this loses me a client. But I would lose him shortly anyway, so I took Orlo aside and told him in no uncertain terms that he would die, yes die, if he did not quit. He must quit this very day. I asked his friend, when they were back together, NOT to purchase cigarettes for him when so requested.

Orlo tested YES (positive) to HIV, as expected, and was started on the parasite program. At the next visit he was still smoking. But his friend was relentless in his persuasion and by his third visit Orlo had quit. His friend was very happy. We shared his joy.

Next visit (new file)

His skin looks better, purple spots are fading, but he is feeling no better. His appetite is good. He still has night sweats.

☐ Protein 24 (HIV) NO

☐ Ortho-phospho-tyrosine, hCG (Cancer) NO

☐ Benzene (Solvent) NO

☐ 4 Leishmonias (Parasite) NO

☒ Candida, Nocardia (high), Mycoplasma (Pathogens) YES

☒ Moniezia scolex, eggs (Parasite) YES

Start Rascal.

Eleven days later

He was sick last week, just feeling bad; is staying with friend.

☐ Protein 24 (HIV) NO

☐ Ortho-phospho-tyrosine, hCG (Cancer) NO

☒ Moniezia scolex (Parasite) YES at pancreas, NO at white blood cells

☒ Moniezia eggs (Parasite) YES at pancreas and white blood cells

☐ Moniezia main body (Parasite) NO

☐ Other tapeworm eggs (ALL) NO

Two weeks later

He has bad diarrhea. He has been in the hospital. He has gained 13 pounds. He feels well in spite of being sore and achy. He has been living at home. There is a dog in the house.

☒ Fasciolopsis eggs (Parasite) YES in saliva, semen, spleen, urine

We will take a saliva sample to search under microscope.

☒ Human liver fluke adults (Pathogen) YES

☐ Sheep liver fluke (Parasite) NO

☐ Pancreatic fluke (Parasite) NO

☒ Benzene (Solvent) YES

Off ice cream.

☒ Decane (Solvent) YES

Remaining solvents not tested. He will go off cold cereal. He will go back on the 5 day high dose parasite program. He has been eating hamburgers at restaurants. He will go to stay with friend.

☐ Protein 24 (HIV) NO

☐ Ortho-phospho-tyrosine, hCG (Cancer) NO

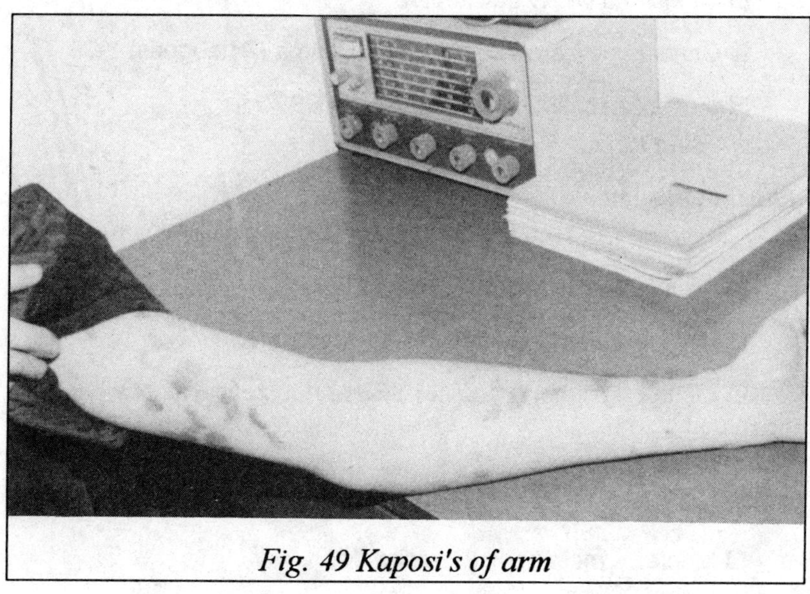

Fig. 49 Kaposi's of arm

Two months later

He looks no better. His arm is covered with purple spots, at least a dozen, some as large as quarters.

☒ Fasciolopsis adult (Parasite) YES at skin

☒ Sheep liver fluke (Parasite) YES at skin

☒ Pancreatic fluke (Parasite) YES at skin

With all three of these large flukes in his skin, it is no wonder he has purple spots.

☒ Necator americanus larva, Taenia pisiformis cysticercus, Taenia solium scolex (Parasites) YES

☐ 4 Leishmanias (Parasite) NO

☐ Protein 24 (HIV) NO

He does not yet have the virus back; perhaps the redia stage is necessary for this; perhaps benzene is essential also.

☐ Benzene (Solvent) NO

☐ Ortho-phospho-tyrosine (Cancer) NO

☒ hCG (Pre-Cancer) YES high everywhere

☒ Propyl Alcohol (Solvent) YES high

Off shampoo and cold cereal. Others not tested.

☒ Arsenic (Toxic Element) YES

Pesticides in house. Must be removed.

☒ Cobalt (Toxic Element) YES

Detergent. Go back to borax and washing soda.

☒ Vanadium (Toxic Element) YES

Gas leak. They will find it immediately.

Summary: We would have liked to show a picture of beautifully recovered skin, but that desire could not be accomplished in time for this book. We admire both Orlo's efforts to comply, and his friend's efforts to save Orlo's life. This has been going on for a number of years, and I hope they succeed.

53* Roy Ferguson	HIV

Roy, age 29, was first seen six months ago regarding his HIV positive status. Two years previously he began to be ill. Last year he had shingles and thrush. He brought with him a considerable number of blood test results, done as recently as a few months ago, showing a CD4 count of 300/mm³ and a CD4/CD8 ratio of 0.18. He also had tested positive to HIV. He appeared healthy.

☒ Protein 24 (HIV) YES in numerous tissues

☐ Ortho-phospho-tyrosine (Cancer) NO

☒ hCG (Pre-Cancer) YES at intestine only

☒ Fasciolopsis (Parasite) YES at thymus and intestine; NO at liver and bone marrow

☒ Benzene (Solvent) YES

This was a very short initial visit, confirming his status. He will start on parasite killing program and stay off the benzene-pollution list. He will eat only fish and seafood for 3 months. He will bring in suspicious products for testing that he is using and are not on the benzene list.

One week later

☐ Protein 24 (HIV) NO

☐ Ortho-phospho-tyrosine, hCG (Cancer) NO

☒ Benzene (Solvent) YES at thymus only

He has been off all products on the benzene list. But he has used Halls Plus™ with liquid center for congestion and has eaten Bryer's™ Strawberry yogurt. He will stop this.

☒ Hepatitis B, Salmonella ent, CMV, Borellia, Shigella flex, Papilloma #4, Influenza, Bacteroid fr, A strep, Strep pn, Chlamydia trach, Measles, Gardnerella vag, Campyl pyl, Mycoplasma, Herpes Simplex 1, Respiratory syn v, B strep, Bacillus cereus, Histoplasma cap, EBV (Pathogens) YES

End box 1. He tested positive for 21 out of 29 pathogens, definitely AIDS. He will take 1 tbs. of L-G 4 times a day and continue the parasite program.

One week later

Neck glands are down, no longer swollen. Energy is slightly up.

☐ Protein 24 (HIV) NO

☐ Ortho-phospho-tyrosine, hCG (Cancer) NO

☐ Benzene (Solvent) NO

☐ Propyl Alcohol (Solvent) NO

☒ Methyl Ethyl Ketone (Solvent) YES

☒ Hexane (Solvent) YES

☐ Solvents (Remainder) NO

He will be more careful to avoid flavored and processed foods.

☒ Regular gasoline (Toxic Element) YES

☒ Mineral oil (Toxic Element) YES

Uses Aubrey™ products, will stop.

☒ Haemophilus inf, Salmonella ent, Borellia, Chlamydia trach, Nocardia, Mycoplasma, B strep, Papilloma #4, Plantar wart, Coxsackie B1 (Pathogens) YES

Note: He still has 10 out of 29 pathogens, a considerable improvement, but still indicative of AIDS.

One week later

His tongue shows a little improvement.

☐ Protein 24 (HIV) NO

☐ Ortho-phospho-tyrosine, hCG (Cancer) NO

☐ Benzene (Solvent) NO

☒ Candida, Corynebacterium dipth, Bordetella pertussis, Corynebacterium xerosis (Pathogens) YES

Only 4 out of 29 pathogens are active.

One week later

Tongue still sore but improved. He feels fine.

☐ Protein 24 (HIV) NO

☐ Ortho-phospho-tyrosine, hCG (Cancer) NO

☒ Taenia pisiformis cysticercus (Parasite) YES at muscles

☒ Taenia solium (Parasite) YES at muscles

He is too fatigued to hold a job.

☒ Mineral oil (Toxic Element) YES

Stop soap and lotion. Use our recipes.

☒ Grain Alcohol (Solvent) YES

He is using our Black Walnut Hull Tincture. His liver can't even oxidize these few drops in an hour! Must put them in warm beverage.

☐ Solvents (Remainder) NO

One week later

He has had no illness; feels quite well. Tongue is about 50% improved.

☐ Protein 24 (HIV) NO

☐ Ortho-phospho-tyrosine, hCG (Cancer) NO

☐ Taenia pisiformis cysticercus (Parasite) NO everywhere

☒ Taenia solium scolex (Parasite) YES at muscle

Start on Rascal; take for 2 bottles.

☐ Benzene (Solvent) NO

☐ Propyl Alcohol (Solvent) NO

☒ Candida, Coxsackie viruses (both), Chlamydia (Pathogens) YES

He is ready for clinical testing for HIV antigen.

One week later:

He has had some lower back pain; will start on our kidney herb recipe.

☐ Protein 24 (HIV) NO

☐ Ortho-phospho-tyrosine, hCG (Cancer) NO

☒ Benzene (Solvent) YES

He suspects a new personal product he is using. He will stop using it.

☐ Propyl Alcohol (Solvent) NO

☒ Aflatoxin (Toxic Element) YES in liver

He will be much more careful to avoid moldy food. I suspect beer. He will do without beer.

☒ Taenia solium cysticercus (Parasite) YES at muscle

Continue Rascal for a third bottle, then for 1 day a week as maintenance. Note: because of the great risk of exposure to benzene-polluted products, Roy will continue follow-ups weekly for a while.

One week later

His clinical test result was NEGATIVE for the HIV antigen. His tongue is improved and less sore, but still deeply furrowed. He has not been ill this week.

☐ Protein 24 (HIV) NO

☐ Ortho-phospho-tyrosine, hCG (Cancer) NO

☐ Aflatoxin (Toxic Element) NO

Has been off peanut butter; keeps his bread in freezer; uses no vinegar.

☒ Candida (Pathogen) YES

We will make a new tongue swab to capture his remaining tongue pathogens on a permanent slide. He is no longer POSITIVE to his earlier slide. Roy is overjoyed at his good results and knowing that his careful adherence to the new lifestyle will protect him.

Summary: Roy was an exemplary client. Fortunately, he was not too ill to take charge of his lifestyle and was able to comply promptly. He never missed an appointment and was an inspiration to us all. He cleared his HIV virus in the first week (probably the first few days) but clearing the AIDS took longer. Once a client has been declared free of disease, it is all too easy to feel overconfident and begin to take small risks. For this reason, we do not recommend the clinical test until six weeks have passed free of the virus. Roy will continue to follow up once a month, sooner if ill.

Finale

I hope you reach the same conclusions as I did from these case histories:

- **HIV is not caused solely by sexual or blood contact** with an infected person. People with no such exposures, even small children and babies, have it. It comes with a parasite which you can pick up easily in your daily routine. It is way too prevalent, and we are all at risk!
- **It is amazing how easy** the HIV virus is to eliminate—*Fasciolopsis buskii* is one of the first to succumb to the parasite killing herbs—but it is just as easy to get reinfected. Nor does getting rid of HIV bring relief, since the thymus has been attacked, immunity has been lost, and AIDS has progressed.
- **Benzene is just as much the problem as HIV**, because it assisted the parasite to seek out the thymus. Worse, it is not suspected that such minute amounts as pollute our foods could accumulate in some persons.
- **If you have HIV you are halfway to having cancer** because the same parasite causes both. All cancer needs to develop now is propyl alcohol.
- **Eliminating HIV does not cure AIDS.** The damage is already done.
- **You can beat AIDS** with a complete program of lifting the burdens on your immune system (dental, diet, body, home). Your body will "miraculously" heal.

One thing that is not clear is why it seems more young people are contracting HIV/AIDS than older people. My explanation, which I am not satisfied with, is that the list of benzene polluted products is used more by younger people.

Also, the homosexual men I see often use lubricants, "rush", and marijuana, all of which are benzene sources.

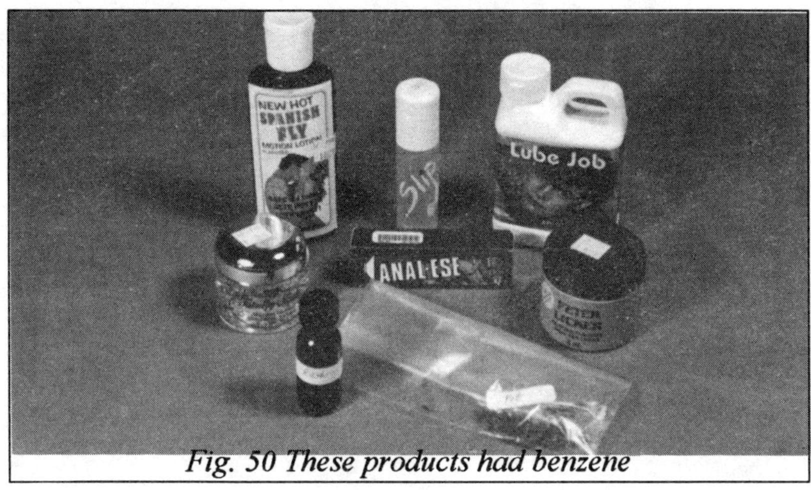

Fig. 50 These products had benzene

The solution stands out clearly. Monitor food and feed for solvent pollution. This would return the parasite to its former status as an <u>intestinal</u> fluke, unable to invade other organs. I hope these case histories have provided the incentive to begin this clean up program.

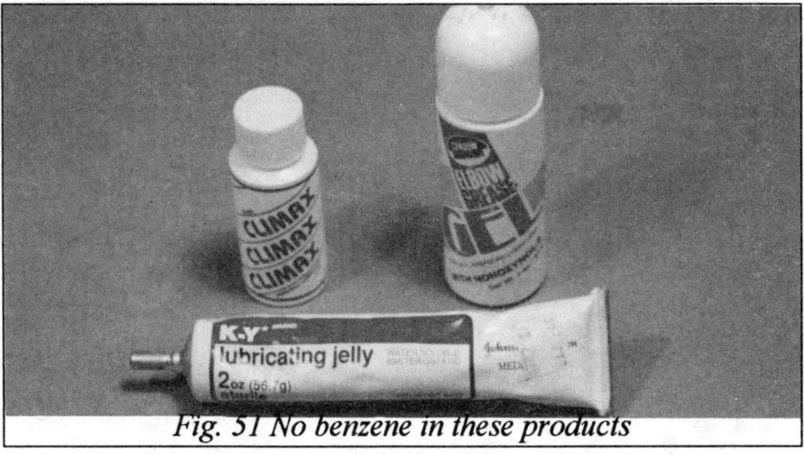

Fig. 51 No benzene in these products

How To Test Yourself

This chapter describes how to make and use the electronic device that lets you do the same tests that I did, and that led to the discoveries in this book.

It is natural to be skeptical that you can accumulate benzene from your toothpaste, or that there is anything toxic in soft drinks, or you should change your house plumbing, or you should remove your gold crowns, or that the new wall-to-wall carpeting must be thrown out. You can look for toxins in all these items for yourself, and you may luckily find that you do not have them!

It is only from years of experience testing every product clients brought in, or that I sampled from the grocery and drug store, that I make generalizations like "all cold cereals have toxic solvents," or "all meat has parasites." But obviously no one can test them all. Maybe your brand is OK! Or perhaps it is not. Unless you test for yourself you must rigorously follow the advice in this book.

Remember these tests can only say **YES** there is something in this food (or water sample or air sample or pill or potion) that my white blood cells (indicating your immune system) are busy removing. Or **NO** my white blood cells are not working on this[33]. And except for very high amounts, it is hard to say how much of a bad effect the toxin is having. But with repeated testing you can even find that out. Suppose your hair spray tests

---

33 Testing in the white blood cells is the best way I have found to both diagnose and predict illness. You will also be taught how to test any other part of the body.

YES (positive) in your immune system five minutes after using it, but not after twenty minutes. This, you may feel, is an acceptable level of toxicity. Or you may find it tests YES even though you washed it out of your hair yesterday. That would be a strong indication that you are accumulating at least some of the toxins from your hair spray in your body, and not only must you not use it, you must find a way to reduce your levels! Again, your own tests will be better than my general advice; but without them, you must follow my advice to get well.

All of the results obtained in this book can be duplicated by a person with skills at the high school level. No knowledge of electronics is required.

When possible, we include Radio Shack catalog numbers to describe materials. This is for convenience only. Equivalents are usually available at any electronics store.

Leads

If you are new to electronics you will need to know what a *lead* is. A lead is simply a wire used to connect two parts electrically. The method of clipping the lead to the component (part) determines its name. An *alligator clip test lead* uses a small metal clothespin for connecting, while a *mini-hook clip lead* is like a small, spring-loaded crochet hook. The mini-hook is best for attaching to a wire, the alligator clip is best for larger connections like to the test surfaces.

Leads come in many different lengths and are carried by all electronics stores.

The testing device consists of four parts

the test surfaces, probe and handhold, speaker, and circuit. These are connected by leads. The first item to construct is the *test surfaces*.

Test Surfaces

You will need two plates to set test samples on. The plates that hold the samples are intentionally separated from the main circuit because, unless you add shielding, the frequencies on the test plates may interfere with the circuit.

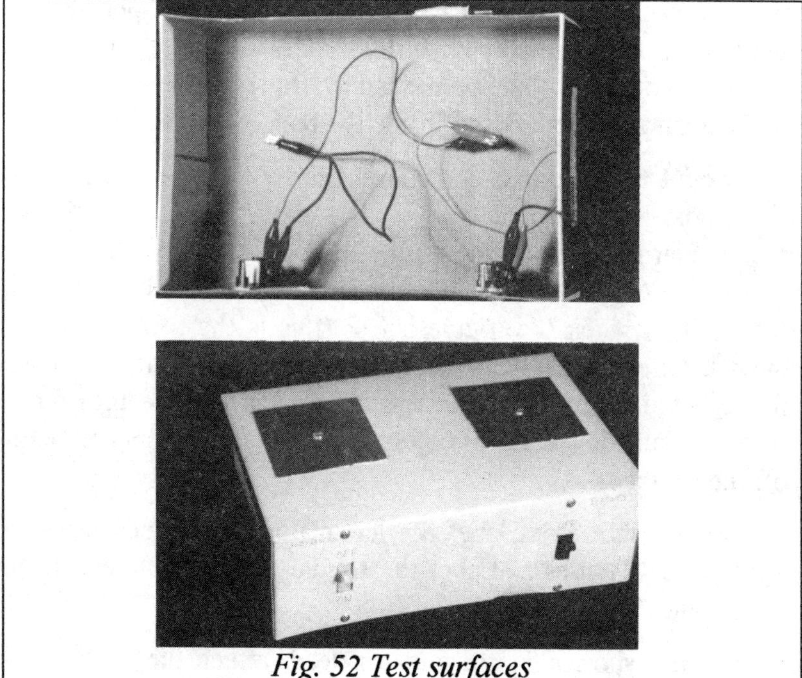

Fig. 52 Test surfaces

Materials needed:

shoe box
aluminum foil
stiff paper
2 bolts and nuts
nail
4 alligator clip test leads (3 very short, 1 about 24 inches)
2 ordinary light switches.

Acceptable:

Cut two 3½ inch squares out of stiff paper such as a cereal box. Cover them with slightly larger squares of aluminum foil, smoothed evenly and tucked snugly under the edges. You have just made yourself a set of open capacitors.

Mount these on the bottom of a shoe box turned upside down. They should be at least two inches apart. Make a hole through each with a small nail, and enlarge with a pencil point until you can fit a small bolt through. Use a washer and a nut to tighten them down. The bolt should be at least one inch long, to make it easy to clip leads to inside the box.

Mount two ordinary light switches on the front side of the shoe box, one in front of each plate. Cut 1 by ½ inch rectangular holes to let the toggle through. Remove the screws that came with the switch, then insert the switch from inside so that OFF is when the toggle is UP (this is the reverse of how most light switches are oriented). Push a pin from the inside through the screw holes, enlarge them, and replace the screws from the outside. If the shoe box is too shallow, flex the "ears" off the switches.

On the shoe box, label the left plate "Substances" and the right plate "Tissues". Label the toggle for each plate with an "OFF" and "ON.

Using a short alligator clip test lead, attach the tissue plate bolt to the tissue switch at one screw terminal. If there are three screw terminals, one will be green for ground–do not use it, use the other two. Attach the other screw terminal on the tissue switch to the substance plate bolt. Attach the substance plate bolt to the substance switch at one screw terminal. Finally attach a long alligator clip test lead to the other substance switch screw terminal. The other end will be attached to the circuit when you build it.

Choose either the "Acceptable" or the "Best" construction technique. You do not have to do both.

Best:

Use a large plastic project box instead of the shoe box. Do not use project boxes with metal lids. If you can not find all plastic boxes, remove the metal top and mount the test plates to the bottom. Use insulating sleeves and solder all connections.

Probe And Handhold

These are what you grasp when testing. The places to attach the probe and handhold are described with the circuit instructions.

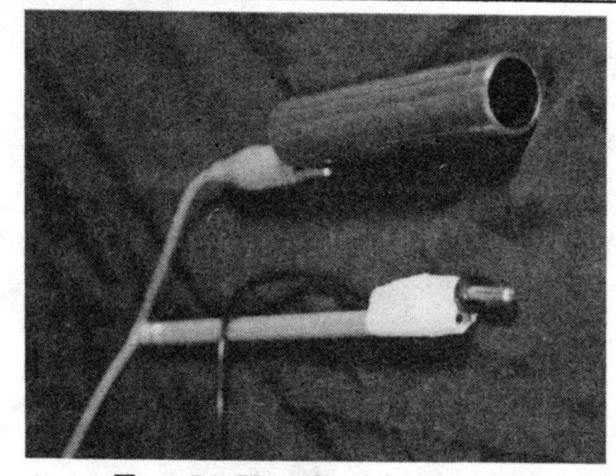

Fig. 53 Handhold and probe

Acceptable

For the probe use an empty ball point pen (no ink) with a metal collar by the point. Connect a two or three foot alligator clip test lead to this collar. For the handhold use a cheap metal can opener (the kind that fills your hand) with a second alligator clip test lead attached.

Best

The Archer Precision Mini-Hook Test Lead Set has a banana plug for the probe on one end and a mini-hook on the other end for easy attachment to the circuit. Tape a long, new pencil to the probe if that makes it easier to hold. The best handhold is simply a 4 inch piece of ¾ inch copper pipe (which a hardware store could just saw off for you) connected to the circuit with a three foot alligator clip test lead.

Item discussed	Radio Shack Cat. No.
banana plug probe	Precision Mini-Hook Test Lead Set (contains two, you only need one) 278-1160A

Speaker

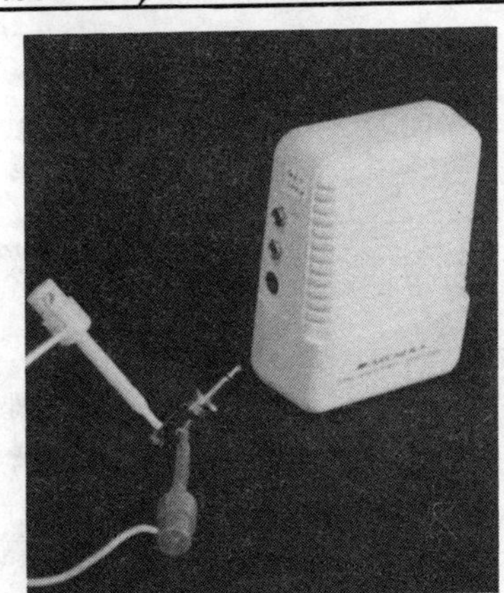

Fig. 54 Attaching the speaker

Hearing is believing. The sound made when you test substances lets you know if you have a YES (positive) or NO (negative). The better the sound quality the easier it is to hear the difference.

The speaker in the *200 in One Electronic Project Lab* (if you select this method of building the circuit) is not satisfactory.

Acceptable

You may hook the circuit up to your stereo system. Make sure you ask an expert to make the attachment. The leads (wires) you need to do this depend on the terminals your stereo has, but the end of the lead to the circuit should have either alligator clips or mini-hooks for easy attachment. Turn the bass all the way down, and the treble all the way up when you use it. Headsets do not work.

Best

The Archer Mini Amplifier Speaker is inexpensive and small (about the size of a transistor radio), making it easy to take with you. It needs a 9 volt battery. Remove the screw at the center back of the speaker using a Phillips screw driver to gain access to the battery compartment. Also get an 1/8 inch phono jack. Plug the phono jack into the receptacle marked "INPUT", and unscrew the plastic housing on the jack to expose the two posts for attaching wires. Each post should have a small hole in it to attach a mini-grabber lead. If there are no holes use alligator clip leads, but slip a piece of plastic tape between the posts to make sure the alligator clips do not touch each other.

Item discussed	Radio Shack Cat. No.
speaker	Archer Mini Amplifier Speaker 277-1008C
1/8 inch phono jack	Two-conductor Phone Plugs 274-286A (package of 2, you only need 1)
AC/DC adaptor (optional)	273-1455C

You are now ready to build the main circuit.

I describe four ways to make a Syncrometer,™ the circuit you can use to test yourself and products:

- **The Easy Way:** buy the *200 in One Electronic Project Lab* by Science Fair, Cat. No. 28-265, at Radio Shack for about $50.00, follow the instructions for connecting *The Electrosonic Human*, then modify the connections as described below
- **The Economical Way:** just buy the parts at Radio Shack for about $35.00, and follow the detailed instructions below (no soldering required)
- **The Rugged Way:** use the parts list, schematic and your electronic expertise
- **The Dermatron Way:** I discovered this method by making some modifications to a commercially available $750.00 ViTel.™ A dermatron (see *Sources*) is a device invented decades ago to measure body resistance (as opposed to skin resistance which is what lie detectors measure). If you own one you already have the circuit, probe, handhold, speaker and test surfaces. You will just be preparing an additional switch.

Select the most suitable method for your level of experience. You don't have to do all four!

The Easy Way Circuit

Build The Electrosonic Human (in the *200 in One Electronic Project Lab* by Science Fair, Cat. No. 28-265, at Radio Shack). It's easy and fun. If your kit has a different catalog number you can expect these connection numbers to be different.

Instead of connecting the probe to terminal T2, just clip it directly to terminal 137, and remove the 137-T2 wire. Similarly, clip the handhold to terminal 76 and remove the 76-26 and 25-T1 wires. This also removes the 4.7K resistor which is not necessary.

Later, when you use the probe to press against your knuckle you may find it painful. In this case try substituting the .005 microfarad capacitor for the .01 microfarad capacitor in the circuit.

Eliminate the Project Lab speaker by removing 53-173 and 54-174. Connect your speaker instead. Positive (the short post, if using the 1/8 inch phono jack) goes to 53, and negative (long post) goes to 54.

Finally, alligator clip the lead from the test plate shoe box to terminal 50.

Turn the control switch on and keep turning the potentiometer to nearly the maximum. (This reduces the resistance.) Make sure you have good batteries installed. Turn the speaker on. Test the circuit by briefly touching the probe to the handhold. The speaker should produce a sound like popping corn. If it does not, check that your alligator clips are not bending the spring terminals so much that other wires attached there are loose. Finally, turn switches OFF.

The Economical Way Circuit

This is a one hour project, have fun building it!

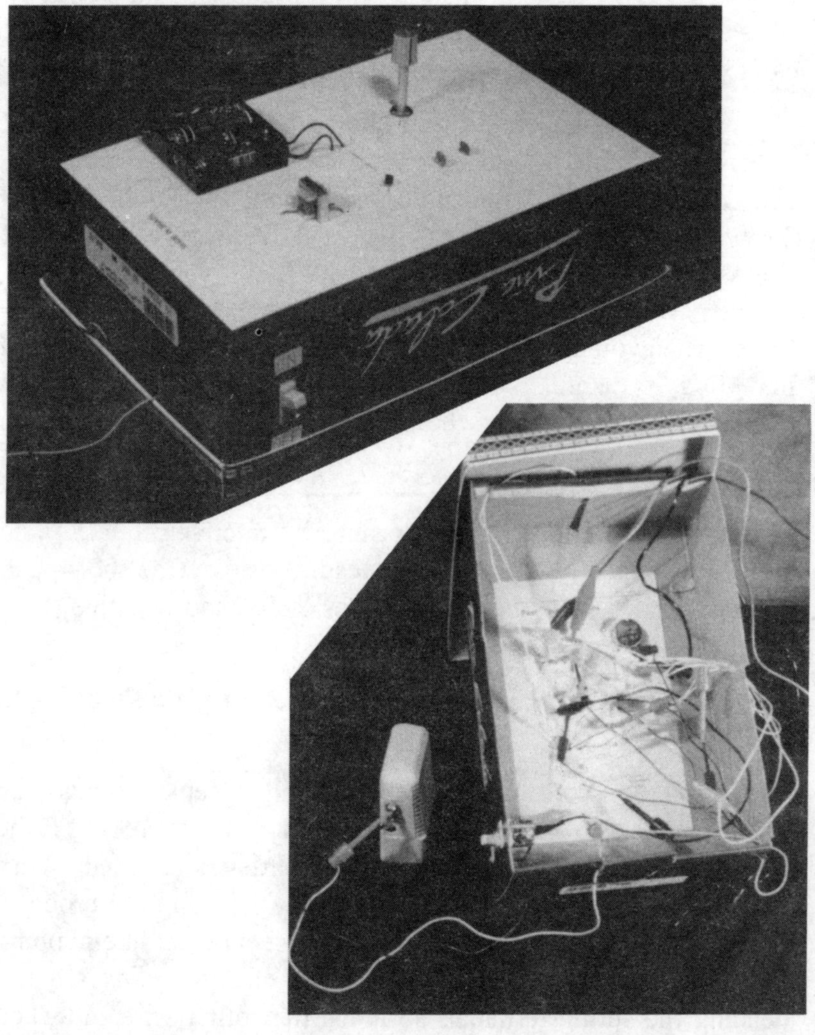

Fig. 55 Finished Economical Way circuit

Materials needed:

shoe box
tape
nail
pointed knife
cheap wire stripper (if needed)
paper clip

Parts List

	Item	Radio Shack Catalog Number
(a)	Ordinary light switch	
(b)	Potentiometer (variable resistor), 50k ohms	271-1716
(c)	Knob to fit the potentiometer	274-428 (package of 2, you only need one, or just wind some masking tape around the shaft in a wad)
(d)	.1 microfarad ceramic disk capacitor	272-1432A
(e)	.0047 microfarad ceramic disk capacitor (.005 will do)	272-130
(f)	MPS2907 PNP silicon transistor or equivalent	276-2023
(g)	Audio output transformer 900 CT: 8 ohm	273-1380
(h)	3 size AA batteries	
(i)	Battery holder for 4 AA's (3 AA batter holder will do)	270-391 has 2 wires coming away from it, one red (for +), one black (for -).
(j)	Microclip test jumpers	278-017 (you need 6 packages of two)

Directions

1. Get a shoe box, save the lid, photocopy the picture in this book and tape it to the bottom (inside) of the box.

Paste This In The Box

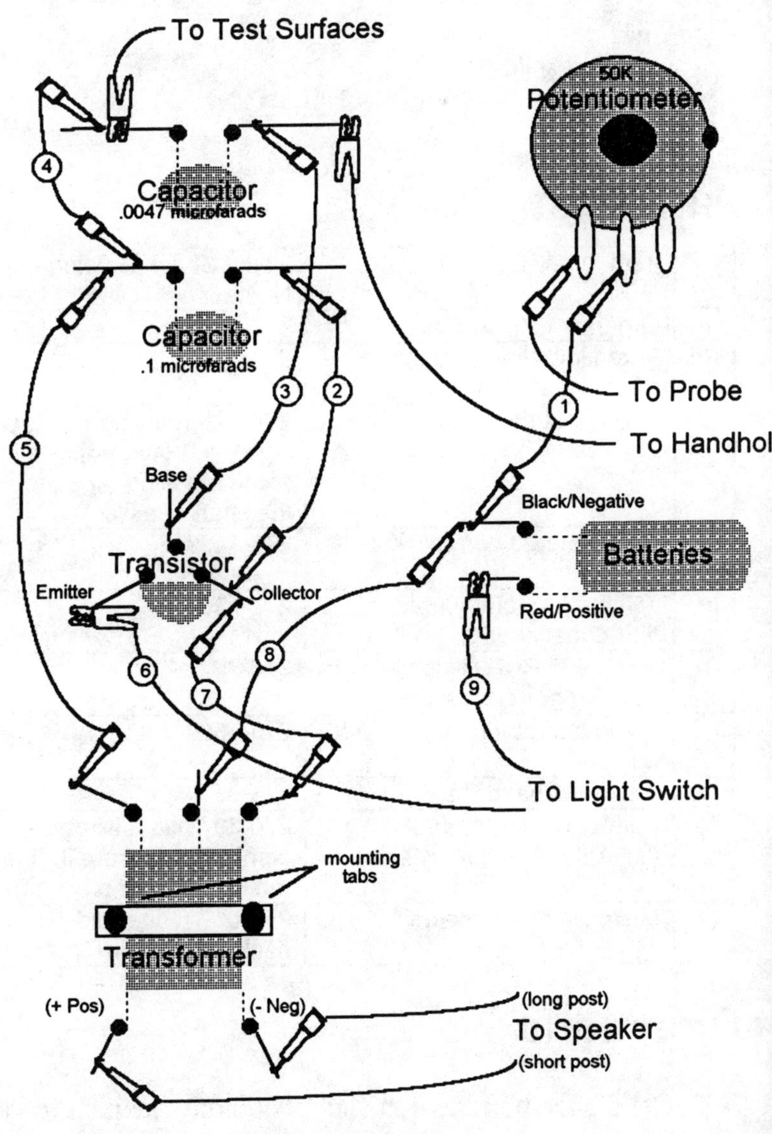

Fig. 56 Parts-layout and connections

2. Mount the light switch (a) just like you did for the test plates on the front of the shoe box. Mount it in the regular way so that ON is UP and label the box clearly. Turn light switch OFF before continuing.

3. Pierce a hole with a large nail or pencil for the shaft of the potentiometer (b), and a smaller hole for the tab on the side of the potentiometer (the tab keeps the potentiometer from rotating when you turn the switch). Remove the nut and washer from the base of the potentiometer shaft, insert the shaft into the hole from the inside of the shoe box. Trim the excess cardboard around the shaft with a knife. Replace the washer, nut, and tighten securely.

4. Attach the knob (c) to the shaft. Use a very small screw driver or pointed knife to tighten.

5. Pierce holes in the box with a pin for the .1 microfarad capacitor (d) and the .0047 microfarad capacitor (e). Push the wires of each capacitor through the holes from the outside. When the ceramic part is almost touching the box, bend the wires inside to keep it in place. The capacitors look very much alike, so be careful not to switch them (open one capacitor package at a time and put the part directly in place, double checking the diagram).

6. Pierce the holes for the transistor (f). Examine the transistor. Hold it in your left hand with the flat side on the left and wires pointing up at you. Notice that the center wire is the "base". Bend the base wire away to the left slightly so you will be able to insert the transistor into the triangle of holes. A diagram on the transistor package tells you that the top wire is the "collector" and the bottom wire is the "emitter". Insert the transistor from the outside of the box so each wire goes where it is supposed to, and bend the wires sideways to secure.

7. Pierce seven holes for the transformer (g). There should be 2 wires on one side and 3 on the other. All wires should have the ends bared and available for connections. If they are not, strip away ¼ inch of insulation and twist the strands together on each wire to keep them neat (practice using the wire stripper, first, on a different piece of wire). Notice that the transformer has 2 little mounting tabs. Push them through the box and bend them down with a knife or screwdriver on the inside to keep the transformer firmly in place or tape the transformer to the outside of the box. Then thread the 5 wires through their respective holes.
8. Prepare the battery holder (i) by cutting the wires to no more than two inches. Bare the ends of the wires for ¼ inch. You will only use three batteries, so in one of the battery slots, fill the space with a paper clip. Straighten one end of the paper clip. Hook the other end to the spring, and thread the straight part through the hole on the other side. Then bend the straight part down on the outside, out of the way.
9. Next, insert three AA size batteries (h) in the holder (i) (note the plus (+) and minus (-) ends are marked on the holder). Notice that one wire is red (for positive) and one is black (for negative). Don't let the bared ends of the two wires touch. Pierce the holes for the battery wires and insert from the outside. Tape the battery holder to the outside of the box. If your batteries get warm remove them and recheck your connections.

Now to connect everything.

10. Use 9 microclip test jumpers (j) to make the nine connections drawn. Note that connection 6 needs an alligator clip lead to the light switch. Pull on each connection after you make it, and stuff the extra wire through a slit made in the side of the shoe box with scissors. Make slits wherever you need them. Then clip the lead from your test plate shoe box to the capacitor where shown. Next attach the probe and handhold where shown. Finally attach the speaker where shown. In the picture there are both mini-hook and alligator clips depicted, but it is not important which kind you use, only that you make secure connections.

11. Test the circuit. Turn the speaker on, and the volume half way. Turn the Syncrometer (light switch) ON. Test the circuit by briefly touching the probe to the handhold. The speaker should produce a sound like popping corn (readjust speaker volume to a comfortable level). If you hear nothing, go over each step carefully. Make sure the batteries are fresh. Recheck all connections, especially ones made to stripped wires. Replace the lid and turn the shoe box over so it sits on its lid.

12. Label the potentiometer. Turn the knob almost fully clockwise. Mark the box where the line on the knob points. Grasp the handhold in one hand and press the probe with your thumb. Listen to the pitch. Now turn the knob almost fully counter-clockwise, mark the box, and listen to this pitch. Whichever pitch is higher label MAX (maximum) on the box.

13. You did it! Turn off the speaker and Syncrometer.

After you have used the Syncrometer for a while you may wish to take your device to an electronics shop and ask someone to mount the components in an all plastic box and solder the connections. This would let you travel with it in your suitcase without mashing it into a jumbled mess of wires.

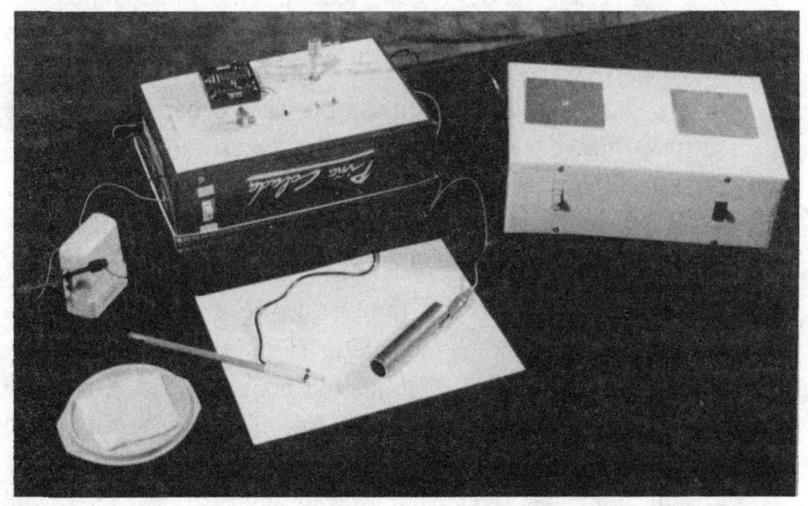

Fig. 57 Economical Way circuit and connections

The Rugged Way Circuit

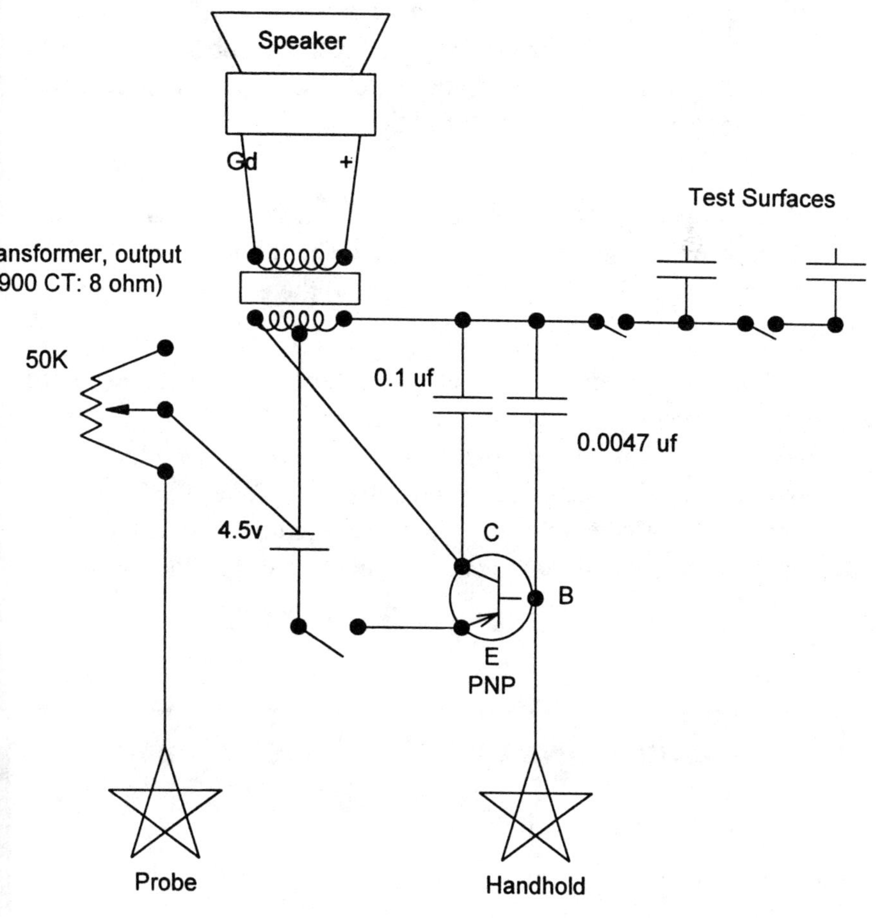

Fig. 58 Schematic

The Dermatron Way

Mount an ordinary light switch in a shoe box as described for The Test Surfaces. This will be called the "tissue switch". Choose one of your test plates as the "substance plate." Your existing switch to that plate is equivalent to the "substance switch." Using an alligator clip, connect the substance plate to one screw terminal on the light switch. Using another alligator clip connect the other screw terminal to your other test surface (the "tissue plate").

You were probably trained to listen for a slight current increase when testing substances. The concept was if the substance was anywhere in the body there would be higher conductance.

You must retrain yourself to listen for something more obvious, *resonance*. Resonance will occur when a substance and a tissue specimen are placed on your test plates that precisely match a body tissue and substance. With the additional information of where the substance has accumulated in the body, you can make much more accurate determinations how problems originate.

You now have the following equipment:

- Electronic circuit with speaker
- Test surfaces
- Probe and handhold

You are ready to learn to use them.

Troubleshooting

The sound you produce when you touch the probe to your damp knuckle should be F on the musical scale. A common problem is producing too low a sound. Don't reduce the size of the copper pipes. Keep all wires as short as possible. Use fresh batteries.

Using The Syncrometer

Fill a saucer with cold tap water. Fold a paper towel four times and place it in this dish. It should be entirely wet.

Cut paper strips about 1 inch wide from a piece of white, unfragranced, paper towel. Dampen a paper strip on the towel and wind it around the large metal handhold to completely cover it. The wetness improves conductivity and the paper towel keeps the metal off your skin.

- Turn the Syncrometer and speaker to ON.
- Start with the substance and tissue switches OFF.
- Test the plate connections, if you haven't done so recently. Touch the handhold to the substance plate briefly, then the tissue plate. There should be no crackle from the speaker. Turn the substance switch ON. Touch both plates briefly again. Only the substance plate should crackle. Now turn the tissue switch ON. Both plates should crackle. Turn both plate switches OFF again. Check your connections once a week.

Pick up the handhold, squeeze it free of excess water.

Pick up the probe in the same hand, holding it like a pen, between thumb and forefinger.

Dampen your other hand by making a fist and dunking your knuckles into the wet paper towel in the saucer. You will be using the area on top of the first knuckle of the forefinger or middle finger to learn the technique. Become proficient with both. Immediately after dunking your knuckles dry them on a paper towel folded in quarters and placed beside the saucer. The degree of dampness of your skin affects the resistance in the circuit and is a very important variable that you must learn to keep constant. Make your probe as soon as your knuckles have been dried (within two seconds) since they begin to air dry further immediately.

With the handhold and probe both in one hand press the probe against the knuckle of the other hand, keeping the knuckles tightly bent. Press lightly at first, then harder, taking one second. Count it out as "a thousand and one." Repeat the probe a half second later at the same location. There is an additive effect. The first probe opens your cells' conductance channels. The second probe tests to hear if they are indeed open.; These are considered the two halves of a single complete probe. All of this takes less than three seconds. Don't linger because your body will change and your next probe will be affected.

Subsequent probes are made in exactly the same way. As you develop skill, your probes will become identical. Plan to practice for one to two hours each day. It takes most people at least twelve hours of practice in order to be so consistent with their probes that they can hear the slight difference when the circuit is resonant.

For reference you may wish to use a piano. The starting sound when you touch down on the skin should be F, an octave and a half above middle C. The sound rises to a C as you press to the knuckle bone, then slips back to B, then back up to C-sharp as you complete the second half of your first probe. If you have a multitester you can connect it in series with the handhold or probe: the current should rise to about 50 microamps. If you have a frequency counter the frequency should hit 1000 Hz.

You should reach C-sharp just before the probe becomes painful. Adjust the potentiometer to make this possible. Mark the box STD (standard) at this setting. We will call this the *standard* state.

Two things change the sound of the probe even when your technique is identical:

1. The patch of skin chosen for probing will change its properties. The more it is used, the redder it gets and the higher the sound goes when you probe. Move to a nearby location when the sound is too high to begin with, rather than adjusting the potentiometer.
2. Your body has cycles which make the sound go noticeably higher and lower. If you are getting strangely higher sounds for identical probes, stop and probe every five minutes until you think the sound has gone down to standard. This could take five to twenty minutes. <u>Learn this higher sound</u> so you can avoid testing during this period. Nervousness or excitement raises the sound. Eating may lower it. A method is given in lesson one to determine whether you are in the standard state for testing.
3. You may also find times when it is impossible to reach the necessary sound without pressing so hard it causes pain. You may adjust the potentiometer if that helps. Or wait for your body to return to standard. Remember to set the potentiometer back to STD later. There will be times when the STD pitch is higher than usual (especially in younger persons). Exchanging the .0047 microfarad capacitor for a .01 microfarad capacitor helps fix this.

All tests are momentary.

This means less than one second. It is tempting to hold the probe to your skin and just listen to the sound go up and down, but if you prolong the test you must let your body rest ten minutes, each time, before resuming probe practice!

For our purposes, it is not necessary to locate acupuncture points.

Syncrometer Resonance

The information you are seeking is whether or not there is resonance in the circuit. If there is the test is YES (positive). You hear resonance by comparing the second probe to the first. You are not merely comparing pitch. Resonance is a tone quality in addition to a higher pitch. During resonance a higher pitch is reached faster; it seems to want to go infinitely high. If there is resonance it will be heard as the probe pressure nears maximum, as a rule.

Remember more electricity flows, and the pitch gets higher, as your skin reddens or your body changes cycle. These effects are not resonance.

Resonance is a small extra hum at the high end of the probe. As soon as you hear it, stop probing. Your body needs a short recovery time (10 to 20 seconds) after every resonant probe. The longer the resonant probe, the longer the recovery time to reach the standard level again.

Using musical notes, here is a NO (negative) result: F-C-B-C# (first probe) F-C-B-C# (compare, it is the same sound). Here is a YES (positive) result: F-C-B-C# (first probe) F-D (stop quickly because you heard resonance). (In between the first and second probe a tissue will be switched in per lessons below.)

It is not possible to produce a resonant sound by pressing harder on the skin, although you can make the pitch go higher. To avoid confusion it is important to practice making probes of the same pressure. (Practice getting the F-C-B-C# tune.)

Lesson One

Purpose: To identify the sound of resonance in the circuit.

Materials: Potentized (homeopathic) solutions. Prepare these as follows: find three medium size vitamin bottles, glass or plastic, with non-metal lids. Remove any shreds of paper sticking to the rim. Rinse well with cold tap water. Then rinse again with filtered tap water.

Pour filtered cold tap water into the first bottle to a depth of about ½ inch. Add 50 little grains of table salt. Replace the lid. Make sure the outside is clean. If not, rinse and dry. Now shake hard, holding it snugly in your hand. Count your shakes; shake 120 to 150 times. Use elbow motion so each shake covers about an eight inch distance. Shaken samples are different from unshaken ones, that's why this is so important. When done label the bottle on its side and lid: SALT #1. Wash your hands (without soap).

Next, pour about the same amount of filtered water into the second and third bottles. Open SALT #1 and pour a small amount, like ¼ to ½ of a teaspoon (do not use a spoon) into the second and third bottles. Close all bottles. Now shake the second bottle the same as the first. Clean it and label it SALT

#2. Do the same for the third bottle. Label it SALT #2 also and set aside for Lesson Three.

These two solutions have unique properties. SALT #1 always resonates. Use #1 to train your ear. SALT #2 shouldn't resonate. Use #2 to hear when you have returned to your standard state.

Method: Place SALT #2 on the substance plate and SALT #1 on the tissue plate.

1. Turn the Syncrometer and speaker ON.
2. Start with both the substance and tissue switches OFF.
3. Make your first probe (F-C-B-C#).
4. Immediately flip the substance switch ON and repeat the probe. Use only one half second to operate the switch. This is why these switches are mounted "upside down", because it is faster to move the toggle down. The result should be a NO (negative). If the second probe sounds even a little higher you are not at the standard level. Wait a few more seconds and go back to step 2.
5. If the first result was NO, you may immediately flip the tissue switch ON. (Again do this within one half second.) This time the circuit was resonating. Learn to hear the difference between the last two probes.
6. The skin must now be rested When SALT #1 is placed in the circuit there is always resonance whether you hear it or not. Therefore, always take the time to rest the skin.
7. How can you be sure that the skin is rested enough? Any time you want to know whether you have returned to the standard level, you may simply test yourself to SALT #2 (just do steps 2, 3 and 4). While you are learning, let your piano also help you to learn the standard level (starts exactly at F). If you do not rest and you resonate the

circuit before returning to the standard level, the results will become aberrant and useless. The briefer you keep the resonant probe, the faster you return to the standard level. Don't exceed one half second when probing SALT #1. Hopefully you will soon hear resonance within that time.

8. This lesson teaches you to first listen to the empty plate, then to SALT #2, then to SALT #1. In later lessons you simply use two probes, substance and substance-plus-tissue, because we assume you checked for your standard level.

Practice hearing resonance in your circuit every day.

White Blood Cells

Checking for resonance between your white blood cells and a toxin is the single most important test you can make.

Your white blood cells are your immune system's first line of defense. In addition to making antibodies, interferon, interleukins, and other attack chemicals, they also "eat" foreign substances in your body and eliminate them. By simply checking your white blood cells for toxins or intruders you save having to check every other tissue in your body. Because no matter where the foreign substance is, chances are some white blood cells are working on removing it.

It took me two years to find this ideal indicator, but it is not perfect. **Tapeworms are a notable exception.** They can be encysted in a particular tissue which will test positive, while the white blood cells continue to test negative. Also, when bacteria and viruses are <u>in their latent form</u>, they do not show up in the white blood cells. Fortunately, in their active form they show up quite nicely. Again, when toxins or invaders are not plentiful, they may not appear in the white blood cells, although they can be found in a tissue.

Making A White Blood Cell Specimen

Obtain an empty vitamin bottle with a flat plastic lid and a roll of clear tape. The white blood cells are not going into the bottle, they are going on the bottle. The bottle simply makes them easy to handle. Rinse and dry the bottle. Make a second specimen on a clean glass slide if available.

Squeeze an oil gland on your face or body to obtain a ribbon of whitish matter (not mixed with blood). Pick this up with the back of your thumb nail. Spread it in a single, small streak across the lid of the bottle or the center of the glass slide. Stick a strip of clear tape over the streak on the bottle cap so that the ends hang over the edge and you can easily see where the specimen was put (see photo). Wipe the lid beside the tape to make sure no white blood cells are uncovered. Apply a drop of balsam and a cover slip to the slide preparation. Both types of preparation will give you identical results. The bottle type of white blood cell specimen is used by standing it on its lid (upside down). The lid is used because it is flat, whereas the bottom of most bottles is not.

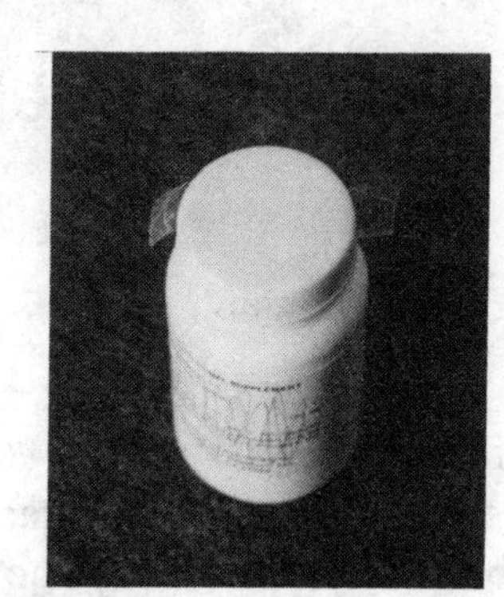

Fig. 59 A White Blood Cell Specimen

Lesson Two

Purpose: To add a white blood cell specimen to the circuit and compare sound.

Method:

1. Turn the Syncrometer and speaker ON.
2. Start with both the substance and tissue switches OFF.
3. Place the white blood cell specimen on the substance plate.
4. Listen to the first probe.
5. Immediately (one half second) turn the substance switch ON and probe again.
6. There should be no difference in sound levels and no resonance.
7. Make sure both plate switches are again OFF.
8. Treat yourself to some junk food. Reserve a piece in a sealed plastic bag.
9. Move your white blood cell specimen to the tissue plate. Place the junk food sample on the substance plate.
10. Listen to the first probe.
11. Immediately (one half second) turn the substance switch ON and probe again. (Remember this should not resonate yet, if you hear any difference you are not at the standard state.)
12. Immediately turn the tissue switch ON and probe a third time. Does this resonate? (If it does, your white blood cells are busy removing the junk food for you.)

Lesson Three

Purpose: To determine your percent accuracy in listening for resonance.

Materials: the SALT #1 and two SALT #2 solutions you made for Lesson One.

Method: move the SALT #1 and SALT #2 labels to the bottom of the bottles so you can not tell which bottle is which.

1. Turn the Syncrometer and speaker ON.
2. Start with both the substance and tissue switches OFF.
3. Mix the bottles up, select one at random, and place it on the substance plate.
4. Make your first probe.
5. Turn the substance switch to ON and make your second probe.
6. Resonance indicates a SALT #1, no resonance indicates SALT #2. Check the bottom. Remember to rest after the SALT #1, whether or not you heard resonance.
7. Repeat steps 3 through 5 a number of times. Work toward getting three out of three correct. Practice every day.

Trouble shooting:

a) If you repeat this experiment and you keep getting the same bottles "wrong", start over. You may have accidentally contaminated or mislabeled the outside of the bottle, or switched bottle caps.

b) If you get different bottles wrong each time, the plates may be contaminated. Wash the outside of the bottles and rinse with filtered water and dry. Wipe the plates very well, too, with filtered water and dry.

c) If all the bottles read the same, your cold tap water is polluted. Change the filter.

Preparing Test Substances

It is possible to prepare dry substances for testing such as a piece of lead or grains of pesticide. They can simply be kept in a plastic bag and placed on the test plate. However, I prefer to place a small amount (the size of a pea) of the substance into a ½ ounce bottle of filtered water. There will be many chemical reactions between the substance and the water to produce a number of test substances all contained in one bottle. This simulates the situation in the body.

Within the body, where salt and water are abundant, similar reactions may occur between elements and water. For example, a strip of pure (99.9% pure) copper placed in filtered water might yield copper hydroxide, cuprous oxide, cupric oxide, copper dioxide, and so forth. These may be similar to some of the reaction products one might expect in the body, coming from a copper IUD, copper bracelet or the copper from metal tooth fillings. Since the electronic properties of elemental copper are not the same as for copper compounds, we would miss many test results if we used only dry elemental copper as a test substance.

Impure Test Substances

It is not necessary to have pure test substances. For instance, a tire balancer made of lead can be easily obtained at an auto service station. Leaded gasoline and lead fishing weights also make good test substances for lead. There is a disadvantage, though, to using impure test substances. You are including the extra impurities in your test. If your lead object also has tin in it, you are also testing for tin. Usually, you can infer the truth by some careful maneuvering. If you have searched your kidneys for leaded gasoline, fishing weights and tire balancers and all 3 are resonant with your kidneys, you may infer that you have lead in your kidneys since the common element in all 3 items is lead. (You will learn how to specify a tissue, such as your kidneys, later.)

Using pure chemicals gives you certainty in your results. You can purchase pure chemicals from chemical supply companies (see *Sources*). Your pharmacy, a child's chemistry set, a paint store, or biological supply company can also supply some.

The biggest repository of all toxic substances is the grocery store and your own home.

You can make test substances out of your hand soap, water softener salt, and laundry detergent by putting a small amount (1/16 tsp.) in a ½ ounce glass bottle and adding about 2 tsp. filtered water. (Or for quick testing just put them dry or wet in a sealed plastic baggie.) Always use a plastic measuring spoon.

Check the items in Toxic Elements (see *The Tests*) to see where they are commonly found. For instance, arsenic is in carpets, stuffed furniture and wallpaper, originating in the pesticide put there. Here are some suggestions for finding sources of toxic products to make your own toxic element test. If the product is a solid, place a small amount in a plastic bag and add a tablespoon of filtered water to get a temporary test product. For permanent use put it in a small amber glass bottle. If the product is a liquid, pour a few <u>drops</u> into a glass bottle and add about 2 tsp. filtered water. Keep all toxic substances in glass bottles for your own safety. Small amber glass dropper bottles can be purchased by the dozen at drug stores (also see *Sources*).

Aflatoxin: scrape the mold off an orange or piece of bread.

Acetone: paint supply store or pharmacy.

Arsenic: 1/16 tsp. of arsenate pesticide from a garden shop.

Aluminum: a piece of aluminum foil or an aluminum measuring spoon. Most aluminum hardware is anodized; this means it has cadmium added to it to prevent tarnishing.

Aluminum silicate: a bit of salt that has this free running agent in it.

Asbestos: a small piece of asbestos sheeting, an old furnace gasket, ¼ inch of a clothes dryer belt that does not say "Made In USA", or a crumb of building material being removed due to its asbestos content (ask a contractor).

Barium: save a few drops from the beverage given to patients scheduled for an X-ray; lipstick that has barium listed in the ingredients.

Benzene: an <u>old</u> can of rubber cement (new supplies do not have it).

Benzopyrenes: a piece of toast, hot dog, or flame cooked food. This substance fades in a day, use it while fresh.

Beryllium: a piece of coal; a few drops of "coal oil" or lamp oil.

Bismuth: use a few drops of antacid with bismuth in it.

Bromine: bleached "brominated" flour.

Cadmium: scrape a bit off a galvanized nail.

Cesium: scrape the surface of a clear plastic beverage bottle.

Chromate: scrape an old car bumper.

Cobalt: pick out the blue and green crumbs from detergent. A sample of cobalt containing paint should also suffice.

Chlorine: a few drops of pure, old fashioned Clorox.™

Copper: ask your hardware clerk to cut a small fragment off a copper pipe of the purest variety or a ¼ inch of pure copper wire.

Ether: automotive supply store (engine starting fluid).

Fiberglass: snip a fragment from insulation.

Fluoride: ask a dentist for a small sample.

Formaldehyde: purchase 37% formaldehyde at a pharmacy. Use a few drops only for your sample.

Gasoline: gas station (leaded and unleaded).

Gold: ask a jeweler for a crumb of the purest gold available or use a wedding ring.

Kerosene: gas station.

Lead: wheel balancers from a gas station, weights used on fishing lines, lead solder from electronics shop.

Mercury: a mercury thermometer (there is no need to break it), piece of amalgam tooth filling.

Methanol: paint supply store (wood alcohol).

Nickel: a nickel coin.

PCB: water from a quarry known to be polluted with it (a builder or electrical worker may know a source).

Platinum: ask a jeweler for a small specimen.

Propyl alcohol: rubbing alcohol from pharmacy (same as propanol or isopropanol). Use a few drops only, discard the rest.

PVC: glue that lists it in the ingredients (poly vinyl chloride).

Radon: leave a glass jar with an inch of filtered water in it standing open in a basement that tested positive to radon using a kit. After 3 days, close the jar. Pour about 2 tsp. of this water into your specimen bottle.

Silver: ask a jeweler for a crumb of very pure silver. Silver solder can be found in electronics shops. Snip the edge of a very old silver coin.

Styrene: a chip of styrofoam.

Tantalum: purchase a tantalum drill bit from hardware store.

Tin: scrape a tin bucket at a farm supply. Tin solder. Ask a dentist for a piece of pure tin (used to make braces).

Titanium: purchase a titanium drill bit from a hardware store

Tungsten: the filament in a burned out light bulb.

Vanadium: hold a piece of dampened paper towel over a gas burner as it is turned on. Cut a bit of this paper into your specimen bottle and add 2 tsp. filtered water.

Xylene: paint store or pharmacy.

This list gets you off to a good start. Since few of these specimens are pure, there is a degree of logic that you must apply in most cases. If you are testing for barium in your breast, a positive result would mean that a barium-containing lip stick tests positive and a barium-free lip stick is negative.

A chemistry set for hobbyists is a wonderful addition to your collection of test specimens. Remember, however, the assumptions and errors in such a system. A test for silver using silver chloride might be negative. This does not mean there is no silver present in your body; it only means there is no silver chloride present in the tissue you tested. You are bound to miss some toxins; don't let this discourage you. There is more than enough that you <u>can</u> find.

The most fruitful kind of testing is, probably, the use of household products themselves as test substances. The soaps, colognes, mouthwash, toothpaste, shampoo, cosmetics, breads, dairy products, juices and cereals can all be made into test specimens. Put about 1/8 tsp. of the product in a small glass bottle, add 2 tsp. filtered water and ¼ tsp. grain alcohol to preserve it. If you test positive to these, then you shouldn't use them, even if you can not identify the exact toxin or pathogen.

Finally, there is the error from the filtered water you are using. Test it by tasting it then searching your white blood cells for it. If you find it there, change the filter and repeat the test. Make a test sample of this water alone.

Lesson Four

Purpose: To determine toxicity of your household products.

Materials: Prepare samples of what you ate at your last meal. Also prepare samples of the soap, shampoo, shaving cream and other products you last put on your body.

Method: Listen for resonance between your white blood cells and the daily foods and products you use.

1. Place your white blood cell specimen on the tissue plate.
2. Place your first sample on the substance plate.

3. Test for resonance.
4. Make two piles. Things that resonate go in the TOXIC pile, things that don't go in the SAFE pile. Don't be surprised if your health brand shampoo "flunks" the test. And if your vitamin C flunks, I hope you write a letter to the manufacturer!

Making Organ Specimens

To test for toxic elements or parasites in a particular organ such as the liver or skin, you will need either a fresh or frozen sample of the organ or a prepared microscope slide of this organ. Meat purchased from a grocery store, fresh or frozen, provides you with a variety of organ specimens. Chicken, turkey, beef or pork organs all give the same results. You may purchase chicken gizzards for a sample of stomach, beef liver for liver, pork brains for brain, beef steak for muscle, sweet breads for thymus, tripe for stomach lining. Other organs may be ordered from a meat packing plant.

Trim the marrow out of a bone slice to get bone marrow. Scrub the bone slice with hot water to free it of marrow to get a bone specimen. Choose a single piece of meat sample, rinse it and place it in a plastic bag. You may freeze it. To make a durable unfrozen sample, cut a small piece, the size of a pea, and place it in an amber glass bottle (½ oz.). Cover with two tsp. filtered water and ¼ tsp. of grain alcohol (pure vodka will do) to preserve it. These need not be refrigerated but if decay starts, make a fresh specimen.

Pork brains from the grocery store may be dissected to give you the different parts of the brain. Chicken livers often have an attached gallbladder or piece of bile duct, giving you that extra organ. Grocery store "lites" provides you with lung tissue. For kidney, snip a piece off pork or beef kidney. Beef liver may supply you with a blood sample, too. Saliva, urine and semen may be your own. Use less than ¼ tsp. of each fluid. Add about 2 tsp. (10 ml) filtered water and a small amount (¼ tsp.) of grain alcohol to preserve them. <u>This dilution of natural fluids is essential to get correct results.</u>

I use ½ oz amber glass bottles with bakelite caps (see *Sources*) to hold specimens. After closing, each bottle is sealed with a Parafilm™ strip to avoid accidental loosening of the cap. However, plastic bags or other containers would suffice.

To make a specimen of skin, use hangnail bits and skin peeled from a callous, <u>not a wart</u>. A few shreds will do. Remember, they must be very close to the test plate when in use; add 2 tsp. filtered water and ¼ tsp. grain alcohol.

Making a Complete Set of Tissue Samples

My original complete set was made from a frozen fish. As it thawed, different organs were cut away and small pieces placed in bottles for preserving in cold tap water and grain alcohol. In this way, organs not available from the grocery store could be obtained. The piece of intestine closest to the anus corresponds to our colon, the part closest to the stomach corresponds to our duodenum. The 2 layers of the stomach and different layers of the eye, the optic nerve and spinal cord were obtained this way.

Another complete set of tissue samples were obtained from a freshly killed steer at a slaughter house. In this way the 4 chambers of the heart were obtained, the lung, trachea, aorta, vein, pancreas, and so forth.

Purchasing a Complete Set of Tissue Samples

Slides of tissues, unstained or stained in a variety of ways for microscope study give identical results to the preparations made by yourself in the ways already described. This fact opens the entire catalog of tissue types for your further study. See *Sources* for places that supply them.

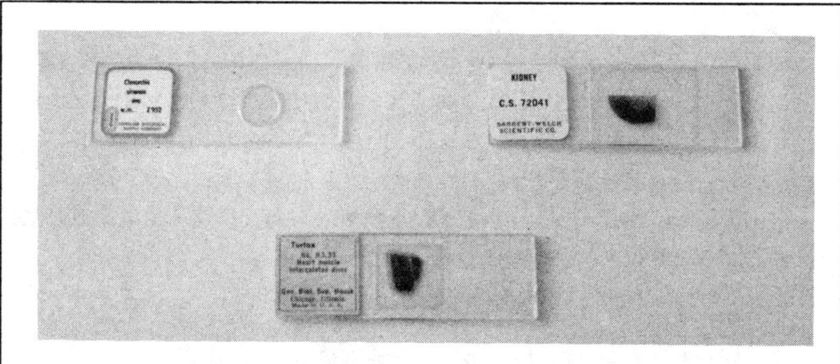

Fig. 60 Some purchased parasite and tissue slides

You now have a set of organ samples, either fresh, frozen, preserved or on slides. You also have a set of test substances, whether chemical compounds, or elements, or products. Your goal is to search in your own organs and body tissues for the substances that may be robbing you of health.

> Keeping yourself healthy will soon be an easy, daily routine.

Body Fluid Specimens

Each of these fluids should be prepared by putting about ¼ tsp. in a ½ oz amber glass bottle. Add about 2 tsp. filtered water and ¼ tsp. grain alcohol for preservation. Undiluted specimens do not work for reasons that are technical and beyond the scope of this book. It is important *not* to shake the specimen, but to mix gently.

Urine. It is desired to have a pure, uninfected urine sample as a tissue specimen. Since this cannot be proved with certainty, obtain several urine samples from different persons whom you believe to be healthy and make several test specimens in order to compare results. Label your specimens Urine A (child), Urine B (woman), Urine C (mine), and so forth.

Semen. A sample from a condom is adequate. Aged specimens (sent by mail, unpreserved and unrefrigerated) work well also. Use one to ten drops or scrape a small amount.

Blood. One to ten drops of blood should be used. A bit of white paper towel for swabbing may be used. Clotted or chemically treated blood is satisfactory. A blood smear on a slide is very convenient.

Milk. Cow's milk is too polluted with parasites and chemicals to be useful. Electronically, a dead specimen is equivalent to a live specimen, so that pasteurization of the milk does not help. A human milk specimen is preferred.

Saliva. Use your own, if you have deparasitized yourself and test negative to various fluke stages. Otherwise find a well friend or child.

Specifying A Tissue On The Syncrometer

All my initial findings were made with a dermatron. The traditional use of a dermatron allows you to identify a substance in your whole body by placing the substance on the plate and comparing the current in the circuit when the empty plate or the loaded plate are added to it. If you are searching for mercury in your body tissues you could put a test specimen of mercury on the dermatron plate and probe acupuncture points to complete the circuit through your body. You would switch between the empty and loaded plates and compare the currents produced. If your body does indeed have significant amounts of mercury in it, the current would be significantly higher with the loaded plate in the circuit. The more mercury that is in you, the higher the current that flows (after allowing for skin reddening and body cycles). The new use of the dermatron, and the primary use of the Syncrometer, allows you to identify a substance in a specific tissue, not just somewhere in your body.

To find mercury in your kidneys or prostate or thyroid gland you must put that tissue specimen in parallel with the open capacitor in the circuit. Any of the specimen types described in the previous section will do. Slides are most convenient. To place the tissue in parallel it must be connected to the test plate on which the mercury sample rests. Dermatron users accomplish this by building a shorting switch (simply putting both items on the same plate may cause interference). Syncrometer users use the test surfaces they have built.

Lesson Five

Purpose: To watch substances travel through your body.

Materials: Prepare a pint of brown sugar solution using filtered water. Use about 1 tsp. for a pint. Do not shake it; gently mix. Make a sample bottle by pouring about ½ inch into a clean used vitamin bottle. Rinse and dry the outside of the sample bottle. Finally wash your hands with plain water.

Method:

1. Prepare a paper applicator by tearing the corner from a white unfragranced paper towel. Fold it to make a wick.
2. Dip the paper wick in the pint of sugar water and apply it to the skin of your inner arm where you can rub freely. Rub it in vigorously for about 10 seconds (otherwise it takes minutes to absorb). Leave the wick on the skin and tape it down with a piece of clear tape about 4 inches long (this increases the time you have to work). Wipe your fingers with a piece of wet towel.
3. Place your skin tissue specimen on the tissue plate and the sugar specimen bottle on the substance plate.
4. Probe for resonance.
5. As soon as you hear resonance, implying that the skin has absorbed the sugar solution (which may take a full minute), replace the skin bottle with one of liver and listen for resonance again. There should be none, yet.
6. Alternate between the skin and liver. Soon the skin will be clear and the liver will resonate. Also check the pancreas to see how quickly sugar arrives there.
7. Check white blood cells and kidneys. It should not appear here (unless it is polluted with a toxin).

8. After five to ten minutes the sugar will be gone from all of these tissues and your experiment is ended. Wash your arm with plain water.

Notice that you have only a few minutes to get all your testing done after the skin has absorbed the test substances.

Lesson Six

Purpose: To verify the propyl alcohol and benzene lists.

Method: Assemble the products named in the propyl alcohol list and benzene list (as many as you can find) and test them.

1. Rub in skin.
2. Test to your propyl alcohol and benzene samples.
3. Wash your arm.
4. Wait until your skin tests negative before testing the next product.

This method can detect as little as 3000 molecules rubbed into the skin. It is a far superior method to even the best chemical methods such as HPLC or gas chromatography. (I determined this by buying a standard solution, which tells the exact concentration. I then repeatedly and accurately diluted it, 1 in 10, for 25 dilutions, <u>without shaking</u>. A measured amount was put on paper, and the skin test applied. One half the amount was assumed to be absorbed. Working from the most dilute, I stopped at my first resonant result, which I calculated at 3025 molecules of iridium chloride. (See Lesson 17 for how you can determine your test sensitivity.)

Even tiny amounts of solvents are toxic! They must not be consumed or be left in our environment.

I have found too many unsuspected products test positive to benzene. This is such a global tragedy that people must protect themselves by using their own tests. Rather than assurances, regulatory agencies should provide the consumer with cheap and simple tests (dip sticks and papers so we need not lug our Syncrometers around). Even if some test should fail, not all tests would fail to find an important pollutant like benzene. It would come to public attention much faster than the present debacle has.

Lesson Seven

Purpose: To test for the presence of aluminum in your brain.

Materials: An aluminum measuring spoon, a tsp. of free flowing aluminized salt, a square inch of aluminum foil, a package of pork brain from the grocery store, kept frozen. Other animal sources will do. A stained slide of cerebrum, cerebellum or other brain tissue, if available.

Method:

1. Cut a piece of brain tissue (about 1 tsp.) and place in a plastic bag.
2. Place the aluminum samples in separate plastic bags. Add filtered water to each, about 1 tbs. Place each bag into another plastic bag to guard against cross contamination. Keep all surfaces and your hands meticulously clean (do not use soap).
3. Place the aluminum sample on the substance plate and the brain sample on the tissue plate.

4. Probe for resonance. If the circuit resonates <u>you</u> have aluminum in <u>your</u> brain.

5. Of course, it would be desirable to have absolute certainty about this. To achieve absolute certainty, you must have <u>nothing other than aluminum</u> in your aluminum specimen. If your aluminum specimen actually has cadmium or copper in it, you are <u>also</u> testing for these in your brain. Test yourself to cadmium or copper, separately. If you don't have these in your brain, the aluminum test result is more likely to be correct. To achieve certainty, purchase a few granules of pure aluminum or an Atomic Absorption Standard from a chemical supply company for your test specimen.

6. Repeat the aluminum test with other aluminum objects if you don't have pure aluminum. If they all resonate, you <u>very, very likely</u> have aluminum in your brain.

7. If you do have aluminum in your brain, notice that <u>you</u> are now a good test subject for aluminum. You can test food and products for aluminum to find out where you are getting it from. Test these items:

    - a teaspoon of cottage cheese or yogurt taken from the top of a container of a foil-capped variety
    - a piece of cream cheese or butter that was wrapped in foil
    - a chip of bar soap or a bit of hand lotion
    - a piece of cake or rolls baked in an aluminum pan
    - a piece of turkey skin or hot dish that was covered with aluminum foil
    - anything baked with baking powder
    - a carbonated beverage from an aluminum can

If any of these resonates with the brain sample or slide in the circuit, they too contain aluminum *or something else that you also have in the brain*! You can distinguish between these possibilities by doing the skin test (previous lesson).

Alternative Lesson:

To test for dental metal in your tissues. Use a piece of amalgam from an old tooth filling. This tests for the rest of the alloys in amalgam fillings as well as mercury. If you can't get a piece of mercury amalgam, use a mercury thermometer (don't break it, just put the bulb on the plate). Choose tissues like kidney, nerves, brain, liver, in addition to white blood cells.

Testing Someone Else

Seat the person comfortably with their hand resting near you. Choose the first knuckle from the middle or first finger just like you do for yourself. Since you are touching this person, you are putting yourself in the circuit with the subject.

To exclude yourself, you need to add inductance to yourself. A coil of about 10 microhenrys, worn next to the skin, works well and is easily made. Obtain insulated wire and wrap 24 turns around a ball point pen (or something about that size), closely spaced. Cut the ends and tape them down securely. Keep it in a plastic bag, even when in your pocket. A commercial inductance of 4.7 microhenrys, worn touching your skin also works well. It can be worn on a string necklace. The inductance acts as an RF (radio frequency) choke, limiting the alternating current that can flow through you while testing another person.

Test your inductor in this way. Repeat Lesson One with the coil next to your body. No resonance, even to SALT #1, should occur. If it does, make the coil bigger. Remove the inductor when you are not testing others.

Surrogate Testing

Use an adult as a surrogate when testing a baby or pet. The pet or baby is held on the lap of the surrogate. A large pet may sit in front of the person. The handhold is held by the surrogate and pressed firmly against the body of the baby or pet. It can be laid flat against the arm, body or leg of a baby and held in place firmly by the whole hand of the adult. The paper covering should be wet. For a pet, the end is held firmly pressed against the skin, such as between the front legs or on the belly. The other hand of the adult is used for testing in the usual way. The adult must wear an inductor for surrogate testing as well as you, the tester.

An ill or bedridden person may be tested without inconvenience or stress. He or she rests their whole hand on the skin of your leg, just above the knee. A wet piece of paper towel, about 4 inches by 4 inches is placed on your leg, to make better contact. You must use an inductor for yourself with this method. You may now proceed to probe on your hand instead of the ill person's.

Lesson Eight

Purpose: To detect aluminum in the brain of another person.

Materials: same as previous lesson, you wear the inductor.

Method:

1. Place the aluminum sample on the substance plate and the brain sample on the tissue plate.
2. Give the other person the handhold. You use the probe. Hold their finger steady in yours.
3. Probe the other person for resonance. The first probe is with substance plate switch ON, second is with both substance and tissue plate switches ON. Resonance implies there is aluminum in the person's brain.
4. Test several samples of aluminum to increase the probability of being right in your interpretation that it is aluminum and not something else with the aluminum that is showing its presence in the brain.

Lesson Nine

Purpose: To test for cancer.

Materials: A pure sample of ortho-phospho-tyrosine (see *Sources*). Place a few milligrams (it need not be weighed) in a small glass bottle, add 2 tsp. filtered water and ¼ tsp. grain alcohol.

All persons with cancer have ortho-phospho-tyrosine in their urine as well as in the cancerous tissue. It is seldom found in other body fluids. Obtain a urine specimen from a friend who has active cancer. Freeze it if you can't prepare it immediately. Keep such specimens well marked in an additional sealed plastic bag. Persons who have recently been treated clinically for cancer are much less likely to have ortho-phospho-tyrosine in the urine.

Urine cannot be considered a chemical in the same way as a sugar or salt solution. Urine is a tissue and has its own resonant frequency as do our other tissues. If combined with another tissue on the test plates, it will not resonate as if a solution of pure ortho-phospho-tyrosine were used. To use urine as an ortho-phospho-tyrosine specimen, you must:

a) Pour a few drops of urine into your specimen bottle

b) Add about 2 tsp. of filtered water

c) Add a few drops of grain alcohol.

Gently mix, do not shake. Rinse and dry the outside of the bottle. Label it "urine-cancer".

Method:

1. Test for cancer by placing the modified urine specimen on the substance plate and a white blood cell sample on the other plate.
2. If you resonate with both samples in the circuit you have cancer. Immediately, search for your cancer in your breast, prostate, skin, lungs, colon, and so forth.
3. To be more certain, test yourself to urine samples obtained from healthy persons. You should not resonate.

As you know by now, you can confirm the cancer by testing yourself to propyl alcohol and the human intestinal fluke in the liver. Next you should eliminate propyl alcohol from use, and start the parasite program. Keep testing yourself for ortho-phospho-tyrosine until it is gone. Also continue to test yourself for propyl alcohol and the intestinal fluke in the white blood cells; make sure they are gone. Test yourself for aflatoxin.

Lesson Ten

Purpose: To test for HIV.

Materials: Purchase a few milligrams of Protein 24 antigen (a piece of the HIV virus core) or the complete HIV virus on a slide (see *Sources*). You may use the vial unopened if only one test specimen is needed. To make more specimens, use about 1 milligram per ½ ounce bottle. Add 2 tsp. filtered water and ¼ tsp. grain alcohol.

Method: Search in the thymus, vagina and penis for the virus because that is where it will reside almost exclusively for the first year or two. If you don't have those tissue specimens, you could search in urine, blood, saliva, or white blood cells, but only a positive result can be trusted. Also search for the human intestinal fluke and benzene in the thymus. Follow the disappearance of HIV after treating for parasites for five days.

Lesson Eleven

Purpose: To test for disease.

Materials: Use slides and cultures of disease organisms.

Homemade preparations of strep throat, acute mononucleosis, thrush (*Candida*), chicken pox, *Herpes 1* and *2*, shingles, warts, measles, yeast, fungus, rashes, colds, sore throats, sinus problems, tobacco virus, and so forth can all be made by swabbing or scraping the affected part. A paper swab or wooden stick works well. Put a small bit on a slide. Let air dry. Add a drop of balsam and a cover slip. Or put the swab in a bottle, add water and alcohol as described previously. Microscope slides of everyday diseases can greatly expand your test set (see *Sources*).

Method: Test yourself for a variety of diseases, using your white blood cell specimen first. Then search in organs like the liver, pancreas, spleen. Notice how many of these common illnesses don't "go away" at all. They are alive and well in some organ. They are merely not making you sick!

Lesson Twelve

Purpose: To test for AIDS.

Materials: Benzene sample, thymus and other tissue samples such as liver, pancreas, penis and vagina. Also a collection of disease specimens such as the ones used in the previous lesson.

Method: Search in the thymus for benzene. If it is positive throughout the day, you are at risk for developing AIDS, although you may not be ill. Search other tissues for benzene. The more tissues with benzene in them the more serious the situation. Immediately search all your body products and foods for benzene. (Use the skin method. If your skin is already full of benzene this test will not work. Go off the benzene list until the skin is free of it, then test.)

Stay off benzene polluted items forever.

Tally up the diseases you tested positive for in Lesson Eleven. Test at least twelve. If you had more than half positive you already have AIDS. (50% is my standard, you may set your own; an ideal standard for defining a healthy person should be 0% positive.)

Lesson Thirteen

Purpose: To test for aflatoxin.

Materials: Do not try to purchase a pure sample of aflatoxin; it is one of the most potent carcinogens known. Having it on hand would constitute unnecessary hazard, even though the bottle would never need to be opened. Simply make specimens of beer, moldy bread, apple cider vinegar and raw nuts using a very small amount and adding cold tap water and grain alcohol as usual.

Method: Label your specimens Mold A, Mold B, and so forth. Test yourself for these. If you have all of them in your white blood cells and liver then you very, very probably have aflatoxin build up. Next, test your daily foods for their presence in your white blood cells. Those that test positive must be further tested for aflatoxin using the skin method. For instance, to test bread, rub some into your skin; wait for it to be absorbed; then test for molds in your skin. Notice the effect of vitamin C on aflatoxin in your liver. Find a time when your liver is positive to aflatoxin. Take 1 gram vitamin C in a glass of water. Check yourself for aflatoxin every five minutes. Does it clear? How long does it take?

Lesson Fourteen

Purpose: To identify a pollutant in a product.

It is important to test your drinking water for lead and cadmium, especially if you have high blood pressure. It is also important to test your home air for arsenic, asbestos, fiberglass, and formaldehyde. And it is important to test every <u>flavored</u> food item or product for benzene and other solvents.

Method: Testing your water:

1. Have ready your test bottles of lead, cadmium, chlorine, PCB and solvents.
2. Test your skin to these pollutants, and also to the water sample. It must be negative before proceeding.
3. Apply some of the water you want to test to your skin and use the skin method previously described.
4. After your skin has absorbed the water, retest each toxic substance in turn. Those that test positive are in the water.

Remember you only have a short time, about 4 minutes, to do all your testing because the white blood cells are rapidly clearing it from your skin. Also remember, it takes several minutes for some substances to be absorbed by the skin. Only after it is absorbed should you test for the individual elements.

Air samples are obtained by setting out a wide mouth jar with ½ inch of filtered water in it overnight. Air pollutants attach to dust which settles and gets trapped in the water. The next day rub the water into the skin and test for radon, asbestos, fiberglass, arsenic, PVC, and household gas.

Alternatively, a dust sample can be obtained directly. Cut a square of paper towel, about two inches by two inches; dampen it and wipe the kitchen table or counter with several long swipes. Place it in a plastic baggy. Add enough water to wet the entire paper.

Lesson Fifteen

Purpose: To test for parasites.

Materials: Use cultures or slides of parasites purchased from biological supply companies. If you have a pet, test yourself to pet saliva. Use a paper swab to collect the saliva; place it in a bottle, add 2 tsp. filtered water and ¼ tsp. grain alcohol or vodka Wash your hands.

Method: If you test positive to your pet's saliva, you have something in common–a parasite, no doubt. Treat yourself for parasites until you no longer test positive. This may not be possible if you carry tapeworm stages which so many of us do. You must search your muscles and liver for these, not the white blood cells since they are seldom seen in the white blood cells. The regular parasite program does not kill these. You must use different herbs found in a product called Rascal (see *Sources*). Take it as the label suggests for 20 to 30 days or until you no longer test positive to your pets' saliva, even in your muscles, liver and intestines. Tapeworm intermediate stages seem to do little harm until opened up by solvent action. After this the body may be invaded by unfertilized eggs and bacteria; search for these.

· Don't neglect to test your pets for parasites (using the surrogate method). Be sure to treat your pet on a daily basis with the pet parasite program (see *Part One*).

Lesson Sixteen

Purpose: To test for fluke disease.

A small number of intestinal flukes resident in the intestine may not give you any noticeable symptoms. Similarly, sheep liver flukes resident in the liver and pancreatic flukes in the pancreas may not cause noticeable symptoms. Their eggs are shed through the organ ducts to the intestine and out with the bowel movement. They hatch and go through various stages of development outdoors and in other animals. But if you become the total host so that various stages are developing in your organs, you have what I term *fluke disease*. You can test for fluke disease in two ways: electronically and by microscope observation.

Materials: samples of parasite stages (eggs, miracidia, redia, cercaria, metacercaria). Body fluid specimens to help you locate them for observation under a microscope.

Purchase cultures or slides of flukes and fluke stages from a biological supply company (see *Sources*).

Method: Test for fluke stages in your white blood cells first. If you have any fluke stages in your white blood cells you may wish to see them with your eyes. To do this, you must first locate them. Place your body fluid samples on the tissue plate, your parasite stages on the substance plate, and test for as many as you can procure, besides adults. After finding a stage electronically, you stand a better chance of finding it physically with a microscope.

Lesson Seventeen

Purpose: To see how sensitive your measurements can be. (How much of a substance must be present for you to get a positive result?)

Materials: filtered water, salt, glass cup measure, 13 new glass bottles that hold at least ¼ cup, 14 new plastic teaspoons, your skin tissue sample, paper towel.

Method: Some of the best measurement systems available today are immunological (such as an ELISA assay) and can detect as little as 100 fg/ml (femtograms per milliliter). A milliliter is about as big as a pea, and a femtogram is 1/1,000,000,000,000,000th (10^{-15}) of a gram!

1. Rinse the glass cup measure with filtered water and put one half teaspoon of table salt in it. Fill to one cup, stirring with a plastic spoon. What concentration is this? A teaspoon is about 5 grams, a cup is about 230 ml (milliliters), therefore the starting concentration is about 2½ gm per 230 ml, or .01 gm/ml (we will discuss the amount of error later).

2. Label one clean plastic spoon "water" and use it to put nine spoonfuls of filtered water in a clean glass bottle. Use another plastic spoon to transfer one spoonful of the .01 gm/ml salt solution in the cup measure to the glass bottle, stir, then discard the spoon. The glass bottle now has a 1 in 10 dilution, and its concentration is one tenth the original, or .001 gm/ml.

3. Use the "water" spoon to put nine spoonfuls of filtered water in bottle #2. Use a new spoon to transfer a spoonful of water from bottle #1 to bottle #2 and stir briefly (never shake). Label bottle #2 ".0001 gm/ml".

4. Repeat with remaining bottles. Bottle #13 would therefore be labeled ".000000000000001 gm/ml." This is 10^{-15} gm/ml, or 1 femtogram/ml.
5. Do the usual skin test with water from bottle #13. If you can detect this, you are one hundred times as sensitive as an ELISA assay (and you should make a bottle #14 and continue if you are curious how good your sensitivity can get). If you can not detect bottle #13, try to detect water from bottle #12 (ten times as sensitive as ELISA). Continue until you reach a bottle you can detect.

Calculate the error for your experiment by assuming you could be off by as much as 10% when measuring the salt or water, making 20% error in each of the 13 dilutions. This is a total error in bottle #13 of 280%, or at most a factor of 3. So bottle #13 could be anywhere from 0.33 to 3 femtogram/ml. So if you can detect water from bottle #13, you are definitely more sensitive then an ELISA, in spite of your crude utensils and inexpensive equipment!

If you want to calculate how many salt molecules you can detect, select the concentration at the limit of your detection, and put 2 drops on a square inch of paper towel and rub into your skin. Assume one drop can be absorbed. If you can detect water from bottle #13, you have detected 510,000 molecules (10^{-15} fg/ml divided by 58.5 gm/M multiplied by 6.02×10^{23} molecules/M divided by 20 drops/ml). Water in bottle #12 would therefore have 10 times as many molecules in one drop, and so forth. Even if your error is as much as a factor of 2 (100%), you can still get a good idea of what you can measure.

Troubleshooting: Taste some filtered water and make sure you do not test positive to it in your white blood cells. If you do, the filtered water is not pure enough, change the filter.

Always extend your set until you get a negative result (this should happen by at least bottle #21). If you always "detect" salt, then you shook the bottle!

Never try to reuse a bottle if you spill when pouring into it. Get another new bottle.

Microscopy Lesson

Purpose: To *observe* fluke stages in saliva and urine with a microscope.

Materials:

a. A low power microscope. High power is not needed. A total of 100x magnification is satisfactory for the four common flukes, *Fasciolopsis, Sheep liver fluke, human liver fluke* and *pancreatic fluke.*

b. Glass slides and coverslips.

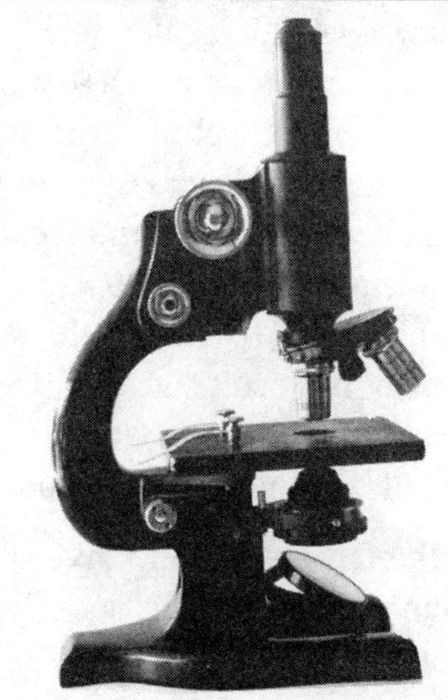

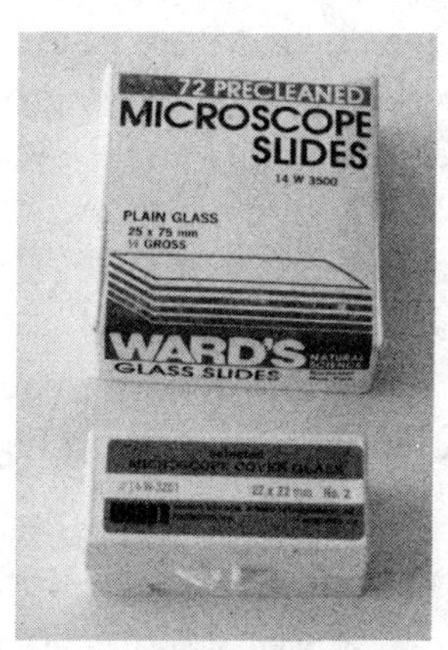

Fig. 61 Microscope, slides and coverslips

c. A disposable eye dropper.

d. For sanitation purposes (wiping table tops, slides, microscope and your hands) a 50% to 70% alcohol solution (not rubbing alcohol!) is best. Dilute 95% grain alcohol 7 parts alcohol plus 3 parts water. Vodka or 56% grain alcohol can be used undiluted. Other varieties of ethyl alcohol are fine.

e. Formaldehyde, 20%. Formaldehyde 37% is commonly available at pharmacies. Dilute this with equal parts of filtered water to get 18½%, which is close enough to 20%, for the purpose of "fixing" (killing) the specimens. Store in a glass bottle in the garage, away from sunlight. Label. Specimens that are fixed properly do not lose their life-like appearance.

f. Iodine solution. This is only useful for the urine specimens. Lugol's iodine and tincture of iodine are both useful. Ask a pharmacist to prepare *Lugol's Iodine Solution* for you, as follows:

- 44 grams iodine crystals
- 88 grams potassium iodide crystals

Dissolve both in 1 liter filtered water (this may take a day of frequent shaking).

Method for saliva:

1. Pour the 20% formaldehyde into a small amber bottle or other receptacle to a depth of about 1/8 inch. Keep tightly closed.

2. The person to be tested is asked to salivate into the bottle so the organisms are immediately "fixed" without undergoing cooling first. The total volume should be about double the original amount of formaldehyde used. Make a mark on the container so the subject knows how

much to produce. The resultant concentration of formaldehyde will be about 10%.

3. Shake the bottle a few times. Set it aside for 24 hours to settle (less if testing is urgent).
4. With a dropper, draw up some of the bottom settlings. Put one drop on a slide and apply a coverslip.
5. View under low power of microscope. Compare objects you observe with specimens obtained on slides from biological supply companies.

Note: Persons with HIV and moderate AIDS will show about one to ten parasite stages per slide. It requires several hours of searching. Persons with HIV and severe AIDS show 10 or more fluke stages per slide; this makes the task of finding them much easier. Persons with terminal untreated cancer have many more fluke stages than relatively well persons.

Method for urine:

1. Prepare bottles of formaldehyde fixative ahead of time. Put about ¼ to ½ inch of 20% formaldehyde in each. Keep tightly closed.
2. Add freshly voided[34] urine from cancer or HIV sufferers to the formaldehyde in approximately equal amounts, resulting in a 10% formaldehyde solution. Shake immediately. Let settle several hours. The sediment has a higher number of fluke stages. Cancer patients with cervical or prostate cancer will show higher numbers of stages in urine than other cancer types.

[34] Urine that has cooled even slightly below body temperature does not show *miracidia* and *redia* in their original shapes.

3. Staining the slide is optional. It helps to outline fluke stages slightly. Prepare Lugol's solution as described above.

   Slides may be stained in either of these two ways:

   - Put a drop of "fixed" urine on a slide. Add a drop of 50% Lugol's (dilute 1:1 with cold tap water). Apply coverslip.
   - Put a drop of "fixed" urine on a slide. Apply coverslip. Add 1 to 3 drops of 50% Lugol's to edge of coverslip and allow it to seep in.

Note: persons who have been treated for cancer or HIV using any of the known drugs may show only 1 to 2 fluke parasite stages per drop of saliva or urine. Very ill persons may show up to 10 parasites per drop (slide). For this reason, you may need to search through 20 or more slides to find flukes.

Taking Pictures Of What You See

You may be unsure of what you see even if you have the microscope slides of labeled flukes and their stages to study and compare. In real life, they vary so much in shape and size that absolute identification is difficult without experience. Unfortunately in a few hours, just as you are getting proficient, your magnificent specimens will be drying out and unfit for observation. To preserve them longer you can paint clear nail polish along the edges.

Or take photographs. To take pictures of what you see under the microscope you will need a photo-micrographic camera, which costs $200.00 and up (see *Sources*). It is easy to use. Remember to label your pictures so you know which slide it came from.

Even photographs, however, do not scientifically prove identity of parasite stages; they must be cultured, live and observed to reproduce their kind. Leave this to scientists.

The Tests

It is seductive to think that the 300+ tests I use are definitive, and by getting rid of the parasites, toxins, solvents, pathogens and kidney stones we are guaranteed good health. But there are far more of each of these than we will ever have samples of. Fortunately, we think we know the major culprits. If you clean these up, then you can expect most, if not all, of your symptoms to go away, including AIDS.

I see mold and solvent pollution as being the number one threat to our health at this time. Molds prevent the liver from detoxifying solvents. Solvents induce parasites to invade animals and tissues that they have never gotten a foothold in before, causing cancer, HIV/AIDS and a number of other modern diseases. In addition they are totally unsuspected, with virtually no federal research dollars being spent on them compared to the grants for viral and bacterial research. Worse yet, our beef and poultry supplies are being overrun by parasites exposing us to new levels of hazard. Even our pets are newly parasitized and can infect us, too!

Although you may think your only goal is to get the human intestinal fluke out of your thymus so that HIV is eliminated, it is just as important to <u>completely</u> clean up your body. This allows you to <u>cure</u> AIDS, and feel better in every way.

HIV

There are a variety of antibody tests which detect whether you have made antibodies to the HIV virus. Obviously, you must have had the virus at some time in the past in order to make the antibodies. And since nobody ever gets rid of the virus once they have it (unless they deparasitize), it is a perfectly adequate diagnostic test.

But if you kill the intestinal fluke and its stages, thereby eliminating the virus, you do not stop making the antibodies. For this reason another type of test is needed. P24, protein 24, antigen is an actual piece of the HIV virus itself. The P24 test, therefore is testing for the actual virus, not antibodies to it. It is like taking a small piece of elephant skin to the zoo to search for elephants. I selected the P24 test to clinically prove the absence of the HIV virus, because the antibody test would remain positive even after the HIV virus is gone. Bear in mind, however, that the P24 test is still a chemical one, and is affected by many other factors which may allow false positives and false negatives to occur. The laboratory test method, of course, tries to take this into account.

My electronic test uses the same P24 antigen, one half milligram dissolved in 3 ml filtered water permanently sealed in a ½ ounce amber glass bottle.

I have also used a slide with lung tissue infected with HIV (see *Sources*) and got identical results.

Cancer

Although there are no true clinical cancer tests, there are more than two dozen markers.[35] Each can identify a particular cancer with reasonable accuracy. Recently, ortho-phospho-

[35] Stewart Sell, M.D., *Diagnostic Uses of Cancer Markers*, The Female Patient, Vol. 9, August 1984.

tyrosine has been found to be reliable for many kinds of human malignancies.[36]

The ortho-phospho-tyrosine sample was prepared by dissolving several milligrams in 10 ml filtered water and kept permanently sealed in a ½ ounce amber glass bottle. The hCG sample was similarly prepared.

Parasites

I test for about 120 different parasites or stages of parasites. (They are divided into Box 1 and Box 2 which you may see referred to in the case histories.) Below is a list of the parasites. They are on slides purchased from biological supply companies. Some are cultures in small vials. Most of them are whole mounts of the adult stage. Some are slides of eggs and other stages.

They are searched for in the white blood cells. This means that encysted forms such as tapeworm cysticercus and Toxoplasma cysts are missed because the immune system is not attacking them. They have to be searched for separately in the tissue suspected (muscles, eyes, etc.).

The importance of testing for a list of parasites is not to cure HIV. *Fasciolopsis buskii*, the human intestinal fluke, has already been identified in my research as the critical HIV parasite. It is the remainder, however, that are undoubtedly contributing to your inability to regain your health. Tracking their demise as you stay on the parasite killing recipe lets you see your progress.

---

[36] Hunter, T., and Cooper, J.A., *Ann. Rev. Biochem*, 54:897, 1985. Also Yarden, Y., *Ann. Rev. Biochem*, 57:443, 1988.

Parasite	Comment
Acanthamoeba culbertsoni	
Acanthocephala	worm
Anaplasma marginale	sporozoa from cows
Ancylostoma braziliense (adult)	hookworm (from dogs and cats)
Ancylostoma caninum	dog hookworm, causes fatigue, anemia, muscle ache
Ancylostoma duodenale male	hookworm
Ascaris larvae in lung	common roundworm of cats and dogs
Ascaris lumbricoides	common round worm of cats, dogs. Brings with it *Bacteroides fragilis* and *Coxasckie* viruses.
Ascaris megalocephala	roundworm of horse
Babesia bigemina	
Babesia canis smear	sporozoa of dog blood
Balantidium coli cysts	
Balantidium sp. trophozoites parasitic ciliate	
Besnoitia	sporozoa in lung
Capillaria hepatica	roundworm in liver, from rats and cats
Chilomastix cysts	from rats
Chilomastix mesnili (trophozoites)	flagellate in intestine (from rat)
Chilomonas	ciliate
Clonorchis metacercariae	human liver fluke stage
Clonorchis sinensis	human liver fluke adult
Clonorchis sinensis eggs	
Cryptocotyle lingua (adult)	fluke of sea gull
Cysticercus fasciolaris	cyst stage of *Taenia taeniaeformis*, tapeworm of pets
Dientamoeba fragilis	a trichomonad, not an amoeba
Dipetalonema perstans	round worm
Diphyllobothrium erinacei (Mansoni) scolex	tapeworm of dogs and cats (head)
Diphyllobothrium latum (scolex)	fish tapeworm (head)
Dipylidium caninum	dog tapeworm
Dipylidium caninum (scolex)	dog tapeworm (head)
Dirofilaria immitis	heartworm of dogs, causes pain over heart, irregular heartbeat in humans
Echinococcus granulosus	small tapeworm (pets)
Echinococcus granulosus (cysts)	small tapeworm, stage
Echinococcus granulosus (eggs)	small tapeworm, stage
Echinococcus multilocularis	tapeworm of pets
Echinoporyphium recurvatum	fluke of poultry
Echinostoma revolutum	flatworm of water foul
Eimeria stiedae	sporozoa of rabbit
Eimeria tenella	sporozoa of large intestine
Endamoeba gingivalis trophozoite	amoeba of gums

Endolimax nana trophozoites and cysts	protozoan
Entamoeba coli cysts	amoeba in small and large intestine
Entamoeba histolytica trophozoites	common amoeba in intestine
Enterobius vermicularis	human pinworm
Eurytrema pancreaticum	common fluke of pancreas (from pigs and cattle), causes diabetes
Fasciola hepatica	sheep liver fluke of mammals, adult
Fasciola hepatica cercariae, eggs, metacercariae, miracidia, rediae	sheep liver fluke stages
Fasciolopsis buskii	human intestinal fluke, adult
Fasciolopsis buskii eggs, miracidia, rediae	human intestinal fluke stages. Brings with it HIV.
Fasciolopsis cercariae	human intestinal fluke stage. Brings with it HIV.
Fischoedrius elongatus	liver fluke of cats
Gastrothylax elongatus	fluke
Giardia lamblia (trophozoites)	common flagellate in intestine
Giardia lamblia cysts	common flagellate in intestine
Gyrodactylus	a fluke
Haemonchus contortus	large stomach roundworm of domestic animals
Haemoproteus	sporozoa, causes bird malaria
Hasstile sig. tricolor (adult)	rabbit fluke
Heterakis	round worm of chickens
Heterophyes heterophyes	fluke of intestine (from crawfish)
Hymenolepis cysticercoides	small tapeworm of pets
Hymenolepis diminuta	small tapeworm of pets
Hypodereum conoideum	fluke of poultry
Iodamoeba butschlii trophozoites and cysts	small amoeba of colon
Leishmania braziliensis	flagellate
Leishmania donovani	infects spleen and liver (from hamsters)
Leishmania mexicana	protozoa
Leishmania tropica	flagellate, infects skin
Leucocytozoon	sporozoa, causes bird malaria
Loa loa	a heart parasite, causes irregular heartbeat
Macracanthorhynchus	spiny headed worm of pig
Metagonimus	fluke of intestine
Metagonimus Yokogawai	a liver fluke
Moniezia (scolex)	large tapeworm of domestic animal (head)
Moniezia expansa	large tapeworm of domestic animals
Monocystis agilis	sporozoa from earth worm
Multiceps serialis	dog tapeworm
Myxosoma	sporozoa from fish gill
Naegleria fowleri	parasite of brain
Necator americanus	human hookworm

Notocotylus quinqeserialis	fluke of intestine (from muskrat)
Onchocerca volvulus	roundworm
Paragonimus Westermanii adult	lung fluke (from pets)
Passalurus ambiguus	rabbit pinworm
Pigeon tapeworm	
Plasmodium cynomolgi	malaria of monkey
Plasmodium falciparum smear	sporozoa of blood, causes malaria
Plasmodium vivax smear	sporozoa of blood, causes benign malaria
Platynosomum fastosum adult	Cat liver fluke
Pneumocystis carnii	sporozoa of the lung from rat
Prosthogonimus macrorchis (eggs)	fluke
Sarcocystis	sporozoa of muscles
Schistosoma haematobium	blood fluke
Schistosoma mansoni	blood fluke of veins
Stephanurus dentalus (ova)	roundworm
Stigeoclonium	
Strongyloides (filariform larva)	human threadworm, causes migraine headache
Taenia pisiformis	tapeworm of cats
Taenia pisiformis (cysticercus)	tapeworm of cats, stage
Taenia saginata (cysticercus)	beef tapeworm, stage
Taenia solium (cysticercus)	pork tapeworm, stage
Taenia solium (scolex)	pork tapeworm
Toxocara (eggs)	roundworm of cats
Toxoplasma (human strain)	sporozoa of mice, cats, etc.; causes eye disease
Trichinella spiralis (muscle)	roundworm, invades muscles, causes myalgia (from pets)
Trichomonas muris	flagellate of rat
Trichomonas vaginalis	protozoa of genital tract
Trichuris sp.	whipworm
Trypanosoma brucei	blood parasite (from rat)
Trypanosoma cruzi	blood flagellate (from mouse)
Trypanosoma equiperdium	causes sleeping sickness
Trypanosoma gambiense	blood flagellate, causes African sleeping sickness (from rat)
Trypanosoma lewisi	blood flagellate of rat
Trypanosoma rhodesiense	blood flagellate, causes sleeping sickness (from rat)
Urocleidus	a fluke

Toxic Elements

I call a substance "toxic" if it can be found in your white blood cells (the immune system). The concept is that if something is found in the white blood cells, it must be harmful to your body or at least useless. Even if the substance isn't harmful, if it preoccupies your immune system, it is a handicap to your body.

Some of the test items, like aluminum silicate, are compounds, not simply elements. Since there are thousands upon thousands of toxic chemicals in our environment and there would be no way of testing them all, my system of using the elements instead of the compounds is a short cut. For this reason, the test is far from perfect. For example, a person may test positive to aluminum silicate but show no aluminum in the white blood cells. So, if I had tested only for aluminum, I would have missed the problem.

Sometimes, toxic elements are present in an organ, but are not present in the white blood cells. For example, there may be mercury stored in the pancreas, but not be showing in the white blood cells at the time I'm testing. I interpret this as reflecting low levels of the toxin. Ideally, a test would search all your organs, but this would be too time-consuming for my technology.

Most of the toxic elements are metals, heavy metals and lanthanides. But some are not; examples are PCBs and formaldehyde.

Some important elements are missing, like iron, zinc and manganese. This is because I never could find them present in the white blood cells, and I finally gave up searching for them.

The most important thing to do after finding the toxic element in your body is to track down the source of it in your environment. Is it in food, air, drugs, vitamins? To test a pill or food, it is put in a plastic bag with cold tap water added and tested the same way as the elements. To test the air in a person's home, an open glass jar, containing filtered water, is set out for 3 days in the room to be tested. Fine particles and gas molecules stick to dust in the air and fall into the water. The jar is then used like any other test solution.

Alternatively, a dust sample can be obtained by wiping the kitchen table or counter with a dampened piece of paper towel, two inches by two inches square. It is then placed in a plastic baggy.

Most asbestos comes from the clothes dryer belt. Most vanadium comes from a gas leak in the house. Most lead comes from soldered copper plumbing. Most mercury comes from tooth fillings. But there are fascinating exceptions as you will see as you read the case histories.

Below is a list of the 70 or so toxic elements in the test. Most of them were obtained as Atomic Absorption Standard Solutions and are, therefore, very pure. This prevents mistakes in identifying a toxin. They were stored in ½ ounce brown glass bottles with bakelite caps and permanently sealed with plastic film since testing did not require them to be opened. The exact concentration and the solubility characteristics are not important in this qualitative test. The main sources of these substances in our environment are given beside each item.

Toxic Substance	Sources
Aflatoxin B	beer, bread, apple cider vinegar, moldy fruit, nuts
Aluminum	cookware, deodorant, lotions, soaps
Aluminum silicate	salt, water softener
Antimony	fragrance in lotions, colognes
Arsenic	pesticide, "treated" carpet, wallpaper
Asbestos	clothes dryer belt, hair blower, paint on radiators
Barium	lipstick, bus exhaust
Benzalkonium chloride	toothpaste
3,4 Benzopyrene	flame cooked foods, toast
4,5 Benzopyrene	flame cooked foods, toast
Beryllium	hurricane lamps, gasoline, dentures, kerosene
Bismuth	colognes, lotions, antacids
Boron	
Bromine	bleached "brominated" flour
Cadmium	galvanized water pipes, old tooth fillings
Cerium	tooth fillings
Cesium	clear plastic bottles used for beverages
Chlorine	from Chlorox™ bleach
Chromium	cosmetics, water softener
Cobalt	detergent, blue and green body products
Copper	tooth fillings, water pipes
Dysprosium	paint and varnish
Erbium	packaging for food, pollutant in pills
Europium	tooth fillings
Europium oxide	tooth fillings, catalytic converter
Fiberglass	dust from remodeling or building insulation
Formaldehyde	foam in mattresses and furniture, paneling
Gadolinium	tooth fillings
Gallium	tooth fillings
Germanium	with thallium in tooth fillings (pollutant)
Gold	tooth fillings
Hafnium	hair spray, nail polish, pollutant in pills
Holmium	usually found in presence of PCBs
Indium	tooth fillings
Iridium	tooth fillings
Lanthanum	computer and printing supplies
Lead	solder joints in water pipes
Lithium	printing supplies
Lutetium	paint and varnish
Mercury	tooth fillings
Molybdenum	auto supplies
Neodymium	pollutant in pills
Nickel	tooth fillings, metal glasses frames
Niobium	pollutant in pills, foil packaging for food

Palladium	tooth fillings
Platinum	tooth fillings
Polychlorinated biphenyl PCB	detergent, hair spray, salves
Polyvinyl chloride acetate (PVC)	glues, building supplies, leaking cooling system
Praseodymium	pollutant in pills
Radon	cracks in basement cement, water pipes
Rhenium	spray starch
Rhodium	tooth fillings
Rubidium	tooth fillings
Ruthenium	tooth fillings
Samarium	tooth fillings
Scandium	tooth fillings
Selenium	
Silver	tooth fillings
Sodium fluoride	toothpaste
Strontium	toothpaste, water softener
Tantalum	tooth fillings
Tellurium	tooth fillings
Terbium	pollutant in pills
Thallium acetate	pollutant in mercury tooth fillings
Thorium nitrate	earth (dust)
Thulium	pollutant in Vitamin C (Ester-C)
Tin	toothpaste
Titanium	tooth fillings, body powder
Tungsten	electric water heater, toaster, hair curler
Uranium acetate	earth (dust)
Vanadium pentoxide	gas leak in home, candles (not necessarily lit)
Ytterbium	pollutant in pills
Yttrium	pollutant in pills
Zirconium	deodorant, toothpaste

Elements like erbium and terbium have only recently come into use. They were formerly called Rare Earth Elements but now are called *Lanthanides*. There are 15 of them: lanthanum cerium, praseodymium, neodymium, samarium, europium, gadolinium, terbium, dysprosium, holmium, erbium, thulium, ytterbium, lutetium, and promethium.

All except promethium are in my test for toxic elements. You can see from the case histories that we have lanthanides in our bodies, widely distributed. They are in our processed foods, in our supplements and medicines, and in our tooth fillings, whether plastic or metal. Is it a good idea for the human species to eat elements that we know nothing about? Several of them absorb UV (ultraviolet) light. Should we be absorbing UV light in this manner when we already have a biological means (riboflavin, vitamin B2) of doing this that took millions of years to evolve? Some of them have special magnetic properties (gadolinium and samarium). Some of them are phosphors; they give off light when irradiated. A number of them are known to "home in" on cancerous tumors. This is not understood. Why are they in our tablets and capsules? Who is making these polluted products? Evidently, the traditional safeguards against massive pollution don't work. It should be possible to make a test strip that detects Rare Earth Elements as a group, since they have very similar properties. The public must not rely on reassurances by industry or government that food or body products are pure and safe. People must be able to test them for themselves.

Solvents

This is a list of all the solvents in the test together with the main source of them in our environment. These are chemicals, very pure, obtained from chemical supply companies, unless otherwise stated. Those marked with an asterisk (*) were the subject of a recent book *The Neurotoxicity of Solvents* by Peter Arlien-Soburg, 1992, CRC Press.

Solvent	Source
1,1,1, Trichloro ethane* (TCE)	flavored foods
2, 5-Hexane dione*	flavored foods
2 Butanone* (methyl ethyl ketone)	flavored foods
2 Hexanone* (methyl butyl ketone)	flavored foods
2 Methyl propanol	
2 Propanol (propyl alcohol)	see the propyl alcohol list
Acetone	store-bought drinking water, cold cereals, pet food, animal feed
Acetonylacetone (2,5 hexanedione)	flavored foods
Benzene	see the benzene list
Butyl nitrite	
Carbon tetrachloride	store-bought drinking water, cold cereals, pet food, animal feeds
Decane	health food cookies and cereals
Denatured alcohol	obtained from pharmacy
Dichloromethane* (methylene chloride)	store-bought orange juice, herb tea blends
Gasoline regular leaded	obtained at gasoline station
Grain alcohol	95% ethyl alcohol obtained at liquor store
Hexanes*	decaffeinated beverages
Isophorone	flavored foods
Kerosene	obtained at gasoline station
Methanol (wood alcohol)	colas, artificial sweeteners, infant formula
Mineral oil	lotions
Mineral spirits	obtained from paint store
Paradiclorobenzene	mothballs
Pentane	decaffeinated beverages
Petroleum ether	in some gasolines
Styrene*	styrofoam dishes
Toluene*	store-bought drinking water, cold cereals
Trichloroethylene* (TCEthylene)	flavored foods
Xylene*	store-bought drinking water, cold cereals

Pathogens

Pathogens are mostly bacteria and viruses, but also may include molds and yeasts. Most of them are on slides, some are preserved cultures, all are purchased from biological supply companies (see *Sources*). They are safe for you to handle.

Bacteria or Virus	Comment
Adenovirus	causes common cold
Alpha streptococcus	respiratory infection
Bacillus anthracis	causes anthrax in cattle
Bacillus cereus	
Bacillus megaterium	soil
Bacterium acnes	causes acne
Bacteroides fragilis	always found with Ascaris
Beta streptococcus	causes respiratory infection
Blepharisma	
Bordetella pertussis	"whooping cough"
Borellia burgdorferi	Lyme disease
Campylobacter fetus smear	stomach and vein disease
Campylobacter pyloridis	stomach and vein disease
Candida albicans (pure powder)	common yeast, causes thrush
Capsules of bacteria (capsular stain)	
Caulobacter vibrioides	
Central spores (bacillus smear)	
Chlamydia trachomatis	eye disease
Clostridium acetobutylicum	soil
Clostridium botulinum	causes food poisoning
Clostridium septicum (human blood)	
Clostridium tetani	causes tetanus
Corynebacterium diptheriae	causes diphtheria
Corynebacterium xerosis	causes stiffness
Coxsackie virus B-1	always found with Bacteroides fragilis
Coxsackie virus B-4	always found with Bacteroides fragilis
Crithidia fasciculata	
Cytomegalovirus (CMV) antigen	
Cytophaga rubra	
Diplococcus pneumoniae	respiratory illness
Eikanella corrodens	
Enterobacter aerogenes	intestinal bacterium
Epstein Barre virus (EBV)	fatigue
Erwinia carotovora	
Escherichia coli (E. coli)	intestinal bacterium
Gaffkya tetragena	causes respiratory infections

Gardnerella vaginalis	ovarian and genital tract infection
Haemophilus influenzae	bacterial meningitis, infects joints
Hepatitis B antigen	
Herpes simplex 1	causes "cold sores"
Herpes simplex 2	causes genital herpes
Herpes Zoster	"shingles"
Histomonas meleagridis (liver)	
Histoplasma capsulatum	
Human papilloma plantar wart #4	wart
Human papilloma virus #4	wart
Influenza A and B (flu shot)	
Klebsiella pneumoniae	causes pneumonia
Lactobacillus acidophilus	
Leptospira interrogans	spirochete, causes arthritis
Measles antigen	
Mumps antigen	
Mycobacterium tuberculosis (infected nodule)	causes tuberculosis
Mycoplasma	chronic cough
Neisseria gonorrhea	causes gonorrhea
Neisseria sicca	soil
Nocardia asteroides	Parkinson's Disease, heart disease
Proteus mirabilis	urinary tract pathogen
Proteus vulgaris	in oxalate kidney stones
Pseudomonas aeruginosa	found in open wounds
Respiratory syncytial virus	
Salmonella enteriditis	intestinal infection, pollutes dairy
Salmonella paratyphi	
Salmonella typhimurium	causes food poisoning, pollutes dairy
Serratia marcescens	occurs in water, soil, milk
Shigella dysenteriae	causes diarrhea, pollutes dairy
Shigella flexneri	depression, pollutes dairy products
Shigella sonnei	
Sphaerotilus natans	
Spirillum serpens	
Staphylococcus aureus	skin bacterium which is common cause of infections, tooth abscesses, heart disease
Staphylococcus epidermidis	infects skin and mucous membranes
Streptococcus lactis	occurs in milk
Streptococcus mitis	lung infection, tooth infection and cavities, abscesses
Streptococcus pneumoniae	causes pneumonia and inner ear disease
Streptococcus pyogenes	one of most common causes of infections
Streptococcus sp. group G	causes sore throats
Terminal spores bacillus smear	
Tobacco mosaic virus	occurs in tobacco
Treponema pallidum	causes pain over overies

Trichomonas vaginalis	genital tract infection
Troglodytella abrassari	
Veillonella dispar	

Kidney Stones

In this test we search in the kidney for seven kinds of crystals or stones.

Stone	Comment
Cysteine	sulfur containing
Cystine	sulfur containing
Dicalcium phosphate	also causes common arthritis, hardening of arteries, spurs
Monocalcium phosphate	also causes common arthritis, hardening of arteries, spurs
Tri-calcium phosphate	also causes common arthritis, hardening of arteries, spurs
Oxalate	cause of lower back pain 95% of the time
Uric acid	also causes gout and arthritis

Stones begin as tiny crystals, much too tiny to be seen by X-ray. They get deposited in the tiny tubules that make up the kidney, partly blocking the flow of liquid. This leads to "water holding" in your tissues. As more crystals are formed, they begin to deposit in other organs, too, such as joints of feet and hands and the interior of arteries, causing hardening. The usual symptoms are low back pain, pain running down the leg, foot pain, hand pain and gout.

Oxalic acid crystals cause pain in the lower back. Uric acid causes pain in the toes. The phosphates cause pain in the other joints (arthritis). But crystals do not cause pain by themselves. Bacteria find these nutritious deposits, and ultimately, it is they and their refuse that cause pain.

By causing partial blockage, these deposits prevent heavy metals from passing out through the kidneys. Mercury and nickel from tooth fillings are constantly being excreted through the kidney tubules. But as the kidneys get older and the deluge of toxic compounds gets higher, the toxins just attach themselves to the deposits already there. Soon, a pile-up of toxins occurs in the kidney.

The treatment is the same for all persons. It is a combination of herbs and nutritional substances, which, together, can dissolve all the 7 kinds of stones. The recipe is quite long. The reason for this is so the individual kinds of stones don't have to be dissolved separately. This recipe dissolves all the stones in three weeks.

Notice that some very sick or elderly people are told to take half a dose only. Persons with a history of kidney stones, who know they have large stones, are also told to drink half a dose daily. Persons with sensitive stomachs may not tolerate these herbs; they could try killing their parasites first.

It is fair to say that we <u>all</u> develop kidney stones; although they may remain very tiny and cause no pain. It is a healthful practice to go on the Kidney Stone Recipe (see *Recipes*) twice a year, regardless of symptoms.

Gallstones

We all have gallstones, so I do not test for this anymore.

Stone	Comment
Cholesterol crystals (encased in bile)	Accumulate in your liver bile ducts.

The Liver Cleanse is recommended many times in the Case histories. This will get rid of gallstones, without surgery!

See *Recipes*.

Blood Tests

There are many blood tests that can be performed by a clinical laboratory. In the case histories I do not list all that were done (I typically ordered about 100), but only the ones that I thought significant. Here are some I refer to in the case histories:

Test	Comment
Alk. Phos.	Alkaline phosphatase, bone enzymes. Goes up with bone disease, cancer.
Amylase	An enzyme produced by the pancreas. It should not be in the blood.
Atyp lymphs	Atypical lymphocytes. Misshaped.
Baso	Basophils, a variety of white blood cells. When over 1% is suggestive of cancer.
Blasts	Immature white blood cells.
BUN	Blood urea nitrogen. Body waste - controlled by kidneys.
Ca125	A cancer marker for ovarian cancer.
Calcium	When low (9.0 mg/dl), lets tissues seep.
Chloride	
Cholesterol	High amounts are indicative of blocked bile ducts in the liver, preventing excretion. Low levels reflect liver problems.
CO2	Carbon dioxide. Goes up with air pollution problems.

Creatinine	Body waste derived from our muscles - controlled by kidneys and should be 1.0 mg/dl or less.
Eos	Eosinophils. Variety of white blood cell; increase with parasitism and allergies. Should be less than 3% of white blood cells.
Estrogen	A major women's hormone. Should not be higher than 100 pg/ml, except in pregnancy.
FBS	Fasting blood sugar (glucose). Blood sugar level measured in the morning in the fasted state. Should be under 100 mg/DL; controlled by islets of Langerhans in pancreas.
Ferritin	A form of iron that is usually high in cancer sufferers
GGT, SGOT, SGPT	Liver enzymes, go up with liver damage.
Hemoglobin	The oxygen carrying part of the red blood cell.
Iron	Should be about 100 mcg/dl.
LDH	Lactic dehydrogenase, goes up with cancer, and with muscle stress such as heart stress.
Lymphs	Lymphocytes. The white cells whose job it is to eat and destroy viruses, and make antibodies. Should be about 25% of white blood cells.
MCV	Mean cell volume (average size of red blood cells). When over 100 suggests pernicious anemia. Corrects itself when Ascaris and hookworm are killed.
Monocytes	Rise when you are sick.
Phosphates	Should be less than 4 mg/DL in adults. Higher levels show bone dissolution is occurring. Children should have higher levels.
Platelet count	Goes up with parasitism. Should be 250 thou/cu mm. Over 400 thou/cu mm is extremely high. Causes blood to clot.
Potassium	Should be no less than 4.4 meq/L.
PSA	Prostate specific antigen. A prostate cancer "marker"; it should be less than 4.1 ng/ml.
RBC	Red blood cell count. Below 5 million per cubic mm is low for a man, below 4.3 million is low for a woman.
Seg	Segmental white blood cells. Those white cells whose job it is to eat and destroy bacteria. There should be about 70%.
Total protein	Blood protein made by the liver; sum of albumin and globulin. Does not reflect protein in diet.
Triglycerides	Blood fat - goes up with kidney problems.
Uric acid	Muscle waste. Goes up with kidney problems.
WBC	White blood cell count. Low levels are below 5,000 per cubic mm.

Recipes

Read old recipe books for the fun and savings of making your own nutritious food. Change the recipes to avoid processed ingredients. Here are some I found:

Beverage Recipes

Anything made in your own juicer is fine. Experiment with new combinations to create different flavorful fruit and vegetable juices. Consider the luxury of preparing gourmet juices which satisfy your own individual palate instead of the mass-produced, polluted varieties sold at grocery stores.

Lemonade

1 cup fresh lemon juice, 1 cup honey, 1½ quarts filtered cold tap water. Bring honey and water to a boil if you plan to keep it several days. Then add lemon juice and store in the refrigerator.

Fresh Tomato Juice

Simmer for ½ hour: 12 medium-sized raw, ripe tomatoes, ½ cup water, 1 slice onion, 2 ribs celery with leaves, ½ bay leaf, 3 sprigs parsley. Strain these ingredients. Season with: 1 tsp. salt (aluminum-free), ¼ tsp. paprika, ½ tsp. honey. Serve thoroughly chilled. Makes about 4 servings.

Fresh Pineapple Juice

Peel a pineapple. Throw away all soft or discolored parts. Cut it into cubes. Extract the juice by putting the pineapple through a food grinder or a blender. There will be very little pulp. Strain the juice and serve it on ice with sprigs of mint. Makes about 1½ cups of juice. Mix the pulp with an equal amount of clover honey and use as topping for homemade ice cream (below), pancakes, or waffles.

Maple Milk Shake

For each milk shake, blend or shake together: 1 glass of cold boiled milk and 2 tablespoons maple syrup.

Yankee Drink

Mix together 1 gal. water, 3 cups honey, ½ cup fresh squeezed lemon juice, and 1 tsp. ginger.

Hot Vanilla Milk

Add one inch of vanilla bean and one tsp. honey to a glass of milk and bring to a near boil. You may add a pinch of cinnamon or other pure spice.

Red Milk

Equal parts fresh carrot juice (use a juicer) and sterilized milk. Save the carrot pulp for salads.

My Own Soda Pop

Excellent for stomach distress. Put 1 tsp. citric acid, 2 tbs. vegetable glycerine (see *Sources*), 2 tbs. honey, and 1 lemon, juiced by hand, into a quart jar and fill with cold water. Refrigerate until ready to use. Then add 1 tsp. baking soda and shake a few times, keeping the lid tight. Pour over a few ice cubes. Many variations are possible: other fruit concentrates, made in the blender, can be used along with some lemon juice; for example, 2 blended whole apples, blended pineapple, orange or strawberries. Always add a bit of lemon to give it zip. You may add a pinch of ginger or other pure spice.

Note: The amount of sodium in ½ tsp. baking soda is .476 grams. If you have heart disease, high blood pressure, or edema, use potassium bicarbonate instead. Ask your doctor what an acceptable amount of sodium or potassium bicarbonate is. I would suggest limiting yourself to one glass of Soda Pop a day, even if you do not have heart disease.

Another Note: the citric acid kills bacteria, while the carbonation brings relief.

My Own Super C-Pop

An excellent way to get lots of vitamin C into a child and relieve stomach distress at the same time. Squeeze 1 slice of lemon and 1 whole orange into an 8 ounce bottle that has a tight lid. Add 1 tsp. vitamin C powder (also known as ascorbic acid), ¼ tsp. citric acid, and 2 tbs. vegetable glycerine (you may also experiment with honey for sweetness). Fill the bottle to the top with cold water. Then add ½ tsp. baking soda and close tightly. Shake briefly and serve immediately.

About honey:

Because honey contains *ergot*, a fungus, it must be detoxified first. Add ¼ tsp. vitamin C per pint at time of purchase and stir well.

Food Recipes

Despite the presence of aflatoxins, benzopyrenes and solvents in many foods, it is possible to have a delicious and safe diet. Many AIDS patients need to gain weight, and with the emphasis in today's society on losing weight, consider yourself lucky in this respect. Help yourself to lots of butter, whipping cream, whole milk, half n'half cream, avocados, and olive oil. Make your own preserves and baked goods, including breads. Remember, when you are recovering from a major illness such as HIV/AIDS, it is essential not to diet to lose weight. You must wait two years after you are recovered to try to lose weight.

Aflatoxins and solvents have been found in store-bought breads, vinegars (except for distilled white vinegar), nuts, grains, and fruit juices. It is best to bake your own bread, and now we are lucky to have an easy way of doing it. Buy a bread maker which does everything. All you need to do is add the ingredients and turn it on. In the morning you can have warm, fresh, homemade, aflatoxin-free and solvent-free bread! Modify recipes to eliminate items which may have toxins. Always add vitamin C to the bread recipe to retard mold. Freeze the bread you buy; don't just store it in the refrigerator. Never toast bread—it forms benzopyrenes. French toast made in the frying pan is safe.

Beer, fresh from the can or bottle, contains aflatoxins, besides alcohol. Stop drinking it. Order cold water and a slice of lemon in gathering places.

Buy nuts very cautiously. Every brown spot is toxic. Soak them in vitamin C water (¼ tsp per pint) or use in baking. Buy fresh made peanut butter and add lots of vitamin C to the jar, after warming it to allow thorough mixing.

Use your refrigerator carefully.

Molds, developed in the refrigerator, produce aflatoxins. Mold spores, from a spoiling orange, will blow away and settle on other food in the refrigerator. For this reason, keep all your food covered. Mold spores blow about in the air, much as yeast does. Yeast and mold spores are omnipresent. Undoubtedly, this is how they get inside the bread wrapper right in the bakery to mold your bread days later.

Leave fruit and vegetables in their original packaging instead of dumping them into the refrigerator bin. When one begins to spoil, throw it away; don't try to salvage part of it. Don't buy dozens of anything, unless you can use them in a few days.

Keep the refrigerator walls and shelves wiped clean every week with a paper towel dampened with plain water or baking soda or borax or 5-10% food grade alcohol.

Daily Foods

Dairy products should contain at least 2% fat to give you the proper amount of calcium.

Remember to sterilize dairy products

If you have low immunity due to cancer or AIDS, you must sterilize milk, buttermilk, yogurt and cottage cheese.

Things that can't be sterilized by boiling may only be used in baked or cooked dishes.

Change brands every time you shop to prevent the same pollutants from building up in your body.

If frying or cooking with fat, use <u>only</u> olive oil, butter or lard. Mix them for added flavor in your dishes. <u>Never use margarine, Crisco™ or other hydrogenated fats.</u> <u>Do not cook over flames or toast.</u>

Eat lots of **fresh fruits and vegetables**. Wash them off <u>only</u> with cold tap water, not commercial food "wash". Scrub hard with a stiff bristled brush.

Be sure to drink plenty of **plain water** from your cold faucet throughout the day, especially if it is difficult for you to drink it with your meals. If you don't like the taste of your own tap water, try to get it from a friend with newer plumbing. Use a 2½ gallon polyethylene water jug from a grocery store to transport it. Never drink water that has been through a water softener or copper plumbing or has traveled through a long plastic hose.

You may improve your tap water with an inexpensive filter pitcher. This removes chlorine and small amounts of metal toxins. It is not reliable for removing your plumbing toxins such as lead, cadmium or copper. No filter can clean up these toxins.

Two Granolas

Because commercial **cold cereals** are very convenient, but have solvents, here are two replacements.

7 cups rolled oats (old fashioned, not quick)
1 tsp. salt
1 cup wheat germ (fresh, not defatted)
½ cup honey
½ cup sunflower seeds, immaculate quality
½ cup milk (no need to sterilize or add iodine, it is being baked)
½ cup melted butter
1 cup raisins

Mix dry ingredients together. Mix liquid ingredients and add gradually, while tossing until thoroughly mixed. Place in large ungreased pans and bake in slow (250°F) oven. Stir occasionally, baking until brown and dry, usually 1-2 hours. Store in airtight container.

6 cups rolled oats
½ cup raw wheat germ
1 cup sesame seeds
1 cup sunflower seeds (raw, unsalted)
1 tsp. cinnamon
½ cup melted butter
½ cup honey

Preheat oven to 225°F. Toss all ingredients in mixing bowl. Spread thinly on a baking sheet and bake 20-25 minutes. Stir often in order to brown evenly. When golden, remove and let cool. Makes 12 cups.

Sweetening and Flavoring

Sugar, syrup and jam. Although I have not tested enough of these to know how polluted they may be, I am prejudiced against them from a health standpoint. So here are some substitutes that I know are safe. (I know candies are not safe, but that is not due to the sugar.)

Brown sugar. three varieties tested revealed no molds or alcohols or benzene.

Maple syrup. Add vitamin C to newly opened bottle, ¼ tsp. to retard mold.

Honeys. Get at least 4 flavors for variety: linden blossom, orange blossom, plain clover and local or wild flower honey. Add vitamin C to each new jar (¼ tsp per pint).

Fruit syrup. Use one package frozen fruit, such as cherries, blueberries or raspberries. Let thaw and measure the amount in cups (it might say on the package). Add an equal amount of clover honey to the fruit. Also add ¼ tsp. vitamin C powder. Mix it all in a quart canning jar and store in the refrigerator. Use this on pancakes, cereal, plain yogurt and homemade ice cream too. Use to make your own flavored beverages in a seltzer maker or to make soda pop.

Note for diabetics

Diabetics must not use artificial sweeteners. Nor can they use all the sweeteners listed. Try stevia powder instead (see *Sources*).

Preserves

Keep 3 or 4 kinds on hand, such as strawberry, pineapple, and pear. Clean and chop the desired fruit. If you use a metal knife, rinse the fruit lightly afterwards. Add just enough water to keep the fruit from sticking as it is cooked (usually a few tablespoons). Then add an equal amount of honey, or to taste and put in sterile jars in refrigerator. Make marmalade the same way, slicing the fruit and peel thinly. Always add vitamin C powder to a partly used jar to inhibit mold.

Salad Dressing

½ cup olive oil
¼ cup white distilled vinegar or fresh lemon juice
1 tsp. thyme

Combine the ingredients in a clean salad dressing bottle. (Baking soda and very hot water is the best way to wash away traces of the old oil.) Shake. Refrigerate. The basic recipe is the oil and vinegar in a 2:1 ratio. After mixing these, add any pure spice desired.

Soups

All home made soups are nutritious and safe, provided you use no processed ingredients (like bouillon), or make them in metal pots. Use herbs and aluminum-free salt to season.

Fish and Seafood

Any kind of fish or seafood is acceptable, provided it is well-cooked. Don't buy food that is already in batter. The simplest way to cook fish is to poach it in milk. It can be taken straight from the freezer, rinsed, and placed in ¼ inch of milk in the frying pan. Heat until it is cooked. Turn over and repeat. Throw away the milk. Serve with fresh lemon and herbs.

Baked Apples

Stem and core carefully, this is where 99% of the pesticide is. Cut in bite-size pieces, add a minimum of water and cook or bake minimally. Add a squirt of lemon juice when done. Serve with cinnamon, cream and honey.

Ice creams

from the grocery store are loaded with benzene and other solvents. Fortunately there are ice cream makers that do everything (no cranking)! Or try our recipe which uses a blender. Be sure not to add store bought flavors.

5 Minute Ice Cream

(Strawberry) Use 2 half pints of whipping cream, 1 package of frozen strawberries (about 10 oz.), and 1/2 cup clover honey. Pour frozen strawberries into blender. Pour whipping cream and honey over them. Blend briefly (about 10 seconds), not long enough to make butter! Pour it all into a large plastic bowl. Cover with a close fitting plastic bag and place in freezer. Prepare it a day ahead. Try using other frozen fruits, such as blueberries and cherries. Keep a few berries out of the blender and stir them in quickly with a non-metal spoon before setting the bowl in the freezer. There are many ice cream recipes to be found in old cook books. Avoid those with raw eggs or processed foods as ingredients. You may add nuts if you rinse them with vitamin C water first.

Cookies, cakes and pies

Bake them from scratch, using unprocessed ingredients. Use simple recipes from old cook books.

Seven Day Sample Menu

Because processed foods have many toxins, you must cook as much from scratch as possible. So for convenience sake, keep your meals simple in preparation. You may want to prepare ahead and refrigerate your dressings and toppings. Or you could make a hot soup for dinner, refrigerate, and eat the leftovers for lunch. Don't save leftovers more than two days. Make sure they are covered. Try baking several potatoes at one time, refrigerate and put them in a salad the next night. Variety is the spice of life, so combine the allowed foods in the most creative ways you can imagine. And don't forget herbs and spices; learn to use them from old cook books.

	Breakfast	Lunch	Dinner
Day 1	Granola and honey with milk, half n'half or whipping cream 1 cup fresh squeezed fruit juice Water Milk	Vegetarian sandwich Soup Milk Water	Orange roughy fish Fresh green beans with butter Baked potato with baked cheese or fresh chives Pie (homemade) Milk 1 cup fresh squeezed or frozen vegetable juice Water
Day 2	Egg Fried potatoes 1 glass milk Peppermint herb tea Fresh orange juice	Homemade bagel or bread Baked cream cheese Tomato 1 cup vegetable juice Water Milk	Homemade bean or lentil soup Dinner roll and butter Salad Homemade dressing Ice-cream (homemade) Water
Day 3	Cream of Wheat™ cooked with raisins and milk Pear Peppermint herb tea ½ cup milk Water	Tuna sandwich with olives and butter Soup Milk Water	Baked sweet potato with butter and sweetening. Fresh broccoli Bread and butter Strawberries and whipping cream 1 cup vegetable juice Milk Water
Day 4	French toast with maple syrup and butter Homemade grapefruit juice Milk Water	Baked cottage cheese with chopped pineapple or chives and fresh ground pepper ½ cup vegetable juice Bread and butter Water	Sautéed shrimp Fresh asparagus Potatoes, mashed or fried ½ cup vegetable juice Water Milk
Day 5	Cooked cereal 1 glass milk Fresh chopped fruit with whipping cream and honey 1 glass water	Cooked potatoes with fresh chopped parsley and butter ½ cup vegetable juice Baked apple Water Milk	1 can sardines or salmon in easy-open can (can openers shed metal) Salad of lettuce, tomato, olives, avocado with homemade dressing Bread with butter Ice cream ½ cup vegetable juice Water Milk

Day 6	Egg and homemade biscuit with honey and butter Homemade yogurt with fruit topping Fruit juice Water	Butter and avocado sandwich Sliced tomato ½ cup vegetable juice Milk Water	Gourmet pizza: homebaked bread topped with olive oil, sliced tomato or homemade sauce, sardines or anchovies, chopped vegetables, garlic and onion Salad Milk Water
Day 7	Pancakes or waffles Banana or chopped fruit with cream Milk Water	Salmon sandwich (from flip top can) ½ cup vegetable juice Milk Water	Stir-fry vegetables: broccoli, carrots, cabbage, in olive oil and butter Bread and butter Pie (optional) Milk Water

Remember to take 100 mg or more of B_2 (see *Sources*) with each meal. Sick persons need 300 mg with each meal.

Too Sick To Cook, Too Tired To Eat

Pick three meals from the sample menu that need no cooking and eat them every day.

Recipes for Natural Body Products

You can use just borax (like 20 Mule Team Borax™) and washing soda (like Arm & Hammer Super Washing Soda™) for all types of cleaning including your body, laundry and your house! You don't need all of those products you see in commercials for each special task!

Even if you have dry skin or difficult hair or some other unique requirement, just pure borax will satisfy these needs. A part of every skin problem is due to the toxic elements found in the soaps themselves. For instance aluminum is commonly added as a "skin moisturizer". It does this by impregnating the skin and attracting water, giving the illusion of moist skin. In fact you simply have moist aluminum stuck in your skin which your immune system must remove. While borax won't directly heal your skin or complexion, it does replace the agents that are causing damage, so that healing can occur.

Anti Bacterial Borax Soap

Buy borax and a plastic funnel at the grocery store. Find a suitable large bottle such as a fruit juice container or gallon water jug. Pour the borax powder into the bottle to a depth of an inch or so.

Fill to the top with water and shake a few times. Let settle. Pour off the clear part into dispenser bottles. This is the soap!

Keep a dispenser by the kitchen sink, bathroom sink, and shower. It does not contain aluminum as regular detergents and soaps do, and which contributes to Alzheimer's disease. It does not contain PCBs as many commercial and health food varieties do. It does not contain cobalt (the blue or green granules) which causes heart disease and draws cancer to the skin. Commercial detergents and non-soaps are simply not safe. Switch to homemade soap, washing soda and borax soap for all your tasks! Borax inhibits the bacterial enzyme *urease* and is therefore antibacterial. It may even clear your skin of blemishes and stop your scalp from itching.

For Laundry

Borax (½ cup per load). It is the main ingredient of non-chlorine bleach and has excellent cleaning power without fading colors. It can be combined with washing soda for extra cleaning power. Your regular laundry soap may contain PCBs, aluminum, cobalt and other chemicals. These get rubbed into your skin constantly as you wear your clothing. For bleaching (only do this occasionally) use original chlorine bleach (not "new improved" or "with special brighteners", and so forth).

For Dishes

Don't believe your eyes when you see the commercials where the smiling person pulls a shining dish out of greasy suds. Any dish soap that you use should be safe enough to eat because nothing rinses off clean. Regular dish detergents are now polluted with PCB's. They also contain harmful chemicals. Use borax plus washing soda (equal amounts) for your dishes.

In The Dishwasher

Use 2 tsp. borax powder pre-dissolved in water. Use vinegar in the rinse cycle.

In The Sink

Use a dishpan in the sink. Use ¼ cup borax plus ¼ cup washing soda and add a minimum of water. Also keep a bit of dry washing soda in a saucer by the sink for scouring. Don't use any soap at all for dishes that aren't greasy and can be washed under the faucet with nothing but running water. Throw away your old sponge or brush or cloth because it may be PCB contaminated.

Shampoo

Borax liquid soap is ready to use as shampoo. It does not lather but goes right to work removing sweat and soil without stripping your color or natural oils. It inhibits scalp bacteria and stops flaking and itching. Hair gets squeaky clean so quickly (just a few squirts does it) that you might think nothing has happened! You will soon be accustomed to non-lathery soap. Rinse very thoroughly because you need to leave your scalp slightly acidic. Take a pint container to the shower with you. Put ¼ tsp. citric (not ascorbic) acid crystals (see *Sources*) in it. For long hair use a quart or more of rinse. Only citric acid is strong enough to get the borax out. After shampooing, fill the container with water and rinse. Rinse your whole body, too, since citric acid is also anti-bacterial. All hair shampoo penetrates the eye lids and gets into the eyes although you do not feel it. It is important to use this natural rinse to neutralize the shampoo in your eyes. (Some people have stated that citric acid makes their hair curlier or reddens it. If this is undesirable, use only half as much citric acid.) Citric acid also conditions and gives body and sheen to hair.

Hair Spray

I haven't got a recipe that holds your hair as well as the bottle of chemicals you can buy at the store. Remarkably a little lemon juice (not from a bottle) has some holding power and no odor! Buy a 1 cup spray bottle. Squeeze part of a lemon, letting only the clear juice run into the bottle. Fill with water. Keep it in the refrigerator. Make it fresh every week. Spraying with just plain water is nearly as good! For shinier hair, drop a bit of lemon peel into the bottle.

Homemade Soap

A small plastic dishpan, about 10" x 12"
A glass or enamel 2-quart sauce pan
1 can of lye, 12 ounces
3 pounds of lard (BHT in it is OK)
Plastic gloves
Cold tap water

1. Pour 3 cups of very cold water (refrigerate water overnight first) into the 2-quart saucepan.
2. Slowly and carefully add the lye, a little bit at a time, stirring it with a wooden or plastic utensil. (Use plastic gloves for this; test them for holes first.) Do not breathe the vapor or lean over the container or have children nearby. Above all: USE NO METAL. The mixture will get very hot. In olden days, a sassafras branch was used to stir, imparting a fragrance and insect deterrent for mosquitoes, lice, fleas, ticks.
3. Let cool at least one hour in a safe place. Meanwhile, the unwrapped lard should be warming up to room temperature in the plastic dishpan.
4. Slowly and carefully, pour the lye solution into the dishpan with the lard. The lard will melt. Mix thoroughly, at least 15 minutes until it looks like thick pudding.
5. Let it set until the next morning; then cut it into bars. It will get harder after a few days. Then package. This is a year's supply!

Liquid Soap

Make chips from your homemade soap cake. Add enough hot water to dissolve.

Skin Sanitizer

Make up a 5 to 10% solution of food grade alcohol. Food grade alcohols are grain (ethyl) alcohol or vodka. Find a suitable dispenser bottle. Mark it with a pen at about one tenth of the way up from the bottom. Pour 95% grain alcohol (190 proof) to this mark (for 50% grain alcohol or vodka make your mark one fifth of the way up). Add water to the top. Keep shut. You may add a chip of lemon peel for fragrance.

Use this for general sanitizing purposes: bathroom fixtures, knobs, handles, canes, walkers, and for personal cleanliness (but use chorine bleach for the toilet bowl). Always clean up after a bowel movement with wet toilet paper. This is not clean enough, though. Follow with a stronger damp paper towel. This is still not clean enough; use a final paper towel with skin sanitizer. After washing hands, sanitize them too, pouring a bit on one palm and put finger tips of the other hand in it, scratch to get under nails, repeat on other hand. Rinse with water.

Deodorant

Your sweat is odorless. It is the entrenched bacteria feeding on it that make smells. You can never completely rid yourself of these bacteria. The strategy is to control their numbers. Here are several deodorants to try. Find one that works best for you:

Vitamin C water. Mix ¼ tsp. to a pint of water and dab it on. Follow with a dab of cornstarch.

Citric Acid water. Mix ¼ tsp. to a pint of water and dab it on. Follow with a dab of cornstarch.

Only a few drops of these acids under each armpit are necessary. If these acids burn the skin, dilute them more. Never apply anything to skin that has just been shaved!

Baking soda. Dab a bit under the arms after your morning shower.

Lemon juice. This acid is not as strong, use what you need.

Pure alcohol (never rubbing alcohol). The food grade alcohols are grain alcohol and vodka. Dab a bit under each arm and/or on your shirt or blouse. If it burns, dilute it with water. Be very careful not to leave the bottle where a child or alcoholic person could find it. Pour it into a different bottle! Follow with a dab of cornstarch.

Pure zinc oxide. You may ask your pharmacist to order this for you. She or he may wish to make it up for you too, but do not let them add anything else to it. It should be about 1 part zinc oxide powder to 3 parts water. It does not dissolve. Just shake it up to use it. After you get it home, you can add cornstarch to it to give it a creamy texture. Heat 3 tsp. cornstarch in 1 cup of water, to boiling, until dissolved and clear. Cool and add some to the zinc oxide mixture (about equal parts). Store unused starch mixture in the refrigerator. Only make up enough for a month.

Alcohol and zinc oxide. This is the most powerful deodorant. Apply alcohol first, then the zinc oxide. Then a dab of cornstarch.

Plain cornstarch. Dab it on. This is many people's favorite.

Remember that you need to sweat! Sweating excretes toxic substances, especially from the upper body. Don't use deodorant on weekends. Go to the sink and wipe clean the armpits like our grandparents did. These homemade deodorants are not as powerful as the commercial varieties—this is to your advantage.

Brushing Teeth

Go buy a new toothbrush. Your old one is soaked with toxins from your old toothpaste. Use baking soda out of the box if you have any metal fillings. Put a pinch in a glass, add water to dissolve it. Use food-grade hydrogen peroxide (see *Sources*) if you have only plastic fillings. Dilute it from 35% to 17½% by adding water (equal parts). Store hydrogen peroxide only in polyethylene or the original plastic bottle. Use 4 or 5 drops on your toothbrush. It should fizz nicely as oxygen is produced in your mouth. Your teeth will whiten noticeably in 6 months.

Before brushing teeth, floss with monofilament nylon fish line, two to four pound test. Both waxed and unwaxed floss is polluted with mercury and thallium. Floss and brush only once a day. If this leaves you uncomfortable, brush the extra times with plain water and a second "water-only" toothbrush. Make sure that nothing solid, like powder, is on your toothbrush; it will scour the enamel and give you sensitive teeth, especially as you get older and the enamel softens. Salt is corrosive–don't use it for brushing metal teeth. Plain water is just as good.

For Dentures

Use salt water. It kills all germs and is inexpensive. Salt water plus grain alcohol or food-grade hydrogen peroxide makes a good denture soak.

Mouthwash

A few drops of food grade hydrogen peroxide added to a little water in a glass should be enough to make your mouth foam and cleanse. Don't use hydrogen peroxide, though, if you have metal fillings, because they react, you could use Lugol's Iodine. Don't use regular drug store variety hydrogen peroxide because it contains toxic additives (see *Sources*). Never purchase hydrogen peroxide in a bottle with a metal cap.

For persons with metal tooth fillings, use baking soda or just plain hot water. A healthy mouth has no odor! You shouldn't need a mouthwash! If you have breath odor, search for a hidden tooth infection or cavitation.

Foot Powder

Use cornstarch poured into a salt shaker. You may also try arrow root or potato starch. For foot fungus use equal parts cornstarch and zinc oxide powder.

Contact Lens Solution

A scant cup of water brought to a boil in glass saucepan. After adding ¼ tsp. aluminum free salt (Hain Sea Salt) and boiling again to kill mold, pour into a sterile canning jar. Refrigerate. Freeze some of it.

Lip Soother

For dry, burning lips. Heat 1 level tsp. sodium alginate plus 1 cup water until dissolved. After cooling, pour it into a small bottle to carry in your purse or pocket (refrigerate the remainder). Dab it on whenever needed. If the consistency isn't right for you, add water or boil it down further. You can make a better lip soother by adding some *lysine* from a crushed tablet, vitamin C powder, and a vitamin E capsule to the alginate mix. If you have a persistent problem with chapped lips, try going off citrus juice and not drinking beverages with ice.

Massage Oil

Use olive oil. It comes in very light to heavy textures. Pick the right one for your purpose. Alginate or cornstarch mixtures can be used instead of, or added to, oil.

Skin Healer Moisturizer Lotion

1 tsp. sodium alginate
1 cup water

Make the base first by heating these together in a covered, non-metal pan until completely dissolved. Use low heat–it will take over an hour. Use a wooden spoon handle to stir. Set aside. Then make the following mixture:

¼ tsp. Vitamin C (ascorbic acid) (You may crush tablets)
¼ tsp. lysine (crush tablets)

2 tbs. pure vegetable glycerine
2 Vitamin E capsules (400 units or more, each)
1 tsp. apricot kernel oil (olive oil will do)
1 tbs. lemon juice from a lemon or ¼ tsp citric acid (this is optional)
1 cup water

Heat the water to steaming in a non-metal pan. Add vitamin C and lysine first and then everything else. Pour into a pint jar and shake to mix. Then add the sodium alginate base to the desired thickness (about equal amounts) and shake. Pour some into a small bottle to use as lip soother. Pour some into a larger bottle to dispense on skin. Store remainder in refrigerator. (See *Sources* for sodium alginate, vegetable glycerine and apricot kernel oil. Sodium alginate is also available in capsule form at some health food stores.)

Other Skin Healers

Vitamin C powder (ascorbic acid, not the same as citric acid). Put a large pinch into the palm of your hand. With your other hand pick up a few drops of water from the faucet. Rub hands together until all the powder is dissolved and dispensed. It may sting briefly. Do this at bedtime, especially for cracked, chapped hands. Include lips if they need it.

Vitamin E oil. the vitamin E oil listed in *Sources* was not polluted at the time of this writing, but for the future it would be safer to rely on capsules. Snip open a capsule and rub into skin.

50% Glycerine. Dilute 100% vegetable glycerine with an equal amount of water. This is useful as an after shave lotion.

Vitamin C liquid. Mix ¼ tsp. vitamin C powder in one pint water (crushed tablets will do). This is useful as an after shave lotion and general skin treatment.

Apricot Kernel Oil. This is a very light oil, useful as an after shave lotion and general skin treatment.

Combining several of these makes them more effective.

Dry skin has several causes: too much water contact, too much soap contact (switch to borax), low body temperature, not enough fat in the diet, or parasites.

Sunscreen Lotion

Purchase PABA (see *Sources*) in 500 mg tablet form. Dissolve 1 tablet in grain alcohol or vodka. Grind the tablet first by putting it in a plastic bag and rolling over it with a glass jar. It will not completely dissolve even if you use a tablespoon of the alcohol. Pour the whole mixture into a 4 ounce bottle of homemade skin softener. Be careful not to get the lotion into your eyes when applying it. A better solution is to wear a hat or stay out of the sun. Remember to *take* PABA as a supplement, too (500 mg, one a day).

Nose Salve

(When the inside of the nose is dry, cracked and bleeding.)

Pour ½ tsp. pure vegetable glycerine into a bottle cap (emollient glycerin from a pharmacy will do). Add ½ tsp. of water.

Applicator: use a plastic coffee stirrer and twist the end into some cotton wool salvaged from a vitamin bottle. Dip it into the glycerin mixture and apply inside the nose with a rotating motion. Do both nostrils and then throw it away. Make a new applicator for each use.

Corn Starch Skin Softener

1 tsp. lysine powder or 8 tablets, 500 mg each
1 tsp. Vitamin C powder (ascorbic acid); or 8 tablets, 500 mg each
3 tsp. pure cornstarch from grocery store

Vitamin E, 1 capsule 400 mg
¼ tsp. apricot kernel oil (optional)
1 cup water

Heat starch in water until boiling and clear. Add other ingredients and stir until dissolved. Cool. Pour into dispenser bottle. Keep refrigerated when not in use. Apply after washing dishes and after showering.

Quick Corn Starch Skin Softener

4 tsp. cornstarch
1 cup water

Heat together until boiling and clear. This is the base; all by itself, it will do a nice job of coating and moisturizing the skin. For extra healing action add:

1/8 tsp. ascorbic acid powder (crush 1 Vitamin C tablet, 500 mg)
1/8 tsp. lysine (a 500 mg tablet)
1 Vitamin E perle

Dissolve the additions all together in a tablespoon of hot water before adding. After cooling, pour into a suitable dispenser bottle.

After Shave

Vitamin C. ¼ tsp. vitamin C powder, dissolved in 1 pint water.

Apricot kernel oil.

Vegetable glycerine. Equal parts glycerin and water or to suit your taste.

Personal Lubricants

Heat these together: 1 level tsp. sodium alginate and 1 cup water in a covered non-metal pan until completely dissolved. Use very low heat and stir with a wooden spoon. It takes a fairly long time to get it perfectly smooth. After cooling, pour into a small dispenser bottle. Keep the remainder refrigerated.

Or, mix and heat 4 tsp. cornstarch and 1 cup water until completely dissolved in a covered saucepan. Use non-metal dishes and a non-metal stirring spoon. Cool. Pour some into dispenser bottle. Refrigerate remainder. This is many person's favorite recipe.

People Wipes

¼ tsp. powdered lysine (you may crush tablets)
¼ tsp. Vitamin C powder (you may crush tablets)
¼ cup vegetable glycerine
1 cup water

Prepare wipes by cutting paper towels in quarters. Use white, unfragranced towels that are strong enough to hold up for this use. Fold each piece in quarters again and stack in a plastic zippered baggie. Pour the fluid mixture over the stack and zip. Store a bag full in the freezer to take on car trips. If you want to keep them a month or more, add 1 tbs. grain alcohol or vodka to the recipe.

Recipes For Natural Cosmetics

Eyeliner and Eyebrow Pencil

Get a pure charcoal pencil (black only) at an art supply store. Try several on yourself (bring a small mirror) in the store to see what hardness suits you. You may need to dip the pencil in water or oil first. Bring a wet napkin or oily napkin (olive oil) with you for testing. Don't put anything on your *eyelids*, since this penetrates into your eye. To check this out for yourself, close your eye tightly and then dab lemon juice on your eyelid. It will soon burn! Everything that is put on skin penetrates. Otherwise the nicotine patch and estrogen patch wouldn't work. Not even soap belongs on your eyelids! Charcoal pencils are cheap. Get yourself half a dozen different kinds so you can do different things.

Lipstick

Beet root powder (see *Sources*)
100% vegetable glycerine

Combine 1 tsp. vegetable glycerine and 1 tsp. beet root powder in a saucer. Stir until perfectly smooth. Then add ½ tsp. of vitamin E oil. Snip open vitamin E capsules or buy vitamin E oil (see *Sources*). Thick olive oil can be substituted. Apply liberally with your finger or a lipstick brush. Do not purse or rub your lips together after application. Store in a small plastic container. To make the lipstick stay on longer, apply 1 layer of lipstick, then dab some corn starch over the lips, then apply another layer of lipstick. Store your supply in the refrigerator, tightly covered in a plastic bag.

Face Powder

Use cornstarch from the original box. You may also try arrow root starch or potato starch.

Blush (face powder in a cake form)

Add 50% glycerin to cornstarch in a saucer to make a paste. Slowly add beet root powder to the desired color. Use a few drops of black walnut extract to darken it (here you can use the extract available at health food stores and save your tincture for killing parasites). Or try darkening it with a bit of baking soda. A drop of food grade alcohol will also darken it. To make 50% glycerin, add equal parts of glycerin and water.

Recipes For Household Products

Floor Cleaner

Use washing soda from the grocery store. You may add borax and boric acid (to deter insects except ants). Use white distilled vinegar in your rinse water for a natural shine and ant repellent.

Furniture Duster and Window Cleaner

Mix equal parts white distilled vinegar and water. Put it in a spray bottle.

Furniture Polish

A few drops of olive oil on a dampened cloth. Use cold tap water to dampen.

Insect Killer

Boric acid powder (not borax). Throw liberal amounts behind stove, refrigerator, under carpets and in carpets. Since boric acid is white, you must be careful not to mistake it for sugar accidentally. Keep it far away from food and out of children's reach. Buy it at a farm supply or garden store (or see *Sources*). It will not kill ants.

Ant Repellent

Spray 50% white distilled vinegar on counter tops, window sills and shelves and wipe, leaving residue. Start early in spring before they arrive, because it takes a few weeks to rid yourself of them once they are established. If you want immediate action, get some lemons, cut the yellow outer peel off and cover the peels with grain alcohol in a tightly closed jar. Let stand at least one hour. Use 1 part of this concentrate with 9 parts water in a spray bottle. Mix only as much as you will use because the diluted form loses potency. Spray walls, floors, carpets wherever you see them. The lemon solution even leaves a shine on your counters. Use both vinegar and lemon approaches to rid yourself of ants.

Flower and Foliage Spray

Food-grade hydrogen peroxide. See instructions on bottle.

Moth Balls

I found this recipe in an old recipe book. Mix the following and scatter in trunks and bags containing furs and woolens: ½ lb. each rosemary and mint, ¼ lb. each tansy and thyme, 2 tbs. powdered cloves.

Health Improvement Recipes

Quassia Tea

1/8 cup quassia chips to 3 cups water. Simmer 20-30 minutes. Pour off 1/8 cup now and drink it fresh. Refrigerate remainder. Drink 1/8 cup 4 times/day, until ½ cup of chips is used. Flavor with black cherry extract.

Black Walnut Hull Tincture

The black walnut tree produces large green balls in fall. The walnut is inside, but we will use the whole ball, uncracked, since the active ingredient is in the green outer hull.

Find a few walnuts with a patch of green still in the hull; the more green area, the better. Wash free of dirt and place them in a glass canning jar. You may freeze them in a zippered plastic bag if you can't get to making the extract immediately. (Simply refrigerating them does not keep them from turning black and useless.)

Fill the jar to cover the walnuts with a 50% alcohol solution. The exact percentage is not critical. But it must, of course, be food-grade alcohol, like whiskey or vodka. In some states you can buy grain alcohol, which is 95% alcohol. This should be diluted with water, equal parts of alcohol and water, to get the 50% solution you want. If you buy a lower concentration, add less water.

Put a plastic baggie over the top and then the lid. Let the jar stand in the kitchen for 2 days. Then pour the liquid into a glass bottle. **This is concentrate**. You must add an equal amount of water to get the finished product. This is your Black Walnut Hull Tincture. The best quality is a pale greenish brown. The darker tincture has less green hull to start with and has poorer quality. But it all works! One ball makes a pint: enough for 20 persons.

For alcoholic persons: put the green balls into a small non-metal saucepan. Cover them with cold tap water. Heat to boiling, covered. Turn off heat. Let stand, untouched, for 1 day closely covered. Pour into a glass bottle. It will be darker than the tincture. Do not dilute. Refrigerate what you will use in two days and freeze the rest.

For use: Pour your tincture or extract into a glass dropper bottle. Add a pinch of vitamin C to preserve potency.

Kidney Stone Cleanse

¼ cup dried Hydrangea root
¼ cup Gravel root
¼ cup Marshmallow root
4 bunches of fresh parsley
Goldenrod tincture (leave this out of the recipe if you are allergic to it)
Ginger capsules
Uva Ursi capsules
Vegetable glycerine
Black Cherry Concentrate
Vitamin B6, 250 mg
Magnesium oxide tablets, 300 mg

Measure and set the roots to soak, together, in 10 cups of filtered water, using a non-metal container and a non-metal lid (a dinner plate will do). After four hours (or overnight) heat to boiling and simmer for 20 minutes. Drink ¼ cup as soon as it is cool enough. Pour the rest through a bamboo strainer into a sterile pint jar (glass) and several freezable containers. Refrigerate the glass jar.

Boil the fresh parsley, after rinsing, in 1½ quarts of water for 3 minutes. Drink ¼ cup when cool enough. Refrigerate half the remainder and freeze the other half. Throw away the parsley.

Dose: each morning, pour together ¾ cup of the root mixture and ½ cup parsley water, filling a large mug. Add 2 tbs. black cherry concentrate and 20 drops of goldenrod tincture and 1 tbs. of glycerin. Drink this mixture in divided doses throughout the day. Keep cold. <u>Do not drink it all at once</u> or you will get a stomach ache and feel pressure in your bladder. If your stomach is very sensitive, or you know you have kidney stones, or are over 70, start on half this dose.

Save the roots after the first boiling, storing them in the freezer. When your supply runs low, boil them a second time, but add only 6 cups water and simmer only 10 minutes.

You may cook the roots a third time if you wish, but the recipe gets less potent. If your problem is severe, only cook them twice. Also take:

- Ginger capsules: one with each meal (3/day).
- Uva Ursi capsules: one with breakfast and two with supper.
- Vitamin B6 (250 mg): one a day.
- Magnesium oxide (300 mg): one a day.

Take these supplements just before your meal to avoid burping.

Some notes on this recipe: this herbal tea, as well as the parsley, can easily spoil. Heat it to boiling every fourth day if it is being stored in the refrigerator; this resterilizes it. If you sterilize it in the morning you may take it to work without refrigerating it (use a glass container).

When you order your herbs, be careful! Herb companies are not the same! These roots should have a strong fragrance. If the ones you buy are barely fragrant, they have lost their active ingredients; switch to a different supplier. Fresh roots can be used. Do not use powder.

- Hydrangea (*Hydrangea arborescens*) is a common flowering bush.
- Gravel Root (*Eupatorium purpureum*) is a wild flower.

- Marshmallow root (*Althea officinallis*) is mucilaginous and kills pain.
- Fresh parsley can be bought at a grocery store. Parsley flakes and dried parsley herb do <u>not</u> work.
- Goldenrod herb works as well as the tincture but you may get an allergic reaction from smelling the herb. If you know you are allergic to this, leave this one out of your recipe.
- Ginger from the grocery store works fine; you may put it into capsules for yourself (size 0, 1 or 00).

There are probably dozens of herbs that can dissolve kidney stones. If you can only find several of those in the recipe, make the recipe anyway; it will just take longer to get results. Remember that vitamin B6 and magnesium, taken daily, can prevent oxalate stones from forming. But only if you stop drinking tea. Tea has 15.6 mg oxalic acid per cup[37]. A tall glass of iced tea could give you over 20 mg oxalic acid. Switch to herb teas. Cocoa and chocolate, also, have too much oxalic acid to be used as beverages.

Remember, too, that phosphate crystals are made when you eat too much phosphate. Phosphate levels are high in meats, breads, cereals, pastas, and carbonated drinks. Eat less of these, and increase your milk (2%), fruits and vegetables. Drink at least 2 pints of water a day.

Cleanse your kidneys at least twice a year.

[37] Taken from *Food Values* 14ed by Pennington and Church 1985.

You can dissolve all your kidney stones in 3 weeks, but make new ones in 3 days if you are drinking tea and cocoa and phosphated beverages. None of the beverage recipes in this chapter are conducive to stone formation.

Gallstone (Liver) Cleanse

Cleansing the liver of gallstones has nothing to do with HIV/AIDS, but everything to do with gaining your health back. It dramatically improves digestion, which is the basis of your whole health. You can expect your allergies to disappear, too, more with each cleanse you do! Incredibly, it also eliminates shoulder, upper arm, and upper back pain. You have more energy and an increased sense of well being.

> Cleaning the liver bile ducts is the most powerful procedure that you can do to improve your body's health.
>
> But it <u>should not</u> be done before the parasite program, and for <u>best results</u> should follow the kidney cleanse and any dental work you need.

It is the job of the liver to make bile, 1 to 1½ quarts in a day! The liver is full of tubes (*biliary tubing*) that deliver the bile to one large tube (the *common bile duct*). The gallbladder is attached to the common bile duct and acts as a storage reservoir. Eating fat or protein triggers the gallbladder to squeeze itself empty after about twenty minutes, and the stored bile finishes its trip down the common bile duct to the intestine. There are other substances that can trigger the gallbladder, such as red pepper (cayenne), ginger, and fruit acids. Note fruit juice is the first thing you have after the cleanse.

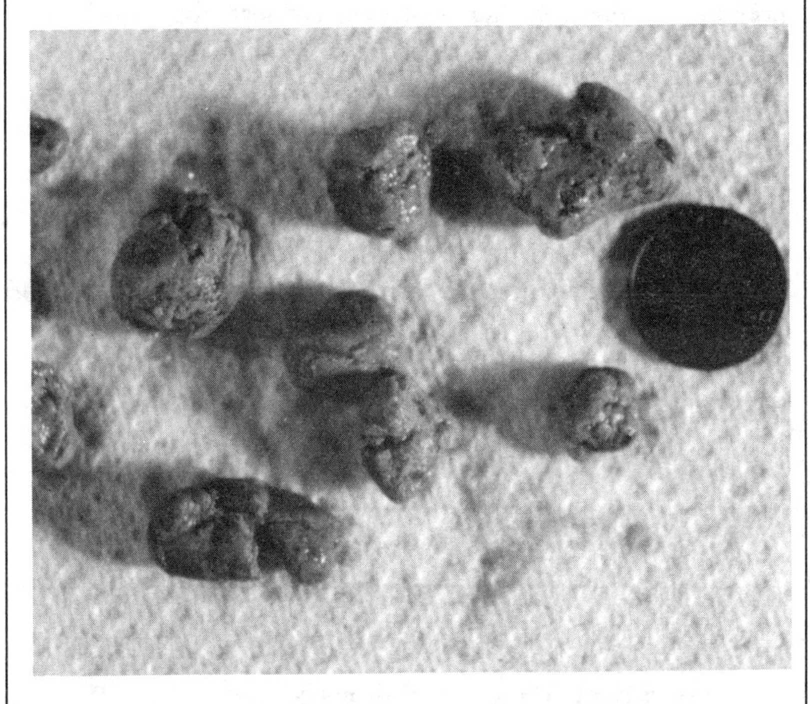

Fig. 62 These are gallstones

For many persons, including children, the biliary tubing is choked with gallstones. Some develop allergies or hives but some have no symptoms. When the gallbladder is scanned or X-rayed nothing is seen. Typically, they are not in the gallbladder. Not only that, most are too small and not calcified, a prerequisite for visibility on X-ray. There are over half a dozen varieties of gallstones, most of which have cholesterol crystals in them. They can be black, red, white, green or tan colored. The green ones get their color from being coated with bile. At the very center of each stone is found a clump of bacteria, suggesting a dead bit of parasite might have started the stone forming.

As the stones grow and become more numerous the back pressure on the liver causes it to make less bile. Imagine the situation if your garden hose had marbles in it. Much less water would flow, which in turn would decrease the ability of the hose to squirt out the marbles. With gallstones, much less cholesterol leaves the body, and cholesterol levels may rise.

Gallstones, being porous, can pick up all the bacteria, cysts, viruses and parasites that are passing through the liver. In this way "nests" of infection are formed, forever supplying the body with fresh bacteria. No stomach infection such as ulcers or intestinal bloating can be cured permanently without removing these gallstones from the liver.

Cleanse your liver twice a year.

Preparation. There are 10 drops of "peroxy" (17½% food-grade hydrogen peroxide) in the cleanse recipe to kill bacteria and viruses as they come out of the bile ducts, also 10 drops of Black Walnut Hull Tincture to kill any remaining parasites. These drops could make you feel quite ill by themselves, unless you work your way up to this dose ahead of time:

- Take one drop of peroxy in a beverage with each of your three meals in a day. The type of beverage does not matter; drink it throughout the meal. The purpose is to mix the peroxy thoroughly with your food. When the peroxy contacts bacteria it fizzes, giving a sensation of nausea. If you feel sick, stay at that dosage, or less, until you feel better. The next day increase to two drops with each meal. Increase by 1 drop each day until you are taking 10 drops with each meal (12 for elderly or recently ill people). Stay at this level until you do the cleanse.

- You can't clean a liver with living parasites in it. You won't get many stones, and you will feel quite sick. Get through the first three weeks of the parasite killing program before attempting a liver cleanse. If you are on the maintenance parasite program, do a high dose program the week before.
- Completing the kidney rinse before cleansing the liver is also highly recommended. You want your kidney, bladder and urinary tract in top working condition so it can efficiently remove any undesirable substances incidentally absorbed from the intestine as the bile is being excreted.
- Do any dental work first, if possible. Your mouth should be metal free and bacteria free (cavitations are cleaned). A toxic mouth can put a heavy load on the liver, burdening it immediately after cleansing. Eliminate that problem first for best results.

Liver Cleanse. Things you need:

Epsom salts	4 tablespoons
Olive oil	half cup (light olive oil is easier to get down)
Fresh pink grapefruit	1 large or 2 small, enough to squeeze 2/3 to 3/4 cup juice
Black Walnut Hull Tincture	10 drops
Peroxy	10 drops
Ornithine	4 to 8 depending on your experience with the parasite program, to be sure you can sleep. Don't skip this or you may have the worst night of your life!
Large plastic straw	To help drink potion.
Pint jar with lid	

Choose a day like Saturday for the cleanse, since you will be able to rest the next day.

Take no medicines, vitamins or pills that you can do without; they could prevent success. Stop the parasite program and kidney herbs, too, the day before.

Eat a no-fat breakfast and lunch such as cooked cereal with fruit, fruit juice, bread and preserves or honey (no butter or milk), baked potato or other vegetables with salt only.

2:00 PM. Do not eat or drink after 2 o'clock.

Get your Epsom salts ready. Mix 4 tbs. in 3 cups water and pour this into a jar. This makes four servings, ¾ cup each. Set the jar in the refrigerator to get ice cold (this is for convenience and taste only).

6:00 PM. Drink one serving (¾ cup) of the ice cold Epsom salts. If you did not prepare this ahead of time, mix 1 tbs. in ¾ cup water now. You may add 1/8 tsp. vitamin C powder to improve the taste. You may also drink a few mouthfuls of water afterwards or rinse your mouth.

Get the olive oil and grapefruit out to warm up.

8:00 PM. Repeat by drinking another ¾ cup of Epsom salts.

You haven't eaten since two o'clock, but you won't feel hungry. Get your bedtime chores done. The timing is critical for success; don't be more than 10 minutes early or late.

9:45 PM. Pour ½ cup (measured) olive oil into the pint jar. Squeeze the grapefruit by hand into the measuring cup. Remove pulp with fork. You should have at least ½ cup, more (up to ¾ cup) is best. You may top it up with lemonade. Add this to the olive oil. Add 10 drops Black Walnut Hull Tincture and 10 drops peroxy. Close the jar tightly with the lid and shake hard until watery (only fresh grapefruit juice does this).

Now visit the bathroom one or more times, even if it makes you late for your ten o'clock drink. Don't be more than 15 minutes late.

10:00 PM. Drink the potion you have mixed. Take 4 to 8 ornithine capsules with the first sips to make sure you will sleep through the night. Drinking through a large plastic straw helps it go down easier. You may use ketchup, cinnamon, or brown sugar to chase it down between sips. Take it to your bedside if you want, but drink it standing up. Get it down within 5 minutes.

LIE DOWN IMMEDIATELY. You might fail to get stones out if you don't. The sooner you lie down the more stones you will get out. Be ready for bed ahead of time. Don't clean up the kitchen. As soon as the drink is down walk to your bed and lie down flat on your back with your head up high on the pillow. Try to think about what is happening in the liver. Try to keep perfectly still for at least 20 minutes. You may feel a train of stones traveling along the bile ducts like marbles. There is no pain because the bile duct valves are open (thank you Epsom salts!). GO TO SLEEP.

Next morning. Upon awakening take your third dose of Epsom salts. If you have indigestion or nausea wait until it is gone before drinking the Epsom salts. You may go back to bed. Don't take this potion before 6:00 am.

2 Hours Later. Take your fourth (the last) dose of Epsom salts. Drink ¾ cup of the mixture. You may go back to bed.

After 2 More Hours you may eat. Start with fruit juice. Half an hour later eat fruit. One hour later you may eat regular food but keep it light. By supper you should feel recovered.

How well did you do? Expect diarrhea in the morning. Use a flashlight to look for gallstones in the toilet with the bowel movement. Look for the green kind since this is proof that they are genuine gallstones, not food residue. Only bile from the liver is pea green. The bowel movement sinks but gallstones float because of the cholesterol inside. Count them all roughly, whether tan or green. You will need to total 2000 stones before the liver is clean enough to rid you of allergies or bursitis or upper back pains permanently. The first cleanse may rid you of them for a few days, but as the stones from the rear travel forward, they give you the same symptoms again. You may repeat cleanses at two week intervals. Never cleanse when you are ill.

Sometimes the bile ducts are full of cholesterol crystals that did not form into round stones. They appear as a "chaff" floating on top of the toilet bowl water. It may be tan colored, harboring millions of tiny white crystals. Cleansing this chaff is just as important as purging stones.

How safe is the liver cleanse? It is very safe. My opinion is based on over 500 cases, including many persons in their seventies and eighties. None went to the hospital; none even reported pain. However it can make you feel quite ill for one or two days afterwards, although in every one of these cases the maintenance parasite program had been neglected. This is why the instructions direct you to complete the parasite and kidney rinse programs first.

CONGRATULATIONS

You have taken out your gallstones without surgery! I like to think I have perfected this recipe, but I certainly can not take credit for its origin. It was invented hundreds, if not thousands, of years ago, THANK YOU, HERBALISTS!

This procedure contradicts many modern medical viewpoints. Gallstones are thought to be formed in the gallbladder, not the liver. They are thought to be few, not thousands. They are not linked to pains other than gallbladder attacks. It is easy to understand why this is thought: by the time you have acute pain attacks, some stones are in the gallbladder, are big enough and sufficiently calcified to see on X-ray, and have caused inflammation there. When the gallbladder is removed the acute attacks are gone, but the bursitis and other pains and digestive problems remain.

The truth is self-evident, however. People who have had their gallbladder surgically removed still get plenty of green, bile-coated stones, and anyone who cares to dissect their stones can see that the concentric circles and crystals of cholesterol match textbook pictures of "gallstones" exactly.

L-G Recipe

1/8 cup L-Glutamic acid powder, not glutamine (see *Sources*)
1/8 cup L-lysine powder

Add the above powders to two quarts of cold tap water and heat, covered, till completely dissolved; it will be near boiling. Use a non-metal pan and non-metal stirring spoon. When it cools, freeze most of it, in suitable small bottles. Keep one cup of it handy in the refrigerator, for immediate use. If it develops a white crystalline precipitate at the bottom, it must be shaken up to make sure you get the pure L-G. You may also reheat it to dissolve it again. Since it has no preservatives, you must reheat it every fourth day to kill any growing bacteria.

Dose: take 1 tablespoon 4 times a day (if you are quite ill) on an empty stomach. Take 1 tablespoon 3 times a day (if not so ill) before meals for as long as you feel you have a viral condition. There are no side effects. Use a non-metal spoon.

EXTRA POTENCY. You can make L-G more potent by adding one or more of the following items to your recipe. Add them after the lysine and glutamic acid have dissolved and the mixture is steaming hot.

- 1/8 teaspoon Aspartic acid (see *Sources*).
- 1/2 teaspoon of boric acid. **This is not a food item. Do not exceed this amount.** It is a white powder, easily mistaken for sugar, so keep it out of sight and reach of children. Boric acid is used for simple eye infections and for a good reason. It inhibits the growth of bacteria. Boric acid for topical use can be obtained at a pharmacy. When ½ tsp. is dissolved in two quarts water and you drink 4 tbs. a day, you will be consuming 75 mg of boric acid each day. If you exceed this amount for an extended time (such as months) it could become toxic. This was learned years ago when boric acid was used in the public milk supply and cases of "borism" developed. **Do not give any boric acid to children.**
- 1/16 teaspoon EDTA (ethylene diamine tetra acetate). Presumably, this helps rid the body of the large amounts of mercury, nickel, chromium, and other metals accumulated in the body from your tooth fillings. **Do not exceed this amount.** Ask your pharmacist to provide this for you. **Do not give EDTA to children.**

Mechanism of L-G. L-G travels to your thymus; this much can be observed electronically. Does it stimulate T cell production? Does it do some other vital task? Only further study can answer these questions.

Lugol's Iodine Solution

In some states, and outside the U.S. you can ask your pharmacist to make it up for you. The recipe to make 1 liter/quart is:

44 gm iodine, granular (1½ ounces)
88 gm potassium iodide, granular (3 ounces)

Dissolve the potassium iodide in about a pint of the water. Then add the iodine crystals and fill to the liter mark with water. It takes about 1 day to dissolve completely. Shake it from time to time. Keep out of sight and reach of children. Do not use if allergic to iodine.

White Iodine

88 gm potassium iodide, granular

Add potassium iodide to one quart or one liter cold tap water. Potassium iodide dissolves well in water and stays clear; for this reason it is called "white iodine." Label clearly and keep out of reach of children. Do not use if allergic to iodine.

The Story Of L-G

A tribute to Dr. James Schaffer M.D. of Bloomington, Indiana.

Dr. Schaffer was a pediatrician who devoted 20 years of his life to discovering L-G (lysine-glutamate). He called it "JS14". At any time of day, his office was crowded to the door with parents holding sick children. He was a gruff man but infinitely caring about his patients. On Saturdays and Sundays he worked on his pet product, JS14.

He had discovered that if you grow a culture of ordinary bacteria, *Staphylococcus albus* (a variant of *S. aureus*), found on anybody's skin, they would make a substance of great immune significance.[38] I gleaned this from reading his patent(s) on the culturing technique.[39] He discovered that by adding a little bit of an amino acid, aspartic acid, to the culture, the bacteria would make much more of this mysterious substance than without it. Are these bacteria always making this for us, on our skin, in our intestines? Do these bacteria need a special factor to make it in good quantities for us? These were questions he was trying to answer in his private lab where he worked every spare minute. He would inject some of the culture into mice and then infect them with diseases to see if they got protection from it. Indeed, they did. So he perfected JS14 for human use.

---

[38] James Schaffer, Parker R. Beamer, Philip C. Trexler, Gerald Breidenbach, Dwain N. Walcher, *Proc. Soc. Exp. Biol. Med.* 1963, v112, pp. 561.

[39] Process For Producing Antiviral Substance From Staphylococcus Organisms, US Patent 3,625,833, Inventor James J. Schaffer.

His potent immunity-brew was injected just under the skin where it produced a small bubble. It became known as Dr. Schaffer's Bubble Shot. He used it for children and adults with chronic illnesses caused by *Herpes*, Epstein Barre Virus, Cytomegalovirus, cancer. Later, he used it on porphyria, as well as a mystery disease that nobody could diagnose at that time, which turned out to be HIV/AIDS.

He was getting exceptionally good results and his excitement flowed to those around him. If that excitement had not reached me, I may not have survived to work on cancer and HIV/AIDS. I was suffering from ordinary *Herpes* simplex, but it had spread to the eyes and was spreading through my brain! Once a week I got his Bubble Shot and listened as he updated me on his research. But, occasionally, I would be called by his office to let me know he was ill and could not make the appointment time. I realized this beloved doctor was indeed very ill, and I should learn how to make this immune booster myself.

I did not culture *Staphylococcus aureus*. I studied its molecular structure. It has lysine-glutamate links frequently along the chain of molecules making up its coat. Are our bodies intended to utilize this common skin bacteria after they die in such a way that we would digest these chains to make a superb immune booster for ourselves? Should I begin to experiment with *Staphylococcus aureus* or other "Staphs"? Perhaps such a product was already on the market? So it was! I purchased a kind of L-G and tried it as a bubble shot during those weeks that Dr. Schaffer was ill. My shot did not work well. His return was a great relief. I decided to make the culture broth and learn to culture the bacteria. But Dr. Schaffer was not well enough to teach me the techniques. In desperation I studied the recipe for his cultures from the published reports he gave me. There were large amounts of L-lysine and L-glutamic acid in it. Could they be reacting with each other <u>in the brew</u> to make this potent immune booster? Could this be simulating a part of the *Staph* molecular structure? Perhaps the *Staph* was not even necessary! It was a crazy idea but simple enough to try and throw out if it was wrong. I mixed L-lysine and L-glutamic acid under sterile conditions, and tried this as a bubble shot. It had some effect! I was on the right track! It was not as effective as Dr. Schaffer's bubble shot but perhaps it could be made stronger!

Then it occurred to me that this is merely food. These two amino acids are produced in the stomach and intestine by digesting protein. Are some of us with very low immunity not capable of making this mysterious substance because our stomachs are sick? I studied digestion of these amino acids. A great deal has been published about them. In fact, my stomach had been misbehaving for years. Maybe my stomach and intestines were not able to make it by digesting ordinary food. Perhaps this substance could simply be eaten instead of injected. That was the magic answer! By eating it, the potency was greatly <u>increased</u>. Ordinarily, the potency of chemicals is much lowered by the oral route, but in this case, it was reversed. This discovery came just in the nick of time. Bloomington's beloved Dr. James Schaffer passed away. It is a terrible loss to us all. His research was not completed. His results, his data, were voluminous, but only usable by someone intimately acquainted with it. Our mourning after him has not yet ended.

But I could treat myself: not weekly, as before, but daily! I became well. JS14 and L-G were the decisive factors in fighting my chronic *Herpes* eye infection.

The recipe is simple (see *Recipes*), a gift to you in memory of Dr. James Schaffer. Perhaps it is not the same as his Bubble Shot. Perhaps we will never know. But it came into existence as a result of his Bubble Shot and I am ever grateful.

Sources

This list was accurate as this book went to press in late-1993. Only the vitamin sources listed were found to be pollution-free, and only the herb sources listed were found to be potent, although there may be other good sources that have not been tested. The author has no financial interest in, influence on, or other connection with any company listed, except for having family members in the Self Health Resource Center.

Item	**Source**
Amber bottles, ½ ounce	Drug store, Continental Glass & Plastic, Inc. (large quantities)
Apricot Kernel Oil	Now Foods
Arginine	Now Foods, Jomar Labs
Artemesia (wormwood) seed	R. H. Shumway
Aspartic acid	Jomar Labs, EDOM Labs, a crushed tablet will do.
B Complex	Bronson Pharmaceuticals
Vitamin B_6	Bronson Pharmaceuticals, EDOM Labs
Baking soda (sodium bicarbonate)	Grocery store
Beet root	San Francisco Herb & Natural Food Co.
Belts for clothes dryer	Three that tested negative to asbestos are: Maytag™ 3-12959 Poly-V belt, Whirlpool™ FSP 341241 Belt-Drum Dr. (replaces 660996), and Bando™ V-Belt A-65. Bando American makes other belts, some of which might be the right size for your dryer. Call for a dealer near you, make sure it says "Made In America", not all do.
Black cherry concentrate	Health food store
Black Walnut Hull Tincture	Self Health Resource Center, Say Yes To Life

Borax, pure	Grocery store
Boric acid, pure	Now Foods, health food store, pharmacy
Cascara sagrada	Brasseur's Herbs, health food store
CFH capsules	Brasseur's Herbs
Charcoal capsules	Health food store or drug store.
Chemicals for testing.	Aldrich Chemical Co., Spectrum Chemical Co., ICN Biomedicals, Inc. (research chemicals only, including genistein), Boehringer Mannheim Biochemicals (research only)
Citric acid	Now Foods or health food store
Cloves	San Francisco Herb & Natural Food Co. (ASK for fresh)
Dental information	Health-Wise/Dental-Wise
Dermatron	Synergy Health Systems
Electronic parts	A Radio Shack near you.
Empty gelatine capsules size 00	Now Foods, or your health food store
Ginger capsules	Brasseur's Herbs, Now Foods
Goldenrod tincture	Bioforce of America, Ltd.
Grain alcohol or vodka	Liquor store
Gravel root (herb)	San Francisco Herb & Natural Food Co.
Hain Sea Salt™	Grocery store
Histidine	Jomar Labs
HIV virus on slide	Pneumocystis carnii human lung 92W4856 Wards Natural Science, Inc.
Hydrangea (herb)	San Francisco Herb & Natural Food Co.
Hydrogen peroxide 35% (food grade)	New Horizons Trust
Iodine, pure	Spectrum Chemical Co.
L-glutamic acid powder (This is not glutamine.)	Now Foods, Jomar Labs, or crush tablets from Schiff Bio-Food Products
L-lysine powder	Now Foods, or crush tablets from Bronson's Pharmaceuticals
Lugol's iodine	For slide staining (not internal use) from Spectrum Chemical Co., and farm animal supply store. For internal use must be made from scratch.
Lysine	Bronson Pharmaceuticals
Magnesium oxide	Bronson Pharmaceuticals

Marshmallow root (herb)	San Francisco Herb & Natural Food Co.
Microscope slides and equipment	Carolina Biological Supply Company, Ward's Natural Science, Inc., Southern Biological Supply Company, Fisher-EMD
Microscopes	Carolina Biological Supply Company, Ward's Natural Science, Inc., Edmund Scientific Co.
Milk Thistle	Herb companies. For one example see Thisilyn.
Ornithine	Now Foods, Jomar Labs
Ortho-phospho-tyrosine	Aldrich Chemical Co.
Oscillococcinum	Boiron Borneman
P24 antigen sample	Bachem Fine Chemicals Inc.
PABA (para amino benzoic acid)	Bronson Pharmaceuticals
Peroxy	See Hydrogen peroxide.
Photo-micrographic camera and film	Ward's Natural Science, Inc.
Potassium iodide, pure	Spectrum Chemical Co.
Rascal™	Kroeger Herb Products
Salt (sodium chloride), pure	Spectrum Chemical Co.
Sodium alginate	Spectrum Chemical Co. or health food store
Stevia powder (sweetener)	Health food store
Thallium, homeopathic	Dolisos America, Inc.
Thioctic acid (also called lipoic acid)	Ecological Formulas, Inc., L&H Vitamins
Thisilyn	Brasseur's Herbs
Uva Ursi	Brasseur's Herbs or health food store
Vegetable glycerine	Now Foods or health food store
Vermifuge syrup (for children)	VMF from Brasseur's Herbs
Vitamin B_2 (riboflavin)	Nutrition Headquarters (250 mg), or Bronson Pharmaceuticals (100 mg)
Vitamin C (ascorbic acid) powder only	Bronson Pharmaceuticals
Vitamin D 50,000iu	From dentist, by prescription
Vitamin E capsules	Bronson Pharmaceuticals

Vitamin E Oil	Now Foods
Washing soda (sodium carbonate)	Grocery store
Wormwood Combination capsules	Kroeger Herb Products

Aerobic Life Products
P.O. Box 28802
Dallas, TX 75228
(214) 327-0707
(800) 798-0707

Aldrich Chemical Co.
P.O. Box 355
Milwaukee, WI 53201
(414) 273-3850

Bachem Fine Chemicals Inc.
3132 Kashiwa St.
Torrance, CA 90505
(310) 539-4171

Bando American Inc.
1149 West Bryn Mawr
Itasca, IL 60143
(708) 773-6600

Bioforce of America, Ltd.
P.O. Box 507
Kinderhook, NY 12106
(800) 645-9135

Boehringer Mannheim Biochemicals
9115 Hague Rd.
P.O. Box 50816
Indianapolis, IN 46250

Boiron Borneman
1208 Amosland Rd.
Norwood, PA 19074
(215) 532-2035

Brasseur's Herbs
608 Hudson Ave.
Newark, OH 43055
(800) SAY-HERBS

Bronson Pharmaceuticals
Div. of Jones Medical Industry
1945 Craig Road
P.O. Box 46903
St. Louis, MO 63146-6903
(800) 235-3200 retail
(800) 525-8466 wholesale

Carolina Biological Supply Company
Burlington, NC 27215
(800) 334-5551
Also (919) 584-0381

Continental Glass & Plastic, Inc.
841 West Cermak Rd.
Chicago, IL 60608-4517
(312) 666-2050

Dolisos America, Inc.
3014 Rigel Ave
Las Vegas, NV 89102
(702) 871-7153

Ecological Formulas, Inc.
a division of
Cardiovascular Research Ltd.
1061-B Shary Circle
Concord, CA 94518
(800) 888-4585
(510) 827-2636 (CA)

Edmund Scientific Co.
101 E. Gloucester Pike
Barrington, NJ 08007
(609) 573-6250

EDOM Labs, Inc.
860 Grand Boulevard
P.O. Box T
Deer Park, NY 11729
(516) 586-2266

Fisher-EMD
4901 West LeMoyne Street
Chicago, IL
(800) 628-6793

Health-Wise/Dental-Wise
639 Washington Street
Columbus, IN 47201
(812) 376-8525

ICN Biomedicals, Inc.
Biochemicals Division
P.O. Box 28050
Cleveland, OH 44128
(800) 321-6842 or
(800) 431-2800
(216) 831-3000 Ohio

Jomar Labs
251 East Hacienda Avenue
Campbell, CA 95008
(800) 538-4545

Kroeger Herb Products
(wholesale:)
805 Walnut St.
Boulder, CO 80302
(800) 225-8787
(for retail call:)
Hanna's Herb Shop
5684 Valmont Rd.
Boulder, CO 80301
(800) 206-6722

L&H Vitamins
37-10 Crescent St.
Long Island City, NY 11101

New Horizons Trust
53166 St. Rt. 681
Reedsville, OH 45772
(800) 755-6360

Now Foods
550 Mitchell Rd.
Glendale Heights, IL 60139
(708) 545-9098

Nutrition Headquarters, Inc.
Carbondale, IL 62901

R. H. Shumway
P.O. Box 1
Graniteville, SC 29829
(803) 663-9771

San Francisco Herb & Natural
Food Co.
1010 46th St.
Emeryville, CA 94608
(800) 227-2830 wholesale
(510) 601-0700 retail (Natures
Herb Company)

Say Yes To Life
P.O. Box 510
Gainesville, MO 65655
(417) 679-4145

Schiff Bio-Food Products
Moonachie, NJ 07074

Self Health Resource Center
757 Emory St. #508
Imperial Beach, CA 91932
(619) 429-4408

Southern Biological Supply
Company
P.O. Box 368
McKenzie, TN 38201
(800) 748-8735

Spectrum Chemical Co.
14422 South San Pedro Street
Gardena, CA 90248
(800) 772-8786

Synergy Health Systems
1223 Wilshire Blvd., Suite 321
Santa Monica, CA 90403
(310) 394-6497

Ward's Natural Science, Inc.
5100 West Henrietta Road
Rochester, NY 14692
(716) 359-2502
1-800-962-2660

Abstract/Summary

The human species is now heavily infested with the fluke family of parasites, particularly the intestinal fluke *Fasciolopsis buskii,* but also the sheep liver fluke *Fasciola hepatica,* the pancreatic fluke of cattle *Eurytrema pancreatica,* and the human liver fluke *Clonorchis sinensis.* This increase is due to the establishment of a new "biological reservoir" in cattle, fowl and household pets. In the presence of solvents, these flukes can complete their entire life cycle in the human body, not requiring a snail as an intermediate host, as they usually do. These solvents are isopropyl alcohol, benzene, methanol, xylene, toluene and others which occur as residues in our foods and pollute our body products such as toothpaste, mouthwash, lotions and cosmetics. These solvents are also contaminants of animal feed, and thus are responsible for establishing this new reservoir or source of infection.

Different solvents accumulate preferentially in different organs. Benzene accumulates in the thymus, resulting in damage to the thymus and completion of the life cycle of *Fasciolopsis* in the thymus. A <u>stage</u> in the life cycle of *Fasciolopsis* brings with it the HIV virus. Its preferred tissues of colonization are the thymus and penis in the male and the thymus and vagina in the female. The HIV virus has not yet become a human virus, since it disappears within 24 hours after the last fluke stage has been destroyed. However, it could become a true human virus through mutation, no doubt. For this reason it is of paramount importance to end this new kind of parasitism in humans.

Removal of all solvents from the patient's lifestyle and destruction of all fluke stages as well as elimination of undercooked beef, turkey and chicken in the diet results in quick recovery, generally less than one week, from HIV infection.

HIV/AIDS could be eradicated in a very short time by clearing our food animals and household pets of fluke parasites and by monitoring all food and feed for solvents.

The cause of benzene accumulation (besides direct consumption) by some persons and not by others appears to be due to eating different amounts of *4,5 benzopyrene* (but not 3,4 benzopyrene). 4,5 benzopyrene is present in grilled, broiled (flame heated) foods, even ordinary toast. Vitamin B_2 speeds up benzopyrene detoxification.

Since developmental stages of the intestinal fluke are found in blood, breast milk, the saliva, semen, and urine and can be seen directly in these body fluids using a low power microscope, it follows that this parasite can be transmitted not only through sexual contact and blood, but by kissing on the mouth, breast feeding, and childbearing. However, the recipient would develop HIV/AIDS only if benzene were accumulated in his or her body.

The methods used to obtain all these results are discussed in *How To Test Yourself*. A simple circuit is also described which can be built by a novice and allows anyone to reproduce my results.

Hope For The Future

A decade has passed and no regular research has uncovered the true source of the HIV virus or the true nature of AIDS. Instead, a path similar to cancer research has been chosen, a path leading to expensive drugs and an outlook toward genetic engineering. Meanwhile, the horrible deaths of young persons increase with accelerating speed. **The investigation has failed**, so far, even though:

- it is entrusted to our best researchers in the academic, medical and industrial sectors
- they have private contracts, a monopoly
- there is incredible funding

The investigation could have been successfully pursued by an ordinary person of reasonable intelligence with a High School education and moderate funds, if only legally permitted. Because of this, I recommend that society withdraw the trust, advantages and resources given to the above institutions and lay open the enterprise of advancement in health issues to the non-professional person who shows dedication to the task.

> It should be legal for a lay person to offer to the public any form of non-invasive health analysis, from astrology to magnetics to radionics to homeopathy to using the device described in this book, provided qualifications, methods and fees are disclosed in advance.

We must have FREEDOM to select health solutions for our physical welfare, the same as we have freedom to select religious solutions for our spiritual welfare. Freedom of religion was hard won. Many sincere and intelligent persons opposed it and still oppose it today, because they feel it is not moral to allow people to choose the "wrong" spiritual path. Similarly, the government passes laws to "protect" you from choosing the "wrong" (non-professional) health path. But those laws prevented us from finding the cure for HIV/AIDS. They are obviously unsound. Religious freedom changed the religious structure on earth profoundly; freedom to select health solutions could have a similar impact.

The only reason I publish and do not patent the new technology described in this book is to make *Self Health* possible. Self Health means freedom of health matters—freedom to consult about illness, not only with medical doctors (M.D.'s), but with resources that are illegal now, like health advisors, researchers, technicians, and other physicians. It means freedom to select and order your own tests and get the results. If your ankle is swollen and painful after a fall, and you go to the emergency room, you can not order an X-ray of it although the need is obvious. A doctor must make the order (and you pay the additional doctor's fee). Then you are not allowed to look at it (only doctors can diagnose). And just try to get a copy of your medical records; your doctor will instead insist on mailing them to your next doctor (because you might misinterpret them). The story is the same for blood, urine and hormone tests. Lay people can understand a great deal of this information, and learn even more on their own, if they were only encouraged instead of prohibited.

Because Self Health, by its very concept, undermines the existence of the medical profession as we know it, those espousing Self Health, hopefully soon to be the majority of persons, need to be protected from the legal wrath of medical institutions as they try to retain total control.

Index